W0043461

SHOCK

PATHOGENESIS AND THERAPY

AN INTERNATIONAL SYMPOSIUM

STOCKHOLM, 27th-30th JUNE, 1961
SPONSORED BY CIBA

CHAIRMAN
U. S. von EULER
STOCKHOLM

EDITED BY
K. D. BOCK
BASLE

WITH 120 FIGURES

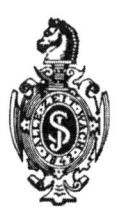

SPRINGER-VERLAG BERLIN HEIDELBERG GMBH

1962

This book has also been published in German under the title
SCHOCK
Pathogenese und Therapie
Ein internationales Symposion

© by Springer-Verlag Berlin Heidelberg 1962
Originally published by Springer-Verlag in 1962
Softcover reprint of the hardcover 1st edition 1962

ISBN 978-3-662-22405-2   ISBN 978-3-662-22403-8 (eBook)
DOI 10.1007/978-3-662-22403-8

Printed by Brühlsche Universitätsdruckerei Gießen

SHOCK
PATHOGENESIS AND THERAPY

AN INTERNATIONAL SYMPOSIUM

STOCKHOLM, JUNE 27th-30th, 1961
SPONSORED BY CIBA

CHAIRMAN

U. S. von EULER
STOCKHOLM

EDITED BY

K. D. BOCK
BASLE

WITH 120 FIGURES

1962
SPRINGER-VERLAG BERLIN HEIDELBERG GMBH

Springer-Verlag · Berlin · Göttingen · Heidelberg

Published in U.S.A. and Canada by
Academic Press Inc. 111 Fifth Avenue, New York 3, N.Y./U.S.A.

This book has also been published in German under the title:
SCHOCK
Pathogenese und Therapie
Ein internationales Symposion

© by Springer-Verlag Berlin Heidelberg 1962
Originally published by Springer-Verlag in 1962
Softcover reprint of the hardcover 1st edition 1962

ISBN 978-3-662-22405-2   ISBN 978-3-662-22403-8 (eBook)
DOI 10.1007/978-3-662-22403-8

Contents

Participants in the Symposium on "SHOCK"

Stockholm, 27th—30th June, 1961

ADAMS-RAY, J., Kirurgiska Avd., Karolinska Sjukhuset, Stockholm (Sweden)
ALLGÖWER, M., Chirurgische Abteilung, Rätisches Kantons- und Regionalspital, Chur (Switzerland)
BACQ, Z. M., Laboratoire de Pathologie et Thérapeutique Générales, Université de Liège, Liège (Belgium)
BEIN, H. J., CIBA Research Laboratories, Basle (Switzerland)
BELLMAN, S., Serafimerlasarettet, Stockholm (Sweden)
BING, J., Universitetets Institut for Eksperimentel Medicin, København (Danmark)
BIÖRCK, G., Serafimerlasarettet, Stockholm (Sweden)
BJURSTEDT, H., Flyg- och Navalmedicinska Avd., Karolinska Institutet, Stockholm (Sweden)
BOCK, K. D., CIBA Research Laboratories, Basle (Switzerland)
BOHR, D. F., Physiology Department, University of Michigan, Ann Arbor (U.S.A.)
BREWIN, E. G., Surgical Unit, St. Thomas's Hospital Medical School, London (Great Britain)
BULL, J. P., Industrial Injuries and Burns Research Unit, Birmingham Accident Hospital, Birmingham (Great Britain)
VON EULER, U. S., Fysiologiska Institutionen, Karolinska Institutet, Stockholm (Sweden)
FINE, J., Department of Surgery, Harvard Medical School, Boston, Mass. (U.S.A.)
FOLKOW, B., Fysiologiska Institutionen, Göteborgs Universitet, Göteborg (Sweden)
GELIN, L.-E., Sahlgrenska Sjukhuset, Kir. Klin. II, Göteborgs Universitet, Göteborg (Sweden)
GILBERT, R. P., Department of Education and Research, Evanston Hospital Association, Evanston, Ill. (U.S.A.)
GREENFIELD, A. D. M., Department of Physiology, The Queen's University of Belfast, Belfast (Northern Ireland)
GREGERSEN, M. I., Department of Physiology, College of Physicians and Surgeons, Columbia University, New York, N. Y. (U.S.A.)
GREGG, D. E., Department of Cardiorespiratory Diseases, Walter Reed Army Medical Center, Washington, D. C. (U.S.A.)
GROSS, F., CIBA Research Laboratories, Basle (Switzerland)
HALPERN, B.-N., Centre de Recherches Allergiques et Immunologiques, Hôpital Broussais, Paris (France)
HÖKFELT, B., Endokrinologiska Avd., Karolinska Sjukhuset, Stockholm (Sweden)
HOWARD, J. M., Department of Surgery, Hahnemann Medical College, Philadelphia, Pa. (U.S.A.)
IMHOF, P., Lory-Abteilung, Inselspital, Bern (Switzerland)
KRAMER, K., Physiologisches Institut der Universität, Göttingen (Germany)

VI   Participants in the Symposium "SHOCK"

KROG, J., Institutt for Eksperimentell Medisinsk Forskning, Universitetet i Oslo, Oslo (Norway)
LILLEHEI, R. C., Department of Surgery, The Medical School, University of Minnesota, Minneapolis (U.S.A.)
MATTHES, K., Medizinische Universitätsklinik, Heidelberg (Germany)
MIGONE, L., Istituto di Patologia Speciale Medica e Metodologia Clinica, Università di Parma, Parma (Italy)
NEIL, E., Department of Physiology, Middlesex Hospital Medical School, London (Great Britain)
NICKERSON, M., Department of Pharmacology and Therapeutics, Faculty of Medicine, University of Manitoba, Winnipeg (Canada)
OSSIPOV, B. K., Department of Clinical Surgery, Central Institute for Postgraduate Study, Moscow (U.S.S.R.)
RUSHMER, R. F., Department of Physiology and Biophysics, University of Washington School of Medicine, Seattle (U.S.A.)
SELKURT, E. E., Department of Physiology, School of Medicine, Indiana University Medical Center, Indianapolis (U.S.A.)
SENNING, Å., Chirurgische Universitätsklinik A, Kantonsspital, Zürich (Switzerland)
SPINK, W. W., Department of Medicine, The Medical School, University of Minnesota, Minneapolis (U.S.A.)
STRÖM, G., Klin.-Fysiol. Avd., Akademiska Sjukhuset, Uppsala (Sweden)
TAKÁCS, L., A Budapesti Orvostudományi Egyetem, II. Sz. Belklinikája, Budapest (Hungary)
TROELL, L., Marinledningen, Fack, Stockholm (Sweden)
UVNÄS, B., Farmakologiska Institutionen, Karolinska Institutet, Stockholm (Sweden)

Opening remarks

By

U. S. VON EULER

I should like to begin by saying how extremely pleased we are that so many of you have been able to attend this symposium. Yesterday I heard some rather favourable comments on the choice of participants at this meeting. I can only say that Dr. GROSS and I have simply picked the best men we knew. This is not precisely a conventional shock symposium, as you may have noticed. In the usual type of symposium on shock, those participating consist almost exclusively of experts on this particular problem. I am very happy that in this instance we have been able to have participants from several adjacent fields, particularly as I think everybody must now admit that the problem of shock has to be solved by joint efforts from many sources. We know that, in addition to surgery and clinical medicine, much information from the fields of physiology, pharmacology, endocrinology, clinical physiology, pathology, and allergy will be needed — not to mention biochemistry and biophysics; and I feel that it is only by uniting our efforts and pooling our knowledge that we may have some hope of arriving at a closer understanding of the pathogenesis and nature of shock. One of the advantages of a small meeting of this kind is that we do not need to give very lengthy accounts of our ideas or of the results on which they are based. Everybody here is a distinguished scientist, and I think this makes for free and frank discussion and brief presentations. On the other hand, I believe that many of us will be grateful for a little more detail as regards technical problems. We cannot each of us be versed in all the details of the technical questions dealt with, and therefore it is always very good to have a few explanatory comments on the techniques used. At least, speaking for myself, I have frequently found that ideas and concepts can be grasped quite quickly, but that one often requires further information on the underlying techniques.

Definition and classification of various forms of shock

By

R. F. RUSHMER, R. L. VAN CITTERS, and D. FRANKLIN

A scientific term is useful when it conveys precise meaning to serve as a reliable tool for communication. The term "shock" is widely used in many different contexts to convey many different meanings and has no universally accepted definition. From the clinical point of view, the term is most commonly used in referring to patients with acute systemic arterial hypotension accompanied by other signs and symptoms. The clinical manifestations vary widely but often include pallor, weakness, sweating, and rapid thready pulse. However, the essential characteristic is a markedly depressed systemic arterial pressure. Thus, the causes of shock must be sought among the factors which determine the pressure in the systemic arteries.

Factors determining systemic arterial pressure. The mean pressure maintained within the systemic arterial system is determined by the balance between the inflow into the system (cardiac output) and the total peripheral resistance. Some of the prominent mechanisms which determine cardiac output and total peripheral resistance are illustrated schematically in Fig. 1.

The cardiac output is the product of the stroke volume and the heart rate. Since the left ventricle may be neither completely filled during diastole nor completely emptied during systole, the stroke volume must be considered as the difference between the diastolic and systolic volumes. The diastolic volume is determined, among other things, by the effective ventricular filling pressure and the resistance to distension offered by the ventricular walls (distensibility). This statement is an oversimplification because the distensibility or compliance of the ventricular walls varies during the various phases of filling and also depends somewhat upon the rate of distension. Control of distensibility by neural or humoral mechanisms, as suggested in Fig. 1, remains controversial but may occur during changes in posture (1).

The effective ventricular filling pressure is determined by the pressure difference inside and outside the ventricle at the end of the diastolic period. The extracardiac pressure as measured either from the pericardial or pleural spaces can be influenced by respiratory activity and by pathological conditions affecting either the pericardium or the lungs. Hemorrhage into the pericardium produces tamponade, which in turn increases extracardiac pressure, restricts ventricular distensibility and leads to marked reduction in systemic

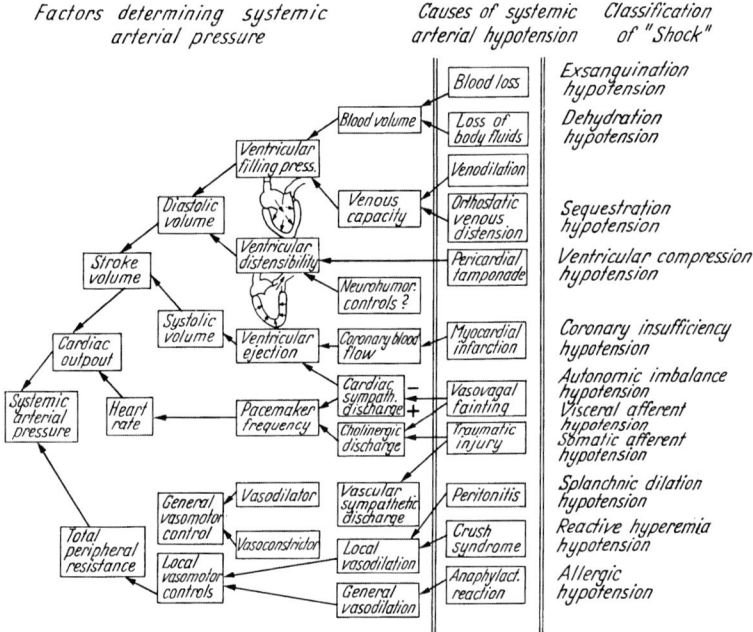

Fig. 1. The reduced systemic arterial pressure is characteristically common to all the various symptom complexes associated with the term "shock". The causes of shock can be classified in terms of the various mechanisms which can influence the level of the systemic arterial pressure. Note that the term "shock" has been used to designate arterial hypotension from virtually every possible cause of systemic arterial hypotension. Each of the causes of arterial hypotension should be assigned a concise name which is clearly defined and established experimentally. If such a list of terms were employed consistently, the term "shock" could be completely abandoned

arterial pressure. The intraventricular pressure is related to central venous pressure, which is largely a reflection of the relationship between the total blood volume and the capacity of the venous system. The total blood volume can be diminished by either blood loss or loss of body fluids. Severe systemic arterial hypotension can be produced by any mechanism which causes sufficient reduction in total blood volume (e. g. internal or external hemorrhage, burns or cholera). As an extreme example, Clarkson et al. (2) recently described a patient who developed cyclical edema and "shock" due to increased capillary permeability on at least 9 occasions before she died from sudden leakage of plasma from the vascular compartment.

The capacity of the venous system is variable and under some kind of control, as evidenced by the ease with which healthy subjects can give up 500 cc. of blood for transfusions. The degree of distension of the venous system as a whole is determined by the smooth muscle in the vein walls, control of which is almost completely unknown. A reduction in total blood volume can be compensated by an appropriate reduction in the capacity of the venous system by contraction of venous channels or venous reservoirs (3). Conversely, a relaxation or distension of the veins or reservoirs can diminish central venous pressure. Generalized venodilation remains questionable (Fig. 1) because we lack methods of measuring the volume of blood in veins or of following venomotor activity under normal control. As an example of local venous distension, soldiers standing at attention for long periods may lose consciousness unless they periodically compress the veins of the legs by voluntary muscular contraction. Although the diastolic volume of the ventricles may be diminished by these mechanisms, stroke volume can theoretically be compensated by greater systolic ejection.

The systolic volume of the left ventricle is determined by the degree of ventricular ejection (i. e. the degree of myocardial shortening). Ventricular ejection involves work output and is dependent upon the availability of adequate coronary blood flow to continuously restore energy lost during contraction (Fig. 1). Acute coronary insufficiency (i. e. acute myocardial infarction) can produce severe systemic arterial hypotension and symptoms commonly associated with the term "shock". The degree of ventricular ejection is normally controlled by the discharge of sympathetic nerves to the myocardium and by the autonomic controls affecting pacemaker activity.

The heart rate is determined by the inherent rate of impulse discharge by the pacemaker as influenced by the balance of sympathetic and parasympathetic discharge to the sino-atrial node (4). Abrupt depression of systemic arterial pressure with loss of consciousness (fainting) is a frequent result of imbalance of autonomic controls. For example, the normal response to a drop in blood pressure is a tachycardia, increased sympathetic discharge to the ventricles and peripheral vasoconstriction; all activated by baroreceptor reflexes. Fainting attacks result from a drop in systemic arterial pressure accompanied by severe bradycardia and peripheral vasodilation (5, 6). Intense stimulation of sensory nerves

1*

within the viscera (visceral afferent fibers) tends to produce such autonomic imbalance. For example, severe fainting reactions with bradycardia can be produced in a large proportion of healthy erect subjects by inserting a needle into an artery (7), by venipuncture or even by the sight of a syringe. During acute fainting reactions, blood flow into extremities is rather abruptly increased, apparently due to the action of sympathetic vasodilator fibers distributed to skeletal muscles (8). The skeletal muscle mass in man may exhibit either vasoconstriction from the administration of norepinephrine or vasodilation from ejection of l-epinephrine. These muscles are also equipped with two types of sympathetic nerves producing either vasoconstriction or vasodilation depending upon the pathway involved. In contrast, stimulation of somatic afferent fibers, particularly somatic pain endings, tends to produce elevated systemic arterial pressure and tachycardia. Destruction of tissue by trauma frequently leads to extreme reduction of systemic arterial pressure, even when the blood loss is slight. This suggests that afferent nerve fibers from the site of the injury may have played a role in this response. The contribution of neural control mechanisms to the clinical syndrome commonly called "shock" is probably greater than is generally recognized, but has not been clearly elucidated (vide infra).

The total peripheral resistance can be adjusted by sympathetic vasomotor nerves to sustain the systemic arterial blood pressure at fairly constant levels in spite of gross changes in cardiac output. Thus, the mean systemic arterial pressure is not greatly altered during exercise when cardiac output may increase several fold. Conversely, a reduction in cardiac output can be compensated by appropriate constriction of peripheral vascular beds. The blood flow through vital organs, such as the heart and brain, is generally believed to be sustained by constriction in other organs which are not so immediately essential to life. Thus, constriction of the vasculature in the skin, skeletal muscle, splanchnic bed and kidneys is the expected reaction to diminished cardiac output. The mechanisms which regulate the distribution of resistance and flow in the vascular beds are indicated by the term general vasomotor control (Fig. 1). Changes in the peripheral vascular beds have been implicated in the low blood pressure of patients with peritonitis (9). In addition, local vasomotor controls are generally pictured in terms of substances which act on local vascular structures producing vasodilation. For example, the grossly exaggerated blood flow during reactive hyperemia is generally explained on the basis of accumulation of vasodilator substances in tissues deprived of blood flow. The greatly depressed systemic arterial pressure in the "crush syndrome" may be related to this mechanism. In contrast, certain humoral substances, such as catechol amines, exert a constrictor action on most vascular beds. The secretion of catechol amines from the adrenal glands has been shown to be elevated during experimentally induced hypovolemia (10). Acute reduction in systemic arterial pressure may accompany serious allergic reactions or anaphylaxis, largely due to peripheral vasodilation.

Classification of shock

Various possible causes of systemic arterial hypotension are listed in Fig. 1. The exact mechanisms by which each of these causes may exert its effect have not been elucidated in all cases. Each factor listed has been assigned prominent or dominant roles in the production of some form of "shock" in human patients. The cardiovascular disturbances produced by these widely different mechanisms could not be reasonably covered by a single term: "shock". Instead, a specific term with precise definition should be consistently applied to each of the different mechanisms.

Should the term "shock" be discarded? Since the term "shock" has been applied to hypotensive states associated with virtually every conceivable mechanism affecting blood pressure (see Fig. 1), the term is not only ambiguous but a serious obstacle to communication. When a group of investigators meet to discuss "shock", misunderstandings are bound to arise on a purely semantic basis, since each may have a different cause or effect in mind.

Scientific communication about "shock" would be greatly clarified by more concise and accurate definitions. Based on the assumption that a characteristic common to all the various conditions called "shock" is a depression of systemic arterial pressure, the various possible causes of systemic hypotension could be used for classification of "shock". Thus, the familiar response to hemorrhage might be labeled *exsanguination hypotension* (or oligemic hypotension). Similarly, the corresponding symptom complex from loss of body fluids could be designated *dehydration hypotension*. Fainting reactions in soldiers standing at attention could be called *sequestration hypotension*, assuming that a shift of blood into dependent extremities is established as the dominant causative factor. Various types of "shock" are listed on the right of Fig. 1 as examples of terms that could be used to specify systemic hypotension caused by different mechanisms. If all the specific causes of systemic hypotension could be verified by carefully designed experiments and then concisely defined and labeled, a group of terms similar to that on the right of Fig. 1 could be evolved to serve as appropriate tools for communication. Under these conditions, the term "shock" could be permanently abandoned in favor of more concise and scientific terminology.

The functional effects of exsanguination

Among all the possible causes of hypotensive states, controlled hemorrhage is the most common experimental model. It appears at the top of the list in Fig. 1. The cardiovascular responses to exsanguination hypotension, and its alleviation, have been studied intensively in many different laboratories. As an example of the kind of analysis which is needed for each different form of hypotensive state, attention is directed to this most popular experimental procedure. By means of an oversimplified hydraulic model, the reactions to exsanguination can be described in three phases: (I) Depletion of venous reservoirs. (II) Depressed systemic arterial pressure. (III) Breakdown of compensatory mechanisms by vicious circles.

Phase I. **Depletion of the venous reservoir capacity.** The quantity of blood contained within the venous system is variable. In 1918 Hooker (*11*) demonstrated that stimulation of a nerve trunk to an isolated segment of the large bowel produced an elevation in venous pressure as measured by a water manometer. Alexander (*12*) demonstrated changes in distensibility of a splanchnic vascular bed. Sjöstrand (*13*) described four different types of reservoirs: (*1*) Pulmonary vessels and heart which take up or release blood due to shifts in balance between right and left ventricular output. (*2*) Areas which take up or release blood without impairing nutrition or function of the tissue, such as cutaneous venous plexus and perhaps venous plexuses in other regions. (*3*) Areas which take up or release blood in response to circulatory readjustments such as larger veins. (*4*) Areas releasing blood in the "alarm" reaction, which may interfere with the function of organs such as the spleen, intestine, liver and kidney.

The functional significance of reservoir capacity can be represented schematically by means of a simple hydraulic model consisting of a pump, a high-pressure conduit system and a series of valves controlling flow through small channels into a low-pressure return system (Fig. 2a). The variability in the capacity of the low-pressure system is represented by bellows, by the collapsible horizontal channel and by the level of fluid in the reservoir just upstream from the pump. If a quantity of blood is removed from the system and the venous reservoir capacity contracts by precisely this amount, the state of the cardiovascular system would be unchanged except for the content of blood on the venous side. The stroke volume, heart rate, cardiac output and the flow through different organs could remain unchanged as long as the venous capacity was compensated by constriction of the reservoirs. If the

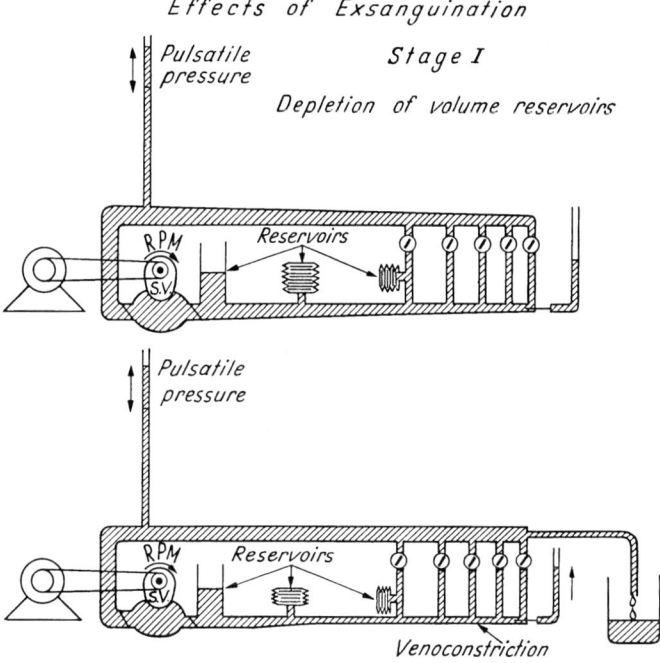

Fig. 2a. The effects of exsanguination (blood loss) can be considered in terms of a simple hydraulic model. In Phase I removal of blood from the system could theoretically be completely compensated by constriction of venous reservoirs—cardiac output, blood pressure and blood flow remaining completely normal

quantity of blood removed exceeded the contraction of reservoirs, the pressure level in the standpipe just upstream from the pump would fall. If the filling pressure descended enough, the stroke volume of the pump would diminish. The quantity of blood loss that can be compensated by contraction of venous reservoirs without reduction in filling pressure or stroke volume is not certain and is probably variable. However, removal of 500 cc. of blood for transfusion is very well tolerated and may represent a reasonable approximation of that state. On the other hand, GAUER, HENRY and SIEKER (14) reported that the central venous pressure diminished on the average by 0.7 cm. of water from withdrawal of 100 cc. of blood in a 70 kg. subject. Spontaneous restoration of filling pressure levels occurred in two stages: a rapid recovery phase followed by a slower return to control pressure in central veins over periods longer than 50 minutes.

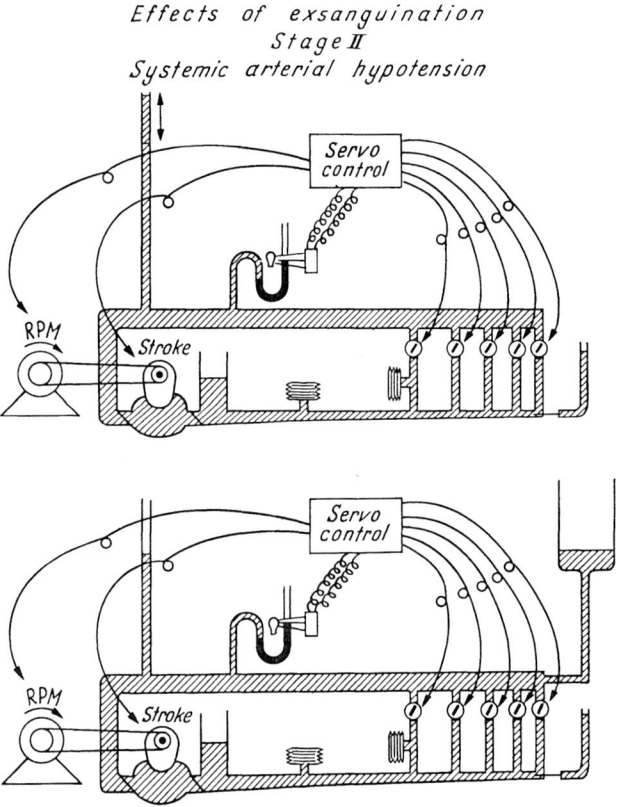

Fig. 2b. In Phase II the systemic arterial pressure is depressed but is partly compensated by a servo control. The hypotension results from reduced cardiac output without corresponding increase in peripheral resistance

Phase II. **Reduction in systemic arterial pressure.** In the schematic model (Fig. 2b), the perfusion pressure is under servo control consisting of a device monitoring the pressure and sending an error signal to a control device capable of instituting appropriate changes in the output of the pump and selective control of the outflow valves. In general, the regulation of systemic arterial pressure is visualized in terms of baroreceptor reflexes affecting heart rate and systolic ejection, more or less simultaneously with appropriate alterations in total peripheral resistance. According to STEAD (15) as much as 40 per cent of the total blood volume may be removed from recumbent humans without fainting. At first systemic arterial pressure becomes progressively lower because of a reduction in cardiac output with the total peripheral resistance tending to remain relatively unchanged as though only the baroreceptor reflexes to the heart were active. More severe hypovolemia, produced by withdrawing 20 ml. of blood per kilogram, was accompanied by reduced right atrial transmural pressure, reduced stroke volume and lower cardiac output in spite of tachycardia (16). These alterations are consistent with the mechanisms indicated in Fig. 1 by which blood loss could cause systemic arterial hypotension. The different vascular beds are not affected equally and the distinctive responses of the various vascular beds to the factors influencing resistance and flow have been recently reviewed by GREEN and KEPCHAR (17). With progressively greater exsanguination, the cardiac output continues to decline and the peripheral resistance increases as flow through the vascular beds in different tissues slows. Thus, ZWEIFACH (18) directly observed almost complete cessation of skin blood flow following removal of about $1/_3$ of the total blood volume from rats. Under similar conditions sluggish or stagnant circulation was seen in skeletal muscle in the abdominal wall of the rat and the tibialis anticus of the cat. By means of dropmeters, CORDAY and WILLIAMS (19) confirmed the concept that resistance to flow through both the kidney and intestine increases greatly following hemorrhage. Impedence to blood flow through these tissues tended to preserve blood flow through the brain and myocardium.

The effects of systemic arterial hypotension on blood flow through various tissues are indicated schematically in Fig. 3a. The lowered mean arterial pressure head diminishes the perfusion pressure through all the tissues. The reduced driving pressure tends to diminish the blood flow through the cerebral blood vessels which have limited capacity for vasodilation. Coronary flow should be curtailed by reduced perfusion pressure, exaggerated by shortened diastolic intervals with tachycardia. So long as the systemic arterial hypotension is neither too severe (i.e. above 40—50 mm. Hg) nor too prolonged, the cardiovascular system may remain in this delicate state of equilibrium for hours. Restoration of the normal blood volume is promptly followed by complete recovery. However, the functional state of the vital organs is so precarious that complete and irreversible collapse can result theoretically in several ways (Fig. 3 b). *Phase III.* **Breakdown of compensatory mechanisms by vicious cycles.** With the cardiovascular system balanced in a state of sustained systemic arterial hypotension, any new factor which further depresses the arterial pressure tends to initiate a vicious

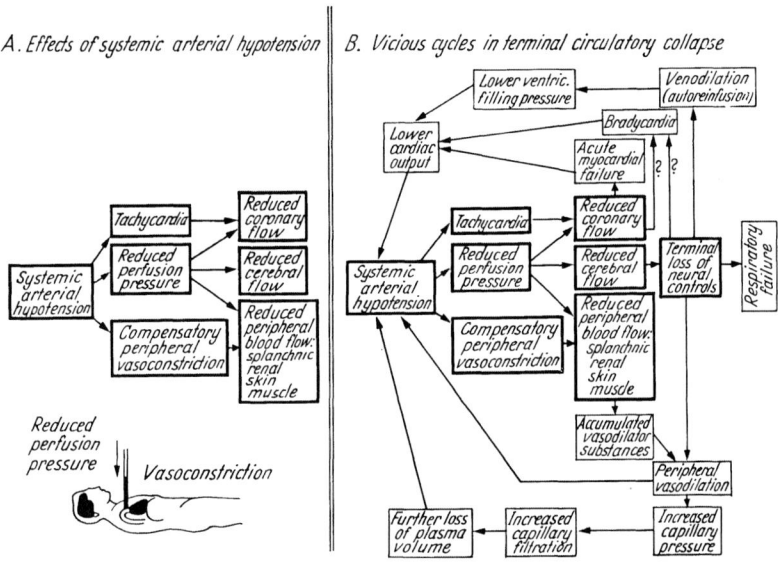

A. Effects of systemic arterial hypotension   *B. Vicious cycles in terminal circulatory collapse*

Fig. 3 A. Systemic arterial hypotension theoretically causes tachycardia, reduced perfusion pressure and compensatory peripheral vasoconstriction. This condition can remain delicately balanced for hours and permit complete recovery with restoration of the blood volume

Fig. 3 B. The terminal events in circulatory collapse may take many different forms depending upon which of many types of vicious cycles are encountered. Note that loss of neural controls plays a central role in several of these different pathways to progressive reduction in blood pressure and death

cycle. For example, insufficient cerebral blood flow frequently leads to depression of the central nervous system, as will be documented below. A common mode of death in such cases is acute respiratory failure. If loss of neural control is manifested by relaxation of the constricted venous reservoirs (Fig. 2 a) the cardiovascular system is not restored to normal function by adding blood to the system. Some animals suddenly develop severe bradycardia or cardiac arrhythmias. This could result either from altered neural control or from inadequate coronary blood flow. Since the mechanism is not at all clear, these mechanisms are queried in Fig. 3 b. The diminished coronary blood flow is coupled with tachycardia, which reduces both coronary flow and myocardial efficiency. The combination could reasonably lead to acute heart failure with reduced cardiac output and further reduction in the arterial pressure. Disastrous vicious cycles can be initiated by vasodilation in the portions of the peripheral vascular system which have been clamped down by compensatory reflex mechanisms. For example, vasodilator substances can theoretically accumulate in ischemic tissues leading to reactive hyperemia. The exact nature of these substances is not known, but they are quite certainly not just reduced oxygen or increased CO_2, pH, lactic acid or other common metabolites. SELKURT (20) demonstrated that experimentally induced ischemia of the intestines was not well tolerated in the absence of liver function and postulated an unknown vasotoxic substance produced by the hypoxic intestine.

A loss of vasoconstrictor activity from cerebral ischemia in the presence of accumulated vasodilator substances could cause peripheral vasodilation, precipitous fall in systemic pressure and death. Increased capillary flow in several anoxic tissues, coupled with increased capillary pressure, could lead to greater capillary filtration, further loss of plasma volume, and further drop in systemic arterial pressure. McRAE et al. (21) directed attention to large quantities of bloody fluid within the bowel of animals dying of "shock". They postulated a terminal loss of plasma fluid into the intestinal lumen, contributing to circulatory collapse and death.

Cardiovascular responses during arterial hypotension in unanesthetized dogs. The importance of the central nervous system in cardiovascular regulation has been repeatedly stressed in recent years (22, 23). Although the systemic arterial pressure can be reduced abruptly and profoundly without producing obvious signs of cerebral dysfunction, reduction in cerebral blood flow becomes apparent when the perfusion pressure drops below some critical level, and cerebral dysrhythmia appears abruptly on the E.E.G. (24, 25). BERTRAND et al. (26) described a patient in whom severe degeneration of the brain might have resulted at least in part from sustained systemic arterial hypotension.

Since the role of the higher levels of the central nervous system cannot be accurately assessed by experiments performed on anesthetized experimental animals, a series of experiments was conducted on seven healthy unanesthetized dogs. In preparation for each study, sensing elements for pulsed ultrasonic flowmeters (27, 28) were mounted on the outside of arteries under aseptic conditions. The animals were fully recovered after one or two weeks. The recording equipment was checked out and the animal

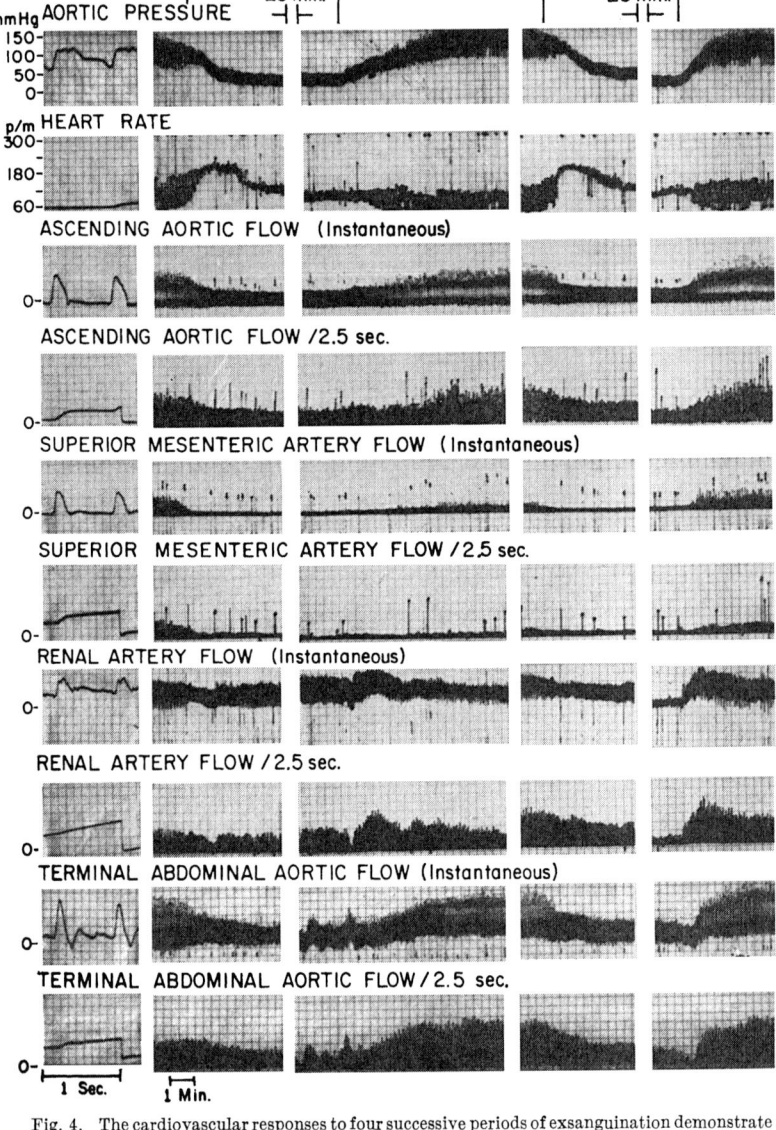

Fig. 4. The cardiovascular responses to four successive periods of exsanguination demonstrate

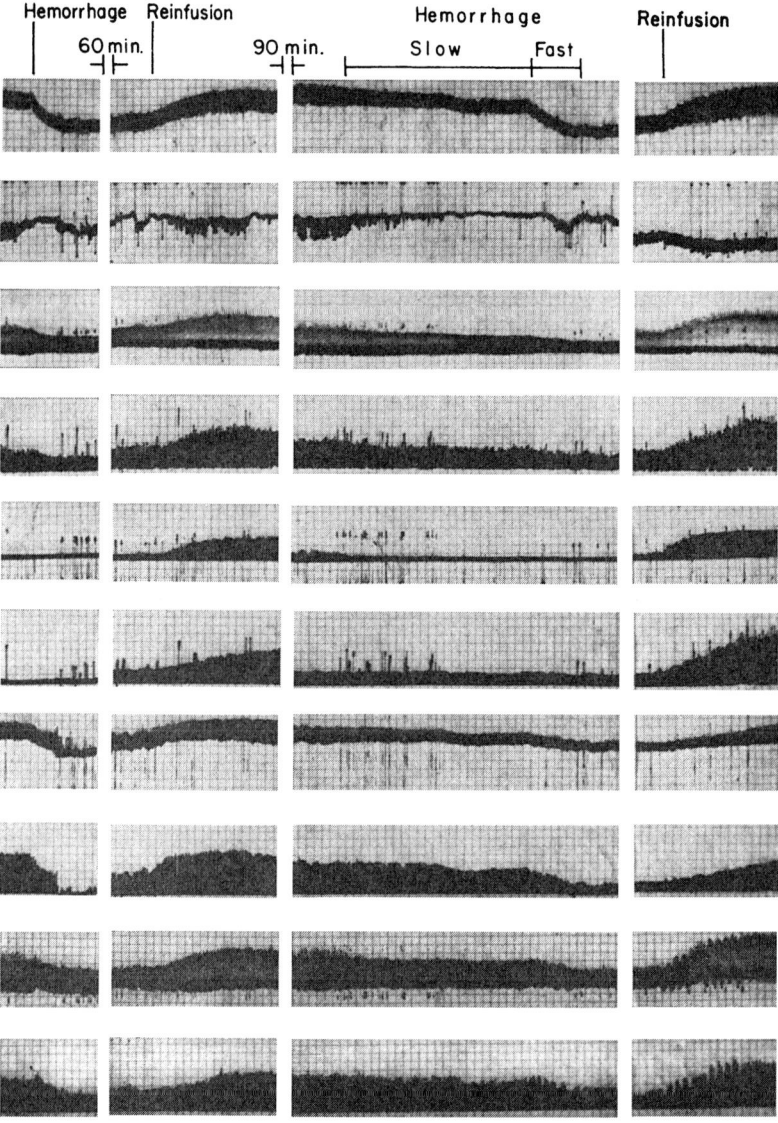

the variety of changes in flow distribution and heart rate in a single unanesthetized dog

was immobilized by securing the front legs and hind legs. Under these conditions a dog with moderate disposition and slight training will lie quietly for hours. Under local anesthetic the femoral artery was canulated with a large-bore polyethylene tube and connected by a T-tube to a Statham pressure transducer and to a reservoir bottle through a heat exchanger. Blood leaving the animal and entering the reservoir was cooled to 4° C, and was rewarmed to body temperature while being reinfused into the dog. The reservoir and tubing were sterilized to further reduce bacterial growth in the blood stored in the reservoir during the experiment. Blood was allowed to run into the reservoir bottle and the height of the fluid level was adjusted to maintain a mean arterial pressure at a predetermined level equivalent to 40 and 50 mm. Hg. The reservoir bottle also acted as a *Windkessel* greatly attenuating the normal pulse pressure fluctuations. Salient features of the cardiovascular adjustments of intact unanesthetized dogs to experimentally induced systemic arterial hypotension are illustrated in Fig. 4. In this experiment, exsanguination and reinfusion were repeated four times in succession to produce systemic arterial hypotension of progressively increasing duration. The reduction in arterial pressure was the same in each instance, but the changes in heart rate, cardiac output, and distribution of blood flow were different. During the first two periods of hypotension, the heart rate accelerated as the blood ran out into the reservoir and then tended to return toward the baseline even though the blood pressure remained depressed. This response was typical and suggested some form of overriding or adaptation of the baroreceptor reflexes. During successive periods of hypotension, the heart rate became faster and the fluctuations in the heart rate diminished. During the fourth period of hypotension, the heart rate remained quite steady at about 200/min. The flowmeter on the ascending aorta continuously monitored left ventricular instantaneous flow velocity and left ventricular output (ascending aortic flow/2.5 sec.), which diminished markedly during each period of exsanguination. The changes in aortic flow were similar during each of the four periods except that the instantaneous flow rates and cardiac output both increased significantly after the final reinfusion. The flow in the superior mesenteric artery diminished to extremely low levels very promptly as the blood loss began and remained low even after the first two reinfusions. After the third and fourth reinfusions, the mesenteric flow increased to levels above the control level. In contrast, the flow to the left kidney displayed marked reduction during the second and third period of exsanguination and moderate or transient changes in the first and last periods. The flow through the terminal abdominal aorta to the hindquarters was distinctly reduced during the first two periods of exsanguination but showed much less effect during the third and fourth periods. Thus, there was no stereotyped cardiovascular response to the controlled reduction in systemic arterial pressure even when repeated in the same dog.

In another dog, some 600 cc. of blood were permitted to enter the reservoir slowly and another 360 cc. entered rapidly (Fig. 5). The heart rate was increased only transiently but the variability was reduced. Both mesenteric and renal blood flow were significantly lower and remained reduced during the period of hypotension. The mean systemic arterial pressure was maintained at about 40 mm. Hg for two hours, by which time blood began to flow back into the dog from the reservoir (autoinfusion of 300 cc. in Fig. 5). When an additional 300 cc. of blood was forceably returned to the animal the arterial pressure rose to approximately the control level. The heart rate abruptly accelerated to about 180 beats per minute after this reinfusion of blood. The superior mesenteric and renal flows increased toward control levels even though the peak flow velocities during each ventricular systole remained depressed. This type of phenomenon might be explained in terms of a smaller ventricular stroke volume associated with tachycardia and associated with some vasodilation in these two vascular beds.

The arterial catheter was clamped to eliminate the *Windkessel* effect and to reveal the full arterial pulse pressure. Both the mean pressure and the systolic pressure declined progressively. The final increment of blood (360 cc.) was returned to the animal, temporarily restoring arterial pressure. In spite of the restoration of the total blood volume, the systemic arterial pressure continued to decline until it was approximately 60/40 mm. Hg. An infusion of Levophed elevated arterial pressure again for a brief period. Acute respiratory failure required artificial respiration, and severe bradycardia appeared soon thereafter. Artificial respiration and a large dose of epinephrine failed to correct the severe hypotension and the animal died. This sequence of events might be considered rather "typical" of hemorrhagic shock. However, the response is not simple. A number of mechanisms can be tentatively identified in the final collapse of the circulation. For example, the blood pressure fell progressively in spite of the fact that the blood volume had been restored. This phenomenon might involve venodilation as suggested in Fig. 3. The blood flow through both mesenteric and renal arteries was increased over that recorded during the sustained hypotension, which suggests some degree of vasodilation of peripheral resistance vessels. On the other hand, the peak flow velocities during each systole were diminished in both renal and mesenteric arteries as though the ejection velocity from the left ventricle were

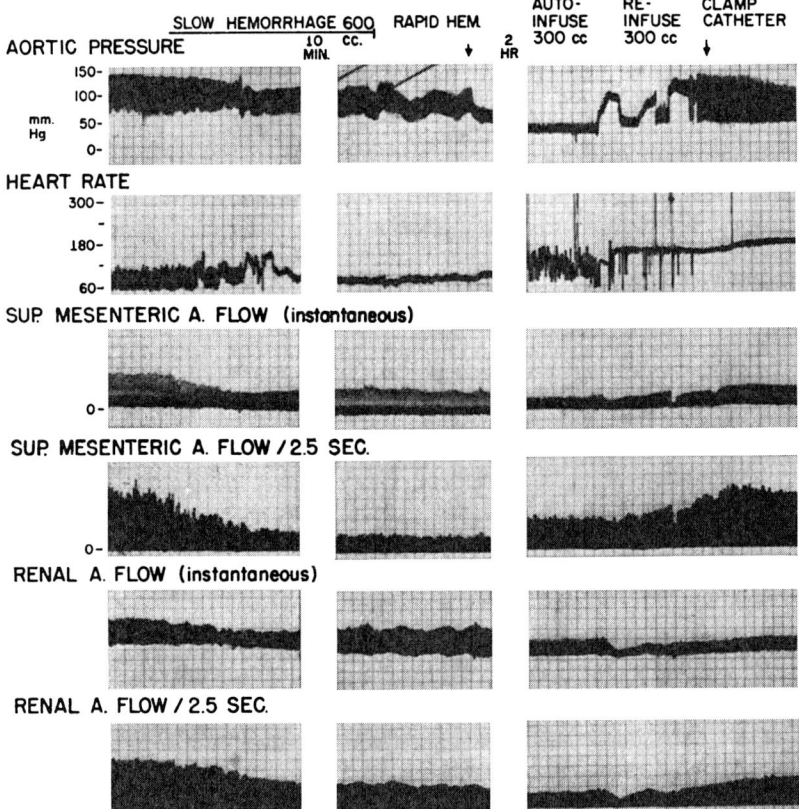

Fig. 5. A rather typical example of "irreversible hemorrhagic shock" in an unanesthetized dog
administration of Levophed, artificial respiration and a large dose of epinephrine.

slowed. Respiratory failure and severe bradycardia occurred in rapid succession at a time when the animal could no longer be aroused. During the initial period of induced hypotension the animal was conscious and would occasionally lift his head and look around, particularly in response to a noise or movement in the room. He could not be aroused at the time of respiratory failure. Tracheal intubation was readily performed without anesthesia.

The corneal reflex and pupillary reflexes were either severely depressed or absent and did not return. The loss of consciousness and sluggish or absent reflexes indicated that the central nervous system was severely depressed. In general, it was noted that

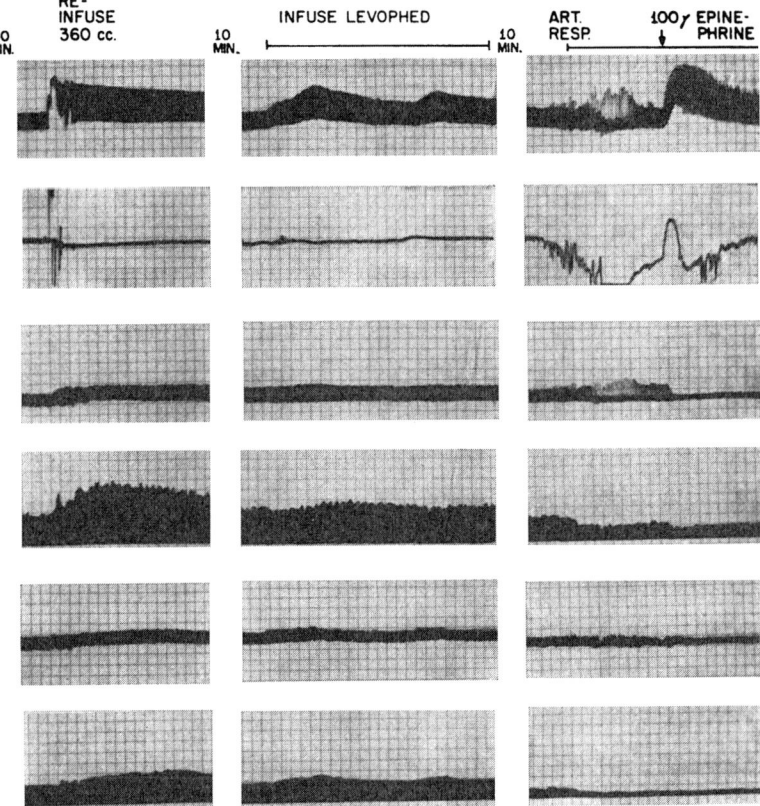

displays progressive fall in systemic arterial pressure in spite of restoration of blood volume, Even in such an experiment the terminal causes of circulatory collapse are complex

respiratory failure, severe bradycardia, rapid autoinfusion or uncontrollable drop in blood pressure were commonly associated with difficulty in arousing the animal and depression of reflexes.

To investigate the state of the central nervous system in the terminal stages of shock, electrodes were implanted in two dogs in diencephalic sites at which stimulation produced very large cardiovascular responses. After one or two weeks for recovery, controlled

18   R. F. Rushmer, R. L. van Citters, and D. Franklin:

arterial hypotension was induced (see Fig. 6). The response of the
animal after sustained hypotension of some 2.5 hours was super-
ficially similar to that illustrated in Fig. 5. However, the superior

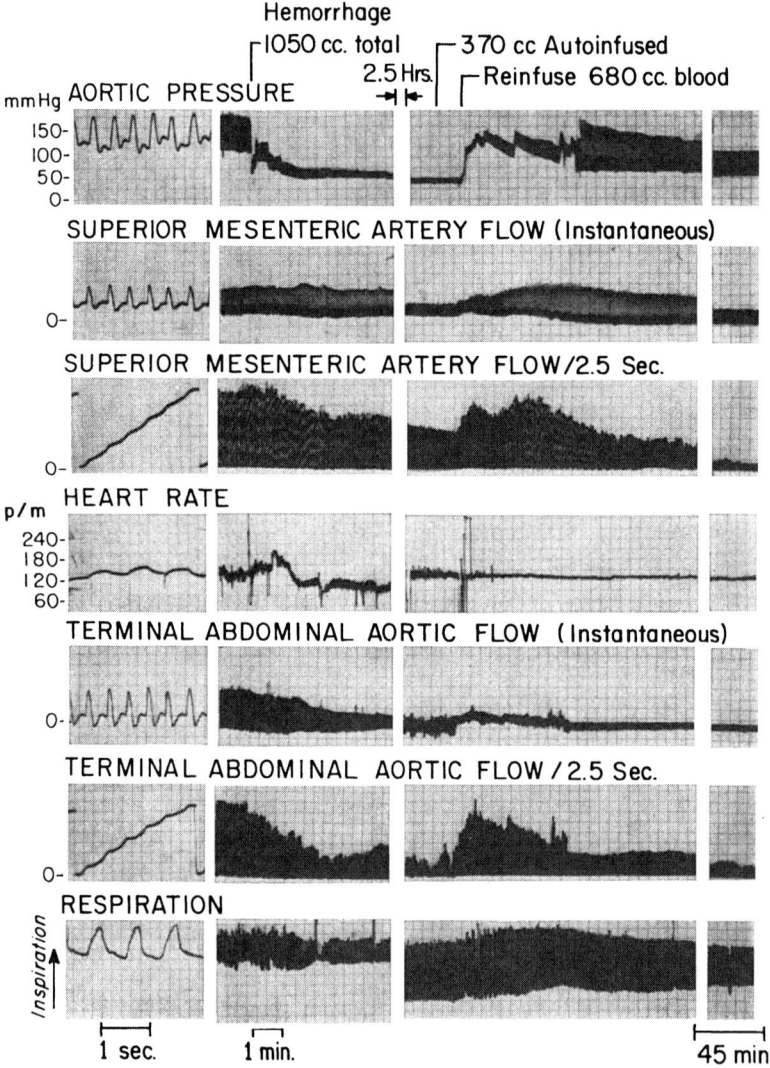

Fig. 6. Depression of the central nervous system is further indicated by greatly
(hypothalamic

mesenteric flow rapidly dropped to very low levels after autoinfusion. About 45 minutes later, the arterial pressure remained low, and respiratory rate increased up to 70 per minute with very small

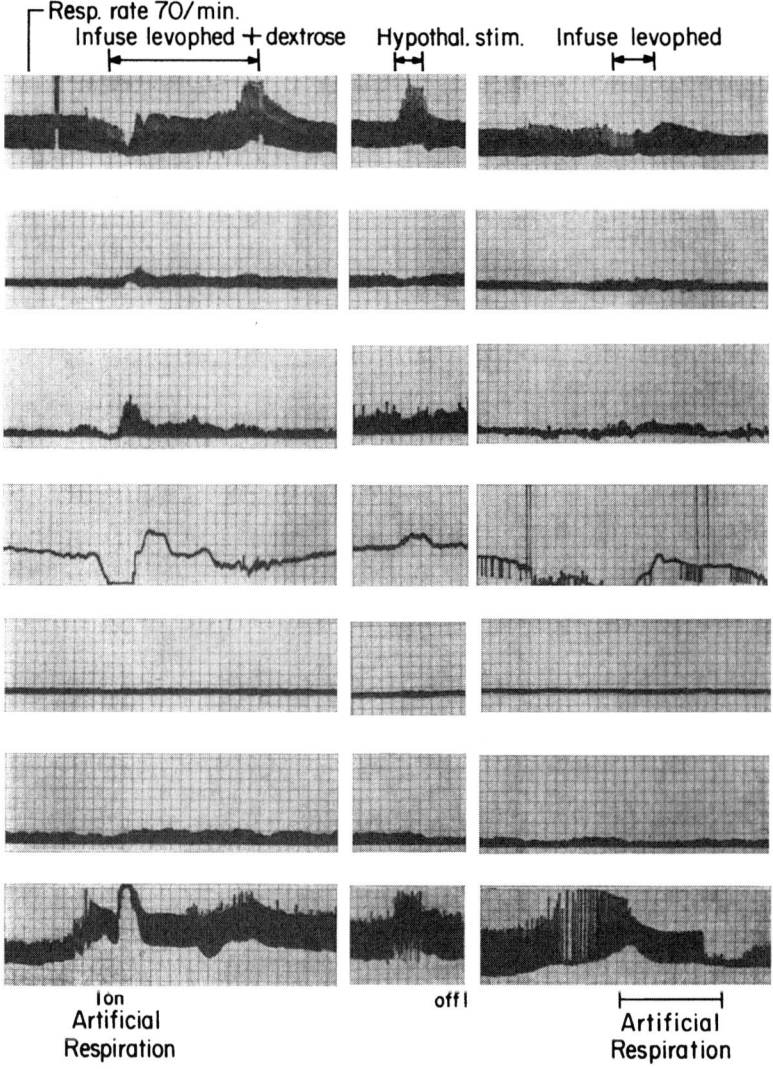

attenuated cardiovascular responses to stimulation of selected sites in the diencephalon stimulation)

2*

tidal volume. Institution of artificial respiration was associated with severe bradycardia, extreme hypotension and a transient increase in mesenteric artery flow. Hypothalamic stimulation produced a slight increase in heart rate and in systolic arterial pressure, presumably by its effect on the myocardium, but failed to influence flow through either superior mesenteric artery or terminal abdominal aorta. In another dog, repeated stimulation of diencephalic sites during the period of the circulatory collapse provided evidence of progressive reduction in the magnitude of the response as the animal became more somnolent; the reflexes became depressed and the circulatory status deteriorated. After the blood pressure was restored by infusion of norepinephrine, the reflexes returned, the animal again spontaneously lifted its head, and stimulation of the same diencephalic site again produced a very pronounced change in peripheral flow.

When systemic arterial pressure is abruptly reduced, a prompt tachycardia should be provoked by baroreceptor reflexes. This tachycardia should be sustained as long as the hypotension persists. In virtually all instances the reduction in systemic arterial pressure was accompanied by transient tachycardia lasting during the period when the blood was being withdrawn. By the time the steady hypotensive levels were reached, the heart rate returned to approximately control levels. This type of response would be seriously obscured in experiments on dogs under anesthesia, which produces cardio-acceleration to levels well over 100/minute during the control period.

Two of the animals died rather suddenly from severe bradycardia without developing uncontrollable systemic arterial hypotension. The mechanism by which bradycardia is produced as a terminal event remains obscure.

Summary

A review of the control of systemic arterial pressure demonstrated that virtually all known mechanisms which can theoretically influence either cardiac output or total peripheral resistance have been assigned a role in the production of "shock". Thus, the term "shock" is not only entirely ambiguous but an impedence to both communication and understanding. Since systemic hypotension is the only consistent characteristic of shock, those factors which can lower systemic pressures should be defined and designated with precise descriptive terms. This symposium could take an important step by discarding the term "shock" throughout the proceedings and by consistently using clear terminology with precise definitions for the various conditions under discussion.

The most common experimental model for systemic arterial hypotension is controlled exsanguination. On a theoretical basis, some unknown quantity of blood could be removed and completely compensated by contraction of the venous reservoir capacity. Under these conditions, the systemic arterial pressures, cardiac output and total peripheral resistance could be normal (Fig. 2a). Further exsanguination leads to systemic hypotension from diminished cardiac output without corresponding reduction in peripheral resistance. With further bleeding, the reduced stroke volume is compensated by acceleration of the heart rate and selective peripheral vasoconstriction through the pressure-controlling servo-system (Fig. 2b). An equilibrium can be established under conditions of systemic hypotension, lasting for hours (Fig. 3a). Replacement of the shed blood promptly restores the circulatory system toward normality. On the other hand, systemic arterial hypotension of too great severity or too long duration can lead to a number of fatal vicious cycles (Fig. 3b). Each of these pathways constitutes a mechanism by which a further reduction in systemic arterial hypotension ultimately causes death.

The final outcome from prolonged systemic arterial hypotension can theoretically take many forms (Fig. 3b). There may be no single result of systemic hypotension just as there is no single cause of hypotension. The importance of the terminal loss of neural control would obviously be obscured in experiments conducted on anesthetized experimental animals. To test the validity of this analysis, systemic arterial hypotension was induced in a series of completely unanesthetized dogs with indwelling instruments to monitor cardiovascular responses.

The terminal stages and types of death take many different forms in unanesthetized dogs subjected to prolonged systemic arterial hypotension. Common among these are severe disturbances in respiratory function, autoreinfusion, uncontrollable depression of systemic arterial pressure, severe bradycardia, and cardiac arrest. In many instances, abrupt deterioration in the condition of the animals was accompanied by loss of corneal and pupillary reflexes associated with failure to arouse on stimulation. These observations all suggest that depression of the central nervous system is a common and important feature in the final circulatory collapse. Since these changes may be obscured in experimental animals subjected to surgical anesthesia, artificial respiration, and operative procedures, definitive studies on these points should be carried out in intact, unanesthetized animals.

References

1. RUSHMER, R. F.: Circulation (U.S.A.) 20, 897 (1959). — 2. CLARKSON, B., D. THOMPSON, M. HORWITH, and E. H. LUCKEY: Transact. Ass. Amer. Physicians 73, 272 (1960). — 3. ALEXANDER, R. S.: Circulation Res. (U.S.A.) 3, 181 (1950). — 4. RUSHMER, R. F.: Amer. J. Physiol. 192, 631 (1958). — 5. BARCROFT, H. and H. J. C. SWAN: Sympathetic control of human blood vessels. vii, 165 pp. Baltimore: The Williams and Wilkins Co. 1953. — 6. SHARPEY-SCHAFER, E. P.: In: Shock and Circulatory Homeostasis. GREEN, H. D., ed. New York: Josiah Macy, Jr. Foundation 1952. p. 115—139. — 7. RUSHMER, R. F.: Amer. J. Physiol. 141, 722 (1944). — 8. UVNÄS, B.: Physiol. Rev. (U.S.A.) 34, 608 (1954). — 9. HARDY, J. D.: J. Surg. Res. 1, 64 (1961). — 10. WALKER, W. F., M. S. ZILELI, F. W. REUTTER, W. C. SHOEMAKER, D. FRIEND, and F. D. MOORE: Amer. J. Physiol. 197, 773 (1959). — 11. HOOKER, D. R.: Amer. J. Physiol. 46, 591 (1918). — 12. ALEXANDER, R. S.: Circulation Res. (U.S.A.) 2, 140 (1954). — 13. SJÖSTRAND, T.: Acta physiol. Scand. 26, 312 (1952). — 14. GAUER, O. H., J. P. HENRY, and H. O. SIEKER: Circulation Res. (U.S.A.) 4, 79 (1956). — 15. STEAD, E. A.: Physiology and methods of measurements of shock. VII. Circulation dynamics

in shock. An address read at the Symposium on Shock at the Army Medical Service Graduate School. May 7, 1951. — 16. FOWLER, N. O., R. SHABETAI, D. ANDERSON, and J. R., BRAUNSTEIN: Amer. Heart. J. **60**, 551 (1960). — 17. GREEN H. D. and J. H. KEPCHAR: Physiol. Rev. (U.S.A.) **39**, 617 (1959). — 18. ZWEIFACH, B. W.: In: Shock and circulatory homeostasis. p. 15—72. GREEN, H. D., ed. New York, Josiah Macy, Jr. Foundation 1952. — 19. CORDAY, E. and J. H. WILLIAMS: Amer. J. Med. **29**, 228 (1960). — 20. SELKURT, E. E.: Amer. J. Physiol. **197**, 281 (1959). — 21. MCRAE, J. M., W. R. WEBB, S. S. LEE, J. D. HARDY, and J. C. GRIFFIN: Surg. Forum (U.S.A.) **9**, 37 (1958). — 22. RUSHMER, R. F. and O. A. SMITH Jr.: Physiol. Rev. (U.S.A.) **39**, 41 (1959). — 23. Proceedings of a symposium on central nervous system control of circulation. EICHNA, L. W., and D. G. MCQUARRIE, eds., Physiol. Rev. (U.S.A). **40**, (Suppl. 4) 1—311, (1960). — 24. STEVENS, H. and J. F. FAZEKAS: Arch. Neurol. Psychiatr. (U.S.A.) **73**, 416 (1955). — 25. FAZEKAS, J. F., J. KLEH, and A. E. PARRISH: Ann. Int. Med. (U.S.A.) **43**, 165 (1955). — 26. BERTRAND, I., F. LHERMITTE, B. ANTOIN, and H. DUCROT: Rev. neurol. (Fr.) **101**, 101 (1959). — 27. FRANKLIN, D. L., D. W. BAKER, R. M. ELLIS, and R. F. RUSHMER: IRE Transact. on Med. Elec. ME-6, 204 (1959). — 28. BAKER, D., R. M. ELLIS, D. L. FRANKLIN, and R. F. RUSHMER: Proc. IRE. **47**, 1917 (1959).

Discussion

GREGERSEN: I have two comments to make and would also like to say at the start that I am strongly inclined toward Dr. RUSHMER's views and presentation. The type of schema he has presented, so useful in teaching, is an excellent starting point in thinking about shock. A similar schema helped to clarify the shock problem, at least in my mind, at the beginning of World War II. As Dr. RUSHMER has emphasised, the diagram helps one to keep in mind that there are many channels through which the vicious cycle can develop and to remember to reduce each experiment or clinical case under study to specific physiological phenomena rather than fall back on using the general term shock. You will recall that, as Dr. WIGGERS pointed out in his monograph ten years ago, the term shock originally referred to the blow causing injury, not to what happened to the organism as a result or to the state produced. I wholly agree that continued use of the term shock tends to block rather than help in useful communication.

Dr. RUSHMER's refined recording techniques seem to me to have great potential for further study of the relations of detailed circulatory events in various parts of the organism in shock-like states. However, I am not quite clear on your technique. You seem to measure linear flow velocity. Am I correct? Is it linear flow or volume flow?

RUSHMER: The original recording is linear flow velocity, which is averaged across the whole flow stream. As a final event in the experiment, each of these flow meters is empirically calibrated *in situ* against known volume flow by both steady flow and pulsatile flow, so that we can then calibrate both in terms of linear flow velocity and volume flow per unit of time.

GREGERSEN: Dr. RUSHMER asked a question: How much blood can be removed before there are changes in heart rate and other vascular reactions? This was the experiment, you remember, that MEEK and EYSTER made in 1921. Their study was not altogether satisfactory, first because they used anaesthetised animals, and secondly, they did not then know the storage function of the spleen in the dog. At my suggestion, Dr. SHU CHIEN in my laboratory repeated these experiments with modern techniques on unanaesthetised, splenectomised dogs. His quantitative evaluation of the compensatory constriction and compensatory dilution in haemorrhage showed that definitive changes in heart rate, etc. begin at 10—15% reduction in blood volume (CHIEN, Amer. J. Physiol. **193**, 605, 1958). I think you will find the answer to your question in his report.

RUSHMER: I came to something like the same conclusion from the fact that one can give up about 500 ml. of blood in a transfusion without difficulty.

NICKERSON: I agree with Dr. RUSHMER that there are a great many different precipitating factors and different sequences of events that can lead to what we often refer to as shock. I hate to add to his diagram, but it appears to me that as it is set out, the primary criterion of shock is decreased systemic arterial pressure. We have come to view systemic arterial pressure as one of the least reliable criteria of the shock state. Severe shock can develop with a high blood pressure, and the circulation can be much improved when the blood pressure is subsequently lowered. This leads to consideration of several factors, one of which is the role of vasoconstriction itself in causing a reduction in the effective circulating blood volume. I wonder if Dr. RUSHMER could include in his diagram the role of a high blood pressure due to vasoconstriction in the development of shock.

VON EULER: I fancy the problem raised now by Dr. NICKERSON could make this discussion go on for a very long time. I rather think we should try and push on.

KROG: I was just wondering: what do you think happens to the big vessels inside the probe? Do you think that vasomotion could invalidate post-experimental calibration?

RUSHMER: We believe that changes in calibre of the artery within the flow section are effectually ruled out by the fact that a layer of scar tissue completely encases the plastic cylinder and holds the vessel rigidly against the walls.

Comparison of various forms of experimental shock

(with special reference to experimental design)

By

J. FINE

Patients in shock do not lend themselves to more than a minimum amount of manipulation. Therefore, if we are to discover the mechanism that leads to death, and to assess the role of individual components in a complex of factors that are so frequently involved, it is necessary to take the problem to the experimental laboratory.

We may begin a consideration of experimental models by defining the clinical state we propose to simulate. The clinical state I shall talk about is one which clinicians see frequently and recognize quite readily. The skin is pale, cold and moist; the pulse is fast; the mean systolic blood pressure is below 80 and falling; and the production of urine has stopped, or is sharply reduced. These are the essential components of the syndrome known as traumatic shock. No other signs need be present, but all of these must be present. In physiological terms this disorder is a state of acute and persisting deficiency of blood flow through the tissues. The rapid development of widespread and far-reaching functional disturbances soon results in death if the condition is not quickly relieved. If it can be relieved, the shock may be defined as reversible. When it cannot be, it is irreversible. Whether it is one or the other depends on the cause, the duration of the shock, and the effectiveness of the available methods of treatment.

We may choose to study features common to all types of shock, such as metabolic acidosis, potassium retention, changes in enzymatic activity, changes in peripheral resistance, decline in oxygen consumption, in cardiac output, or in energy levels. Or we may choose to examine a feature peculiar to a particular type of shock, such as the increased viscosity of the blood in burn or tourniquet shock, the site of action of bacterial toxins in septic shock, or the role of the catechol amines in hemorrhagic shock. Of the various causes of traumatic shock, reduced blood volume produced by hemorrhage is the commonest.

I shall begin this discussion of experimental models with a consideration of hemorrhagic shock, the type which is so widely used experimentally. How shall we design this model? Hemorrhagic shock is usually a relatively simple problem. One stops the hemorrhage and replaces the blood lost. Usually there is a rapid return of the normal state, and that is the end of the problem. This is hemorrhagic shock which we characterize as reversible to transfusion. But occasionally the response to adequate transfusion may not be favorable, and the patient dies. We then are dealing with hemorrhagic shock which is irreversible to transfusion. Why does hemorrhagic shock in certain individuals become irreversible to transfusion, while in others it does not? This is a difficult question to answer. We know that certain factors such as advanced age, prior depleting disease, or undue delay in treating the blood loss may contribute to making the circulation refractory to full replacement of the volume deficiency. But the nature of the injury that causes death is not understood. To study this question we need a model of reversible shock and one of irreversible shock, or better, a model which is reversible at first and in time becomes irreversible.

To produce and to regulate blood loss and to make the necessary experimental manuevers it is most convenient to cannulate the femoral vein and artery. This requires local anesthesia, which all agree does not modify the shock state. A clean, if not sterile, technic is necessary because bacterial contamination of equipment can produce a bacteremia (1). This would introduce a complication which is irrelevant to the objectives of the experiment. We, therefore, insist on meticulous cleansing of glassware, tubing and instruments, followed by prolonged immersion of this equipment in fresh isopropyl alcohol. We also shave the animal's skin, and scrub the shaved area with isopropyl alcohol before making the groin incision. The incision made to cannulate the vessels is not a negligible detail, because bacterial contamination occurs at this site even if the equipment and skin are properly prepared. In our hands, however, the degree of contamination is minimal and does not produce a local or systemic infection. We have found that a rigidly sterile technic does not alter the results and therefore is not necessary (2).

With the foregoing precautions taken we induce bleeding. Intermittent bleeding is cumbersome and unnecessarily time consuming. It serves no better than continuous bleeding to produce a quantitatively reproducible hemodynamic disorder. Hence we allow free bleeding from the cannulated femoral artery into a heparinized reservoir (Lamson technic), elevated above the heart level so as to produce and maintain the lowest mean systolic blood pressure the animal can tolerate for some hours. In the dog this level is between 30—35 mm. Hg. In the rabbit and rat it is between 40—45 mm. Hg. The volume of blood lost into the reservoir in all three species is about 50 ml./kg. Maximum bleed-out occurs in 40—80 minutes and remains maximum for a variable but short interval, after which blood returns to the animal at a variable rate, depending on the state of vascular tone the animal can sustain. Sick or malnourished animals take blood back very much more quickly than healthy ones. Most of those that do this die, even if normal blood volume is restored relatively early. On the other hand, some 10—20% of animals in any large series will take back very little blood, or take it back very slowly; and these survive even if allowed to remain in shock for 6 or more hours (3).

In the average case, if the blood left in the reservoir is rapidly infused after 90—120 minutes of shock, there will be a good and sustained pressor response, and recovery will occur in some 80% of animals. These animals are reversible to transfusion. If, however, shock is allowed to continue, about 40% of the blood lost will have returned to the animal between the 4th and 6th hours. If now the rest of it is rapidly infused, 80% or more of the animals will have a variable pressor response, revert to severe hypotension, and die in spite of the restoration of normovolemia. These animals are irreversible to transfusion (4). No amount of additional blood, nor any other known therapy will revive these animals. Therefore, we have in this model a method which allows us to produce a uniform response in most experiments; i. e. it will provide us with a preparation of hemorrhagic shock which is reversible or irreversible, according to choice. It is a method which is reproducible in quantitative terms of blood volume deficit, as well as of blood pressure and time of exposure to shock.

We emphasize that the model for reversible shock differs from the model for irreversible shock only in terms of the interval prior to transfusion. Thus to find an answer to one of the most fundamental problems in this field of research we need only to discover why the time factor makes all the difference between survival and death.

There are several reasons why we regard this model as preferable for the stated objective. Nearly all other investigators have used anesthetics for convenience in control of the animal's behavior. Anesthetics should not be used for most experimental objectives because they exert their own considerable effects upon the behavior of the vascular system (5). Moreover, they are not necessary. For control of dogs an ordinary dose of morphine an hour or so before bleeding is adequate, and does not notably affect the vascular system (6). We do not favor the Wiggers stepwise technic for producing severe hemorrhagic shock (7), first, because the anesthetic is an irrelevant complication and, second, because the method lacks the flexibility and precision of the reservoir method for controlling the degree of shock. All other methods for producing hemorrhagic shock with which we are familiar are even less precise for quantitative control of the state of shock.

As for the choice of animal, we find it best, as do others, to use different species for different purposes, in order to illuminate the general biologic problem from different points of view. But when choosing a given species, we must make it clear to ourselves, no less than to others, whether or not the pattern of the experiment is intended to have relevance for all mammals. For example, those who wish to study portal hypertension in shock may choose the dog. But in doing so they should avoid the implication that what is being observed is valid for man or the rabbit, neither of which displays the phenomenon as seen in dogs. This special feature of the hemodynamics in the dog does not affect the general course of events in hemorrhagic shock, because an Eck fistula, which wipes out the portal hypertension, does not protect the dog against the development of irreversibility (6). Therefore, for the general purpose of the study of hemorrhagic shock, the dog is very suitable.

We have employed the reservoir technic for the study of the role of various vital organs that might be involved in the development of irreversibility. A large difference in the survival rate, if regularly secured, would carry conviction, whereas a large difference in such terms as a better pressor response to transfusion, or a longer survival time, would not. After observing all the methods at hand that might prevent death which must otherwise occur, we demonstrated that one can prevent the development of irreversibility and death from hemorrhagic shock in three different ways:

1. By maintaining cross-circulation through the liver with a sufficient flow of arterial blood from the beginning of the shock period (8)[1].

2. By oral pre-treatment with non-absorbable antibiotics effective against gram-negative bacteria (9).

---

[1] In considering the possible role of the liver, we used, in addition to the reservoir technic, an arrangement for cross-circulating the liver with an artery of a donor dog, so as to deliver a normal supply of arterial blood to the liver from the beginning of the shock period, while the rest of the animal remains in shock. In this way we could assess the role of the liver in terms of whether or not poor flow through it was responsible for death.

3. By pre-treatment with dibenamine (*10*).

The first of these observations pointed to a key role for the liver. The second demonstrated that a factor derived from intra-intestinal bacteria is also involved in the development of irreversibility. The third, which was first demonstrated by WIGGERS (*11*) and by REMINGTON (*12*), was found in our hands to be effective, like antibiotics, only when given in advance of producing the shock (*10*). It can be argued that the dibenaminized animal cannot serve as a model for comparison with the non-dibenaminized animal, because under dibenamine the blood loss required to produce the selected level of hypotension is substantially less than without its use. SHORR and his colleagues, however, showed that if the bleeding is carried out slowly (*13*), it is possible to impose the same degree of blood loss in both preparations, and yet obtain the favorable effect of the drug. The protective effect of dibenamine, coupled with the fact that the endogenous catechol amines are overactive in shock, strengthened the view proposed in 1935 by FREEMAN (*14*) that adrenergic activity is related to the death from shock.

How can we harmonize these three apparently disparate protective mechanisms? Part of the answer to this question required an experimental model designed to discover whether the liver injury consisted of the collapse of some vital function related to bacteria, e. g. damage to function of the R.E.S.; or whether, according to SHORR, a toxin of tissue origin was generated in the liver (*15*). Our first approach therefore dealt with an evaluation in the shocked animal of the capacity of the R. E. S., the largest part of which is in the liver, to destroy intravenously injected bacteria. The normal, the reversibly shocked, and the irreversibly shocked animal were found to deal differently with a variety of intravenously injected bacteria. Normal animals cleared the blood in 6 hours, and showed no bacteria in the liver or spleen 24 hours later. Reversibly shocked animals also cleared the blood in six hours, but showed a septicemia 24 hours later, and died in 1–4 days with positive post-mortem cultures of the blood, liver and spleen (*16*). Irreversibly shocked animals could not clear the blood in 6 hours, and the blood of about $^1/_2$ of them after 3–4 hours showed bacterial multiplication.

In view of the absence of bacteria in significant numbers in the tissues of living mammals (*17*), it was necessary to consider that differences in tolerance to bacterial products, rather than bacteria themselves, might explain the protective effect of non-absorbable antibiotics in shock. Consequently, further experiments were done to test the tolerance of the animal in hemorrhagic shock to endotoxins. For this purpose rabbits were used instead of dogs, because rabbits are more suitable for quantitative assay of endotoxins than are dogs. These studies showed that the anti-endotoxic capacity was so depleted by 2 hours of shock that as little as a microgram of endotoxin could kill an animal that otherwise would have survived (18).

At about the same time, Shorr and his collaborators, using the Wiggers' technic, had isolated reduced ferritin from the shocked liver and claimed a place for this material as the toxin responsible for irreversibility (19). This claim was made on the ground that the ferritin depressed the sensitivity of the rat's appendiceal mesentery to locally applied epinephrine. Since there is no relevance between the data obtained from such a test and what the ferritin does to the circulatory integrity of the animal from which it was obtained, we do not consider this experiment as a valid model to test for the presence of a substance in the shocked liver which is toxic to its host. Our own procedure to determine the presence or absence of a toxin in the liver was based on the following considerations. If a toxin is present it must be shown to be capable of killing not only a test animal, but the donor animal from which it was obtained, and by the same mechanism in both. Hence the experiment must be in two parts: the first should show that the toxin is present by the fact that it is lethal to a test recipient. It should also show how the toxin kills the recipient, and that death will not occur if the toxin can be eliminated. The toxin should then be isolated and purified. The second experiment should aim to identify the nature and source of the toxin and its biologic properties. For the first part of the experiment we considered that a normal animal is a poor test animal because its detoxifying power may be sufficient to conceal the presence of a small amount of toxin. The test recipient should be an animal with a weak detoxifying power, i. e. one which will survive if not exposed to the toxin but die in the same way as the donor dies if exposed to a small amount of toxin. What kind of animal will fit these requirements ? We have already found the suitable animal. It is a rabbit or dog which has been transfused after 2 hours of hemorrhagic shock, but which will survive if not exposed to a toxin. The experiment was performed as follows. An aliquot of an homogenate of liver from the dog dying of shock, i. e. a dog in shock following an ineffective transfusion, was injected intraperitoneally into a normal dog. The dog survived with almost no untoward signs. The same thing was done to a reversibly shocked dog, i. e. one which would respond well to a transfusion for shock of 2 hours' duration. The result was dramatically different.

Instead of responding as usual with a progressive return of activity and vigor, the transfused recipient reverted to a severe state of shock and developed the typical manifestations of irreversibility, including necrosis and hemorrhage of the intestinal mucosa (20). This was strong evidence of a toxin in the shocked liver. The toxin was then identified as of bacterial origin by the further observation that pre-treatment of the donor of the homogenate with antibiotic protected the recipient from developing irreversibility and death. But surely if there is a toxin of bacterial origin in the liver, why should it not also be in the blood? Accordingly, the experiment performed with liver homogenate was simulated in another experiment in which the assumptions made were the same as in the liver homogenate experiment. We had reason to believe that even very small quantities of toxin in blood might be detected, because we had observed that rabbits recovering from reversible shock were up to one hundred thousand times as vulnerable as normal rabbits to an endotoxin (18). Accordingly, the dog or rabbit dying of severe or prolonged shock was killed by exsanguination. Its blood was tested for toxicity by removing blood from a normal dog or rabbit and promptly replacing it with the same volume of the blood to be tested. In dozens of such tests no harm came to any normal recipient of such blood. The same blood, however, was able to kill dogs or rabbits which were about to be transfused at the end of 2 hours of hemorrhagic shock. As already stated, such animals recover if transfused at this time with their own or a healthy donor's blood. But when part or all of their own blood was replaced with shocked donor blood, the recipient died with all the manifestations of the irreversibly shocked animal, i. e. there was a relapse into deep shock. In the dog a bloody diarrhea developed and continued until death, and the intestinal mucosa was necrotic on post-mortem examination. In the rabbit there were focal hemorrhages in the gut wall. These effects were not observed — i. e. the shocked donor blood was non-toxic — if the donor had been pre-treated with antibiotic (20). Since a non-absorbable antibiotic given orally was as effective as one given parenterally, we concluded that the toxin was derived from the intra-intestinal bacteria. We concluded further that the toxin in the liver homogenate was the same toxin and, therefore, that the entire animal was permeated with toxin. Furthermore, since the liver was a key organ, we concluded that the vital function lost by the liver was the ability of its R. E. system to destroy bacterial toxin. But surely if this is so in hemorrhagic shock, it must be just as true of other kinds of shock, for the R. E. S. must suffer the same kind of injury whenever grossly inadequate peripheral flow persists for long. The same tests were therefore made in other types of shock.

Before discussing the findings, we will pause to consider the models used for the study of other kinds of shock. Are there types of experimental shock other than hemorrhagic shock in which the hemodynamic parameters are sufficiently constant so as to produce predictable patterns of behavior? Traumatic shock has been induced by bullet wounds causing massive injury (21). Such preparations are not suitable because the open wound adds an indeterminate degree of infection to an indeterminate amount of tissue injury. Burns as a tool for the production of experimental hypovolemic shock are also a mixed type of injury, for while the area and depth of tissue burned can be standardized, the consequent bacterial activity cannot be. A simpler type of tissue injury which produces hypovolemic shock is that caused by release of a tourniquet applied to an extremity for a given number of hours. Tourniquet shock is a standardizable lesion because total obstruction to flow in one or both lower extremities for a known period of time is a precisely defined degree of trauma. Shock following release of a tourniquet is a convenient model to study in order to observe the effects of almost pure plasma loss. Data gathered from different experimental animals cannot be compared unless the time of application of the tourniquets is comparable, for the degree of tissue injury is proportional to the duration of the ischemia. Thus, if the tourniquet is removed after 4 hours, replacement of the large amount of plasma lost into the extremity will result in recovery. In the rat or mouse the loss can be made good with salt solution alone, even after many hours of shock (22). In the dog plasma is necessary, and it must be given promptly, or it will fail (23). As a model intended to simulate the clinical state of plasma loss, 4 hour tourniquet shock in the rat or dog should be suitable. It simulates tourniquet injury in man, and it is not unlike the shock that follows the plasma loss which occurs in some patients after ligation of the lower part of the inferior vena cava to prevent pulmonary embolism. Whether it bears comparison with the shock from prolonged compression injury, such as by a landslide or a cave-in, requires more knowledge of the latter condition than is now available. Whereas shock following application of the tourniquet for 4 hours is reversible, shock following 8—10 hours of tourniquet application, in the dog at least, is irreversible unless the extremity is removed, for the capillary leak is so far beyond repair that an attempt to keep ahead of the continuing plasma loss into the area of injury by plasma infusions is futile (23). With antibiotic therapy and continuous infusion of plasma for 36 hours we could not sustain life after stopping the infusions. Even the rare survivor died later from the septic complications of massive necrosis. The process is akin to that of irreversible shock caused by an extensive third-degree burn, in the sense that the tissue injury which allows a continuing loss of plasma is not remediable.

The blood of the dog in tourniquet shock is sterile. But when it is tested for toxicity as described, it is highly lethal. If as little as 50—100 ml. of this blood is given as part of the test recipient's transfusion, blood oozes from the rectum almost at once; the animal remains prostrate after the transfusion, and dies in persistent shock with a hemorrhagic and necrotic mucosa as severe as any observed in endotoxin shock (24). Since there are no gram-negative bacteria in the damaged leg of the donor dog (the gas bacillus is present, but does not produce the local or systemic manifestations of gas-bacillus infection), the toxins are presumably derived from the intra-intestinal flora. This view is supported by the observation that pre-treatment of the donor with a non-absorbable antibiotic renders the donor's blood non-toxic. But whereas reduction of endotoxemia by antibiotics prevents irreversibility in hemorrhagic shock, it cannot do so in tourniquet shock because the hypovolemia cannot be corrected (except by amputation). Therefore, unless the hypovolemia is stopped early enough, by amputation or otherwise, death will occur because the shock persists, and progressive damage to the anti-endotoxic capacity continues to the point where this capacity is lost altogether. Since antibiotics, even if given in advance, do not completely eliminate endotoxin from the intestine, a small amount of endotoxin will be absorbed, and, with virtually no defense, this much can suffice to destroy vascular integrity.

Septic shock is in many respects not unlike tourniquet shock, as the following observations indicate. 15 ml. of a fecal suspension was injected into the peritoneal cavity of a healthy dog. Profound shock developed within 3 hours. There was a large loss of plasma into the peritoneal cavity, the blood pressure fell, the pulse rose, peripheral resistance increased, hematocrit rose as in tourniquet shock, and cardiac output fell to very low levels. In general, all the features of deep shock were present and death occurred in 3—9 hours (25). Massive plasma volume therapy was given and did no good. As in tourniquet shock, the infused plasma ran out at once into the injured area. On the other hand, if the dog was pre-treated with an oral non-absorbable antibiotic, the shock, though equally severe, was not lethal. For after ten hours, without fluid therapy of any kind having been given, the early signs of recovery were in evidence. The blood of the dog not given an antibiotic was as toxic to a test recipient dog as was the blood of the dog in tourniquet or hemorrhagic shock. The blood of the dog given antibiotic was not toxic (24). Hence the endotoxin in the blood was derived primarily from the intra-intestinal flora rather than from the bacteria injected intraperitoneally. This view is supported by the observation that boiling the fecal suspension before injection in no way altered the sequence of events. Failure of the R. E. system to destroy absorbed endotoxin is, therefore, the primary feature in septic shock as it is in the other types. But septic shock differs from tourniquet shock in that it need not be irreversible — for if the endotoxemia is minimized by antibiotics, there is time gained for the hypovolemia to correct itself by the reabsorption of the intraperitoneal fluid. Thus the shock is terminated.

In the foregoing account of experiments on the likenesses and differences of various types of shock we have made three major assumptions. One is that the toxin is endotoxin; 2, that the endotoxin is absorbed from the intestine; and 3, that it is the R. E. S. which destroys endotoxin. The first assumption was shown to be correct by the isolation from the blood of the shocked rabbit and dog of a lipopolysaccharide that is not present in normal plasma. This substance, purified and concentrated, exhibits the same kind of toxicity as the shocked blood given to test recipients. It also exhibits the biologic properties of bacterial endotoxins, such as pyrogenicity and ability to produce the generalized Shwartzman reaction and to induce resistance to a lethal dose of endotoxin (26).

The second assumption was shown to be correct as follows. Rabbits of the same litter, weight and health, whose intestinal flora was free of coliform bacteria, were fed by gavage some 2–3 grams (wet weight) of a strain of P_{32} labelled E. coli 01 11 B_4 which is pathogenic to man, but foreign to the rabbit's intestine. Three hours later half the rabbits were put into hemorrhagic shock for 2 hours, and then transfused with their own blood. After 3 more hours, i.e. 8 hours after feeding the bacteria, all the rabbits were exsanguinated. Blood, liver and kidney were analyzed for dialyzable and non-dialyzable P_{32} activity and for toxicity by the chick embryo test. The endotoxin content of the blood was measured by the hemagglutination inhibition reaction, using an antiserum specific for the strain of bacteria employed. The data demonstrate: 1, that about 1% of the amount of endotoxin fed orally was absorbed by both shocked and normal rabbits; 2, that there was no detectable amount of endotoxin in the blood of the normal rabbit, but that there was a considerable amount of endotoxin in the blood of the shocked rabbit; 3, that the liver and spleen of the shocked and of the normal rabbit contained about equal amounts of the endotoxin; but 4, whereas the liver and spleen of the non-shocked rabbit were not toxic, these tissues as well as the blood of the shocked rabbit were toxic (*27*).

The third assumption, i. e. that the R. E. S. is the organ which destroys endotoxin, was demonstrated to be correct by the following technic. P_{32} labelled endotoxin in plasma was slowly injected into the marginal artery of the spleen of the normal dog. The effluent blood was collected for 10 minutes in one-minute increments of flow. The spleen retained 80% of the injected P_{32}. The blood leaving the spleen in the first minute contained unbound (dialyzable) P_{32}. All effluent bloods as well as the homogenate of spleen were non-toxic. On the other hand, the spleen of dogs which had been exposed to shock for 2 hours before the endotoxin was injected retained only 25% of the amount of P_{32} injected. None of the retained P_{32} was released from the spleen and all tests of blood and spleen showed toxicity. The same was true of the spleen pre-treated with Thorotrast. The normal spleen destroyed the endotoxin within three minutes; the injured spleens were toxic 2 hours after the endotoxin was injected (*28*).

If endotoxin absorbed from the gut is the lethal agent in hemorrhagic shock, what should we expect in animals with a reduced intra-intestinal pool of endotoxin, e.g. rabbits whose intestinal flora is coliform-free or nearly so because of antibiotics in the food? These rabbits tolerate six hours of hemorrhagic shock well, and show no toxin in their bloods. But if *E. coli* (2 gms wet wt.) or 100—200 mg. of its endotoxin is put into the stomach several hours before inducing the shock, this tolerance is lost (*29*). Such tolerance is not to be confused with resistance to 6 hours of hemorrhagic shock which is induced in normal coliform-bearing rabbits by pre-treating them for a week or so with daily small doses of endotoxin (*30*). The tolerance of the coliform-free rabbit to shock is attributable to the small amount of endotoxin in the gut, so that the amount absorbed must be too small to injure the circulation in spite of the weakened R. E. S. The resistance to shock induced in the coliform-bearing rabbit is attributable to a larger R. E. S. capacity to take up and detoxify absorbed endotoxin (*31*).

There is the following evidence to substantiate these statements. If the portal and systemic vein blood of a normal rabbit are collected at the same time, the portal vein blood will be found to contain toxin, while the systemic vein blood will not. If the liver is now injured by injecting Thorotrast, the systemic vein blood also becomes toxic. In the rabbit that is coliform-free the portal vein blood will show a reduced incidence of toxicity, and if this rabbit is fed neomycin beforehand, the incidence of toxicity in the portal and systemic veins is reduced to zero (*32*).

Thus we have justified the three assumptions made, and have obtained further support for the theory that there is one common defect which can account for irreversibility in at least three types of shock. This defect is a weakened endotoxin-detoxifying capacity of the R. E. S., the consequence of which is that endotoxin, which is continuously entering the circulation from the gut, is free to produce irreversible collapse of the peripheral circulatory apparatus.

An irreversible type of peripheral vascular collapse occurs in response to the direct injection of endotoxin. The time it takes to develop depends on the dose and the animal selected for study. The hemodynamic manifestations of endotoxic shock are in most respects the same as those of hemorrhagic shock. In the dog the portal congestion which results from intrahepatic vasoconstriction is much more pronounced than in other animals, so that necrosis of intestinal mucosa with intraluminal bleeding far exceeds in extent and severity what is seen in any other species. As in hemorrhagic shock, these intestinal changes are not a key factor in the lethal outcome, because an Eck fistula prevents the intestinal injury without otherwise altering the general course of events (*33*). The observations on the gut of the dog in shock should not be taken to be valid for other species.

When bacteremic shock, which is a common clinical disorder, is induced by injecting endotoxin-producing bacteria into the experimental animal, there appears to be no need to seek for another source for the endotoxemia. The endotoxin they release, or perhaps other effects of these bacteria, like endotoxin injected directly, injures the R. E. system, so that more endotoxin may then cause lethal shock. In the light of our data on shock from experimental peritonitis, the major source of this endotoxin may not be the injected bacteria, but endotoxin absorbed from the intestine. (Bacteria which are not producers of endotoxin can also produce septic shock. But very little is known about their mechanisms of action.)

To what extent are the foregoing considerations applicable to other types of experimental or clinical shock ? For example, in shock caused by myocardial infarction the deficient volume output of the heart reduces the volume flow through all tissues. In terms of volume flow through tissues this type of shock may be viewed as different from that produced by a prolonged infusion of catechol amines primarily in respect of the point in the circulation where the restriction of flow to the tissues is applied. In the shock produced by clamping or balloon occlusion of the thoracic aorta, or by transient occlusion of the coeliac axis or of the superior mesenteric artery, the interruption of flow is regional, but no less lethal. Death in all of these conditions can be explained in terms of a critical injury to liver or intestine or both. Thus, the shock following occlusion of the superior mesenteric artery for one hour, which is fatal in a few hours, can be prevented by pre-treatment with an oral nonabsorbable antibiotic or by dibenamine. And the shock following ischemia of the liver can damage its R. E. system. Hence, the general hypothesis that the absorption of endotoxin from the intestine and its neutralization by the R. E. system are basic phenomena in lethal shock can be invoked to explain the mechanism of death in these experimental (and clinical) conditions. Other organs might also be involved in the lethal process, but their exclusion requires experiments perhaps like the perfusion experiments already done on the isolated liver and intestine (34).

The usefulness of norepinephrine in shock lies in its ability to improve cardiac output and to increase flow through the brain. But the generalized increase in peripheral vasoconstriction reduces flow through many tissues (35). If one of these is a vital tissue and the flow is already marginal or worse, the administration of adrenergic compounds might be lethal in spite of better cardiac output or better cerebral flow. Hence, even when the use of norepinephrine is justified to improve cerebral or cardiac function, the mixture of its good and bad effects makes it difficult to draw conclusions as to its role in preventing or facilitating the lethal outcome.

In the controversy as to whether the fundamental defect in shock is failure of the myocardium or failure of the peripheral vascular system, the weight of the evidence favors the latter system. Direct observation of the hemodynamics of flow in the peripheral bed has been done chiefly in hemorrhagic shock by CHAMBERS and ZWEIFACH (36). Their description appears to fit the functional data rather well. However, their model for this study is of doubtful validity, for it requires the exteriorization of gut or mesentery or omentum, the immersion and maintenance of these structures in a non-physiologic fluid, in circumstances of bacterial contamination. These and the undesirable physical effects of exposure to strong transilluminating light must mean considerable deviation from the natural conditions under which flow must be taking place. Moreover, BELLMAN could not verify their findings (37). Nor could FULTON and BERMAN (38), who studied flow in the intact cheek pouch of the hamster. The same general criticisms apply to the validity of the technics employed by KNISELEY (39). Even the Clark chamber applied to the rabbit's ear has certain artifactual features. A model which will see what goes on in the peripheral vessels of the intact mammal awaits the development of new methods of visualization.

A theory, such as we propose, to explain the cause of irreversibility must stand examination in the light of all contradictory evidence. Thus, how can we in the light of this theory explain the finding that germ-free rats respond to hemorrhagic shock in the same way as normal rats (40)? The theory does not insist that an animal in a germ-free world should escape death from hemorrhagic shock, since the effects of continuing hypoxia must eventually destroy some vital function. But the germ-free animal, as we know it today, cannot be said to have been reared in a strictly germ-free world, for it is fed a substantial supply of dead bacteria (endotoxin) in its food. Given its poor R. E. system, the amount of endotoxin it absorbs may be sufficient to kill because the shocked animal is hypersensitive to endotoxin (18).

Summary

In this communication the commonest experimental models for the study of traumatic shock have been compared and evaluated in terms of the objectives sought. A major objective of research in this field is to discover why a persisting state of peripheral vascular collapse eventually becomes refractory to all therapy, or why it is refractory from the beginning. For this purpose it is necessary to utilize experimental models which allow a comparison of the reversible and the irreversible states in animals. The importance of use of the right species of animal for a particular objective is also considered. Finally, reasons are given for simplifying the preparation so as to exclude irrelevant or confusing factors, such as anesthetic drugs, and to permit expression of the condition as far as is possible in quantitative terms.

Aided by a grant from the National Institutes of Health, Bethesda, Maryland, and by a contract with the Office of the Surgeon General, United States Army.

References

1. ALTMEIER, W. A. and W. R. CULBERTSON: Progress Reports of Subcommittee on Shock, Div. Med. Sciences, National Research Council, 1957. — 2. FRANK, H. A. et al.: Amer. J. Physiol. 168, 430 (1952). — 3. FINE, J. et al.: The Bacterial Factor in Traumatic Shock. Ann. N. Y.

Comparison of various forms of experimental shock   39

Acad. Sc. **55**, 429 (1952). — 4. FINE, J.: The Bacterial Factor in Traumatic Shock. Springfield, Ill.: Thomas 1954. — 5. ZWEIFACH, B. W., S. G. HERSHEY, E. A. ROVENSTINE, and R. CHAMBERS: Proc. Soc. Exper. Biol. (U.S.A.) **56**, 73 (1944). — 6. BLALOCK, A. and M. F. MASON: Arch. Surg. (U.S.A.) **47**, 326 (1943). — 7. WERLE, C. N., R. S. COSBY, and C. J. WIGGERS: Amer. J. Physiol. **144**, 91 (1945). — 8. FRANK, H. A., A. M. SELIGMAN, and J. FINE: J. Clin. Invest. (U.S.A.) **25**, 1 (1946). — 9. JACOB, S. et al.: Amer. J. Physiol. **179**, 523 (1954). — 10. SMIDDY, F. G., D. SEGEI, and J. FINE: Proc. Soc. Exper. Biol. (U.S.A.) **97**, 584 (1958). — 11. WIGGERS, H. A.: Amer. J. Physiol. **153**, 511 (1948). — 12. REMINGTON, J. W.: Proc. Soc. Exper. Biol. (U.S.A) **69**, 150 (1948). — 13. BAEZ, S., B. W. ZWEIFACH, and E. SHORR: Fed. Proc. (U.S.A.) **11**, 7 (1952). — BAEZ, S.: Report on Adrenergic Blocking Agents in Shock. National Research Council March 22, 1955. — 14. FREEMAN, N.: Amer. J. Physiol. **113**, 384 (1935). — 15. SHORR, E., B. W. ZWEIFACH, and R. F. FURCHGOTT: Ann. N. Y. Acad. Sc. 49, 571 (1948). — 16. SCHWEINBURG, F. B., A. H. FRANK, and J. FINE: Amer. J. Physiol. **179**, 532 (1954). — 17. SCHWEINBURG, F. B. and E. M. SYLVESTER: Proc. Soc. Exper. Biol. (U.S.A.) **82**, 527 (1953). — 18. SCHWEINBURG, F. B. and J. FINE: Proc. Soc. Exper. Biol. (U.S.A.) **88**, 589 (1955). — 19. SHORR, E. et al.: Circulation (U.S.A.) **3**, 42 (1951). — 20. SCHWEINBURG, F. B., P. B. SHAPIRO, E. D. FRANK, and J. FINE: Proc. Soc. Exper. Biol. (U.S.A.) **95**, 646 (1957). — 21. OCHSNER, E., S. JACOB, and A. R. MANSBERGER Jr.: Surgery (U.S.A.) **43**, 703 (1958). — 22. KALETZKY, S. and G. E. GUSTAFSON: Proc. Soc. Exper. Biol. (U.S.A.) **62**, 293 (1946). — 23. FINE, J. and A. M. SELIGMAN: J. Clin. Invest. (U.S.A.) **23**, 720 (1943). — 24. SCHWEINBURG, F. B. and J. FINE: J. Exper. Med. (U.S.A.) **112**, 5, 793 (1960). — 25. FINE, E. D. et al.: Amer. J. Physiol. **182**, 166 (1955). — 26. RAVIN, H., F. B. SCHWEINBURG, and J. FINE: Proc. Soc. Exper. Biol. (U.S.A.) **99**, 426 (1958). — 27. RAVIN, H., D. ROWLEY, C. JENKINS, and J. FINE: J. Exper. Med. (U.S.A.) **112**, 5, 783 (1960). — 28. WIZNITZER, T. et al.: J. Exper. Med. (U.S.A.) **112**, 6, 1157 (1960). — 29. WIZNITZER, T., E. D. FRANK, and J. FINE: J. Exper. Med. (U.S.A.) **112**, 6, 1167 (1960). — 30. SMIDDY, F. G. and J. FINE: Proc. Soc. Exper. Biol. (U.S.A.) **96**, 558 (1957). — 31. BENNET, I. J. Jr. and P. B. BEESAN: J. Exper. Med. (U.S.A.) **88**, 267 (1948). — 32. GREENE, B. et al.: To be published. — 33. FRANK, E. D. et al.: Amer. J. Physiol. **186**, 74 (1956). — 34. LILLEHEI, R. C.: Surg. Forum (U.S.A.) **7**, 6 (1957). — 35. FRANK, E. D. et al.: Amer. J. Physiol. **186**, 74 (1956). — 36. CHAMBERS, R. and B. W. ZWEIFACH: Ann. N. Y. Acad. Sc. **46**, 683 (1960); — Amer. J. Physiol. **150**, 239 (1947). — 37. BELLMAN, S.: Unpublished data. — 38. BERMAN, H. J. and J. FULTON: Unpublished data. — 39. KNISELEY, M. H.: Anat. Rec. (U.S.A.) **65**, 23 (1936); — **106**, 209 (1950). — 40. ZWEIFACH, B. W.: Shock and Circulatory Homeostasis. H. D. GREEN, Ed., Pps. 119—147, J. Macy. Jr. Foundation, 1955.

Possible role of endotoxin in the perpetuation of shock

By

R. P. GILBERT

Dr. FINE has summarized what is, in my opinion, the largest and most significant block of work on shock of the past 15 years. Even those portions which may have to be discarded have served as working hypotheses to stimulate the thought and investigation of many workers. He has offered answers to several perplexing questions:

1. What happens, as a function of time, to render reversible shock irreversible?

2. Is there a final course common to various types of shock, and what is it?

3. Why does stimulation of the R.E.S. induce tolerance to various forms of shock?

4. Is there a toxic factor in shock?

All of this is a unifying concept which I have tried to summarize in Fig. 1. Common to all types of shock is inadequate tissue blood flow with tissue hypoxia, deficiency of substrates, and accumulation of metabolites. This so weakens the R.E.S. that it is unable to detoxify the endotoxin continuously entering the portal circulation from the gut. The circulating endotoxin then increases to the point where it causes its own type of circulatory injury. This produces a vicious circle or positive feedback, with endotoxin causing more shock, which causes more R.E.S. depression and hence more circulating endotoxin. The particular importance of this is that it could be a mechanism to perpetuate shock whether the initiating factor be hemorrhage, trauma, tourniquets, infection or acute myocardial infarction. The items on the right side of Fig. 1 refer to experiments by Dr. FINE's group which bear on the various stages in this system.

Before accepting this schema *in toto*, there is some contradictory evidence which must be explained:

1. Despite the prior dietary ingestion of endotoxin, if endotoxin is the toxic factor, it is hard to understand why germ-free rats should not be more resistant to hemorrhagic shock than normal rats (*1*). It has been stated that they are not more sensitive to endotoxin (*2*) and may, indeed, be less sensitive.

2. Some groups have been unable to demonstrate a protective effect of antibiotics against hemorrhagic shock (3). This may be due to resistant organisms in the gut, but further confirmation is desirable.

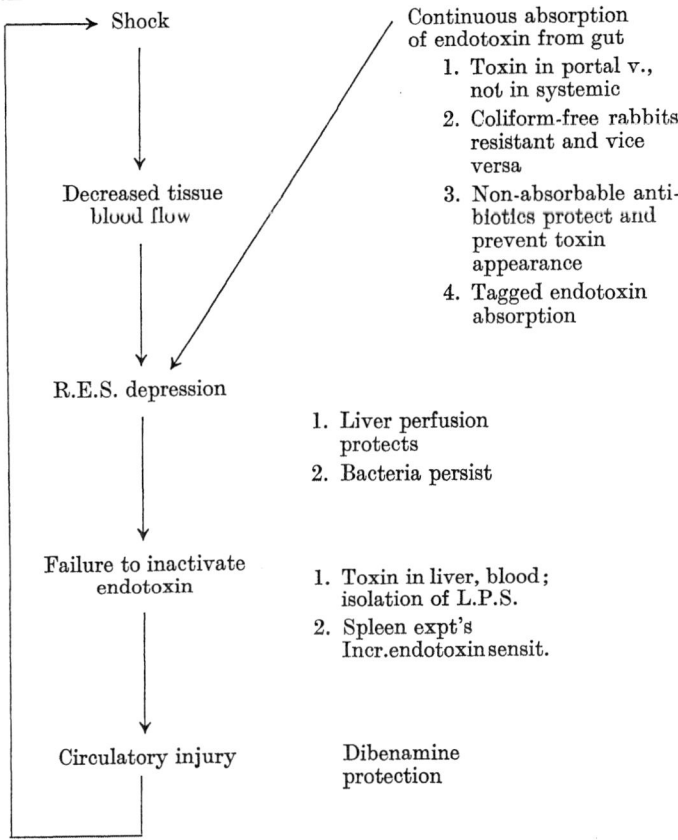

Shock

Continuous absorption of endotoxin from gut
1. Toxin in portal v., not in systemic
2. Coliform-free rabbits resistant and vice versa
3. Non-absorbable antibiotics protect and prevent toxin appearance
4. Tagged endotoxin absorption

Decreased tissue blood flow

R.E.S. depression
1. Liver perfusion protects
2. Bacteria persist

Failure to inactivate endotoxin
1. Toxin in liver, blood; isolation of L.P.S.
2. Spleen expt's Incr. endotoxin sensit.

Circulatory injury
Dibenamine protection

Fig. 1. Outline of Dr. FINE's hypothesis and list of principal supporting experiments

It is possible that there are as yet unidentified toxic substances associated with the endotoxin, and that the R.E.S. depression and endotoxemia is but one more evidence of tissue anoxia.

If endotoxin (or a remarkably similar agency) is common to various forms of shock, how does endotoxin act on the circulation, and does it produce changes similar to those seen in irreversible shock? It affects many "systems" of which we shall hear later from Dr. SPINK. Of present interest is the fact that it does cause hypotension, and thereby can *perpetuate* as well as initiate shock and inadequate tissue perfusion. The central importance of this effect is emphasized by CROWELL's observations. He modified hemorrhagic hypotension in various ways by altering the degree and duration of hypotension, or by giving dibenzyline or pressor drugs, and found that the mortality rate correlated less well with these parameters than with estimates of cumulative oxygen debt (*4*). If chemical repair is to take place, tissue perfusion must be adequate.

The mechanisms by which endotoxin produces hypotension have been reviewed (*5*) and vary considerably between species (*6*). The following effects are important:

1. There is a release of vasoactive agents (e. g., *7—10*), activation of enzymes (*11*), and modification of neural activity.

2. There may be changes in degree and type of activity of endogenous vasoactive substances.

3. Hypotension is due to both a fall in cardiac output and later a fall in total peripheral resistance.

4. Cardiac function is not critically affected, unless perhaps pre-terminally.

5. The total blood volume is normal in the absence of complications, though it may fall later in some species. This is as in irreversible hemorrhagic shock after reinfusion.

6. There is a redistribution or sequestration of blood so that the venous return is diminished. As pointed out by GREEN (*12*), such peripheral pooling is probably responsible for the decreased venous return and cardiac output in the irreversible phase of hemorrhagic shock.

One of the key hemodynamic problems in shock is the mechanism of this pooling. It could, *a priori*, be produced in two ways: 1) a decrease of venous tone, or of all vascular tone with pooling in small vessels, particularly veins; 2) constriction of medium veins, causing a pressure rise in smaller veins and capillaries, dilation of these latter vessels and consequent pooling. This would be aggravated by arterial dilation. It would also cause transudation and hemoconcentration. Possibly both mechanisms are active at different times in the same subject. Also there may be great variation between different vascular beds.

There is microscopic evidence for the first situation in various forms of shock. In addition, there is evidence for a decreasing total peripheral resistance in the eviscerated dog at constant flow after endotoxin (*13*) and in the monkey despite decreasing cardiac output (unpublished data). The second mechanism has been shown to be active in the dog liver (*14*) and lung (*15*) shortly after the injection of endotoxin. There is a trace of it in the isolated perfused dog forelimb after endotoxin. HADDY and others have shown that *various* vasoactive substances can so affect the dog forelimb (*16*). ESTENSEN has found that, in some weighed dog gut experiments at constant pressure, intra-arterial norepinephrine causes a weight gain in association with a rise in small-vein pressure (*17*). This was interpreted as consistent with venous constriction and proximal pooling. ZWEIFACH and co-workers have observed microscopically that epinephrine causes venous constriction and arterial dilation in the rat mesentery preparation after endotoxin (*18*). It is apparent that the mechanism of pooling and the agencies through which it is produced require further study. If it is to be applied to man, much of it must be carried out in primates. If the agency of endotoxin and the mechanisms of sequestration are found to be similar for different species and different forms of shock, it is probable that they also obtain for patients.

Clearly, endotoxin or its reaction products can act to perpetuate shock as seen in the irreversible stage. Any differences are minor. It does, in contrast to irreversible shock, produce hemoconcentration in the dog and a great deal of edema in the intestine, as well as in the lung. It has chemical effects other than those secondary to the hypotension. I would like to ask Dr. FINE what further evidence he would like to see to consider as finally proven its role as a perpetuating factor common to various types of shock.

Summary

The experiments summarized by Dr. FINE, and in particular the isolation of an endotoxin-like substance from the blood of animals in shock, strongly support the hypothesis that endotoxin acts to perpetuate the hypotension of shock, whatever its initiating cause may have been. Against this hypothesis are the facts that 1) germ-free animals have not been shown to be more resistant to hemorrhagic shock and 2) not all workers can confirm the observation that antibiotics protect against hemorrhagic shock.

There is no doubt that endotoxin *could* act to perpetuate hypotension. In most species, it produces hypotension through the mediation of vasoactive substances and through poorly understood effects on the nervous system. The hypotension may be due in part to a drop in the total peripheral resistance (dog, monkey), but is also due to a drop in cardiac output. This is caused by a drop in venous return, which results from a redistribution of blood volume. The mechanisms of this latter effect remain obscure, though in some instances it has been shown to be due to excessive venous constriction with pooling in smaller veins and capillaries.

References

1. Zweifach, B. W., H. H. Gordon, M. Wagner, and J. A. Reyniers: J. Exper. Med. (U.S.A.) 107, 437 (1958). — 2. McNulty, W. P. Jr. and R. Linares: Amer. J. Physiol. 198, 141 (1960). — 3. Hardy, E. G., G. C. Morris, E. M. Yow, B. W. Haynes Jr., and M. E. deBakey: Ann. Surg. (U.S.A.) 139, 282 (1954). — 4. Crowell, J. W.: Fed. Proc. (U.S.A.) 20, 116 (1961). — 5. Gilbert, R. P.: Physiol. Rev. (U.S.A.) 40, 245 (1960). — 6. Kuida, H., R. P. Gilbert, L. B. Hinshaw, J. G. Brunson, and M. B. Visscher: Accepted for publication in Amer. J. Physiol. — 7. Hinshaw, L. B., H. Kuida, R. P. Gilbert, and M. B. Visscher: Amer. J. Physiol. 191, 293 (1957). — 8. Vick, J.: J. Laborat. Clin. Med. (U.S.A.) 56, 953 (1960). — 9. Rosenberg, J. D., R. C. Lillehei, W. H. Moran, and B. Zimmerman: Proc. Soc. Exper. Biol. (U.S.A.) 102, 335 (1959). — 10. Hinshaw, L. B., J. H. Vick, C. H. Carlson, and Y. Fan: Proc. Soc. Exper. Biol. (U.S.A.) 104, 379 (1960). — 11. Spink, W. W. and J. A. Vick: Proc. Soc. Exper. Biol. (U.S.A.) 106, 242 (1961). — 12. Green, H. P.: Conference on Recent Progress and Present Problems in the Field of Shock. To be published. — 13. Hinshaw, L. B., R. P. Gilbert, H. Kuida, and M. B. Visscher: Amer. J. Physiol. 195, 631 (1958). — 14. Weil, M. H., L. D. MacLean, M. B. Visscher, and W. W. Spink: Transact. Ass. Amer. Physicians 69, 131 (1956). — 15. Kuida, H. L., L. P. Hinshaw, R. P. Gilbert, and M. B. Visscher: Amer. J. Physiol. 192, 335 (1958). — 16. Haddy, F. J., J. Molnar, and R. W. Campbell: Accepted for publication in Amer. J. Physiol. — 17. Estensen, R. and R. Gilbert: Accepted for publication in Amer. J. Physiol. — 18. Zweifach, B. W., A. L. Nagler, and L. Thomas: J. Exper. Med. (U.S.A.) 104, 881 (1956).

Discussion

FINE: I am grateful to Dr. GILBERT for his analysis of this paper. He asks what additional evidence I would seek myself in order to prove the hypothesis that endotoxin is a key factor in death from shock, not only in the animal, but also in man. I would first look for endotoxin in the blood, and then see if the endotoxin is responsible for the death, before invoking the loss of some other vital function than the R. E. system as the cause of the death. In this effort, I would be up against a practical technical snag. For to detect the presence of endotoxin in the blood of a person dying of endo-toxaemia may require methods for testing endotoxin that don't exist. To identify endotoxin in very small quantities, say as little as a gamma, we use the chick embryo test of SMITH and THOMAS. For this, we use $^1/_{10}$ ml. of the blood to be tested. Whether it will be valid for man depends on the sensitivity of man to endotoxin. From experience with endotoxins given to man (0 antigen of typhoid, Pyromen, and the like) it appears that man's sensitivity is not very much different from that of the rabbit. WESTPHAL, who is one of the outstanding authorities on endotoxin, says that 0.1—1 mg. of his preparations can sicken a cow. If so, and the same applies to man, one can see that 1 ml. of blood from a person with a lethal endotoxaemia may contain too little for detection by the chick embryo test or any other now available.

GROSS: May I ask Dr. FINE what concentration of endotoxin he found in his dogs ? Have you any idea, when you do a bio-assay in the chick embryo test, what the approximate concentrations of endotoxin are ?

FINE: We have isolated the toxin in the dog's blood and found it to have the properties of endotoxin. We have done the same in the rabbit. In the rabbit, we can do a kind of rough quantitation by the haemagglutina-tion inhibition reaction, when we have an antiserum for a specific endotoxin which has been placed in the gut and has been absorbed into the circulation. Otherwise, all we can say is that we have a detectable amount of endotoxin. This might be less than a gamma or a good deal more, depending on the toxicity of the endotoxin and the sensitivity of the test system.

GROSS: I wonder if you really determine endotoxin or if you determine secondary reaction products which are released by endotoxin in the animal.

FINE: This is all the same to me. From my point of view it matters little whether this test for endotoxin detects endotoxin or the products of endotoxin activity. Those who have developed the tests believe that they do detect endotoxin.

SPINK: I shall have a little more to say later on the problem of endotoxin shock with regard to our own experiments, but one problem that has bothered me during the last ten years or so of clinical observation is the tremendous variability that man shows to endotoxin. In a very empirical and rough way we have measured endotoxin in man by the severity of the bacteraemia that is present. An individual 80 years of age may have his tissues flooded with endotoxin. He has a large number of bacteria in his blood, and yet he does not have shock. We take another individual who has very few bacteria and yet s in profound shock, and it becomes irreversible. I know that Dr. FINE feels that endotoxin is extremely important in the pathogenesis of at least some types of shock. I cannot believe from our own observations, however, that it is the only factor, although it may be a major factor in some forms of shock.

GELIN: What are the toxic substances in crush injuries?

In shock from bacteraemia or sepsis, we know that the shock can be explained by the toxins, or at least this is what we believe. We have tried to

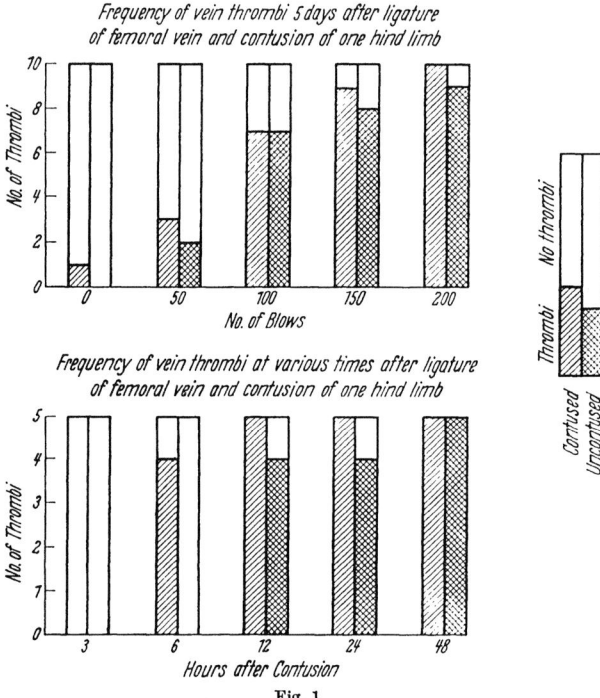

Fig. 1

get an idea about the nature of the toxic substance involved in shock by the following model. We have studied in rabbits the formation of venous thrombi in ligated femoral veins. The upper first two columns in Fig. 1 show that there is evidently no thrombus formation after simple ligation. When we contuse one hind limb, we find that, as the severity of the injury increases, so the number of thrombi increases not only on the contused side, but also on the uncontused side. We think that this must be due to a substance which is liberated from the injured tissue and which is able to produce venous thrombi on both the contused and the uncontused side. A study of the time taken for these thrombi to form reveals the following: After 3 hours, no thrombi are formed. After 6 hours, thrombi are formed only on the contused side, but not on the uncontused side. After 12 hours, however, thrombi are beginning to form on the uncontused side as well. It is during this same time-lag that we can also see considerable amounts of aggregated cells becoming stagnant in the venules.

In a study on the changes in coagulation occurring immediately after crush injury, BERGENTZ and NILSSON showed that the fibrinogen does not start to increase until after 12 hours and that fibrinolytic activity is inhibited. There is an increase in prothrombin, a drop in all coagulation factors, and an increase in the coagulability of the blood during the first 12 hours. We think from these two findings that the primary substance liberated from the injured tissue is tissue-thromboplastin. If thromboplastin is injected into an animal, we find all the signs that are considered to be especially important in traumatic shock, including stasis and aggregation of cells with decreased venous return and the appearance of fat embolism, which is a regular finding in all crush injuries. The formation of crush-induced fat embolism is completed within the first 12—18 hours. We have further reasons for assuming that, after crush injury, there is first an activation of some substance liberated from the injured tissue which is capable of causing aggregation of chylomicrons and formation of white emboli in the capillary bed. It later produces red-cell aggregates, leading in turn to stasis of cells in the venules and to a decrease in cardiac output. This is also in line with AUB's findings relating to the action of *Clostridium welchii* toxin. It is also possible to produce these changes with RUSSELL's viper venom which, among other things, contains lecithinase. I think the possible explanation might be that the toxic substance in traumatic shock first acts on the emulsion stability of the plasma, causing formation of fat droplets and fat emboli, and that it leads secondarily to aggregation of the cells. This toxin is intimately related to the first phase of the coagulation process. Lecithinase is the enzyme which could account for the first phase of shock, increasing the porosity of the endothelium membrane by lysis of the phospholipids in the membranes.

HOWARD: I should like to make two observations relating these experimental models to our experience with patients. First, irreversibility of haemorrhagic shock is a feature of the older patient, not of the young patient. In Dr. FINE's concept, this might imply that the endotoxins were not as deleterious to the young man. The second comment is a question: Is there a syndrome of tourniquet shock in man? Current experience in vascular surgery might justify some doubts on this point. The terminal aorta may be occluded for several hours; its release is usually followed only by a transient drop in blood pressure, which has been interpreted as secondary to the re-opening of a large segment of the peripheral vascular bed. Similarly, arterial occlusion may follow arterial injury. Successful restoration of circulation by means of surgical repair has sometimes been possible after a lag phase of as long as 12—24 hours. Under such circumstances, the early ischaemia may result in muscle necrosis even after restoration of circulation. Even under these conditions, "tourniquet shock" has not been obvious. May I suggest that we take these clinical opportunities to observe whether a tourniquet shock syndrome actually exists in man.

SPINK: Dr. HOWARD has brought up the question that I was going to ask Dr. FINE or anyone else — the question as to the relative importance of endotoxin. One of the observations that we and many others have made is that the young animal of many species is much more tolerant to endotoxin than the older animal. Furthermore, we find that paediatric patients are more resistant to endotoxin with the exception of meningococcaemia. On the other hand, at the neonatal period, infants are very susceptible. So we have two extremes in the human; the neonatal period and the aged are very susceptible to endotoxin. I am wondering whether or not this susceptibility may be related to intolerance to hypoxia with reduced blood flow.

FINE: Relative to Dr. HOWARD's remarks it is appropriate to recall the experiences in World War II of Dr. CHURCHILL and his colleagues in the European theatre, where they did not see irreversibility to haemorrhagic shock of long duration. They were dealing with young men. One would expect these young men to be able to stand up to what a man of 70 in shock from a bleeding peptic ulcer cannot tolerate. Before anyone labels a patient irreversible, one must be sure that the loss has been made good. Recent experience with an instrument that is accurate has shown that we cannot trust our clinical judgment on this score, and we are now convinced of the necessity of reviewing all our data on normovolaemic shock to make sure that this is so on the basis of this new equipment, because the errors of the conventional methods are too great to be trusted.

Dr. HOWARD asks whether the clinical syndrome of tourniquet shock exists in man, and he has cited the example of what happens to a patient after release of a clamp on the aorta. This is not the same thing as putting a tourniquet on the thigh, because there is some collateral circulation, even when the aorta is occluded. The time taken to install an aortic prosthesis produces a lesion different from that occurring in a man who has been pinned underneath a heavy timber load for 24 hours before it is removed. We must compare such injuries in terms of the number of hours of exposure to total ischaemia as well as in terms of the nature of the vascular deprivation.

Dr. SPINK spoke of differences in resistance of the young and old to shock. I would add another point, i. e. the question of the host's defence mechanisms against his own intestinal flora.

HALPERN: We have been working on the reticulo-endothelial system for more than ten years. A quantitative technique for measuring phagocytic and metabolic activity has been developed in my laboratory, which is now universally used. Since I speak as a physiologist, what I have to say is perhaps not really pertinent to the pathological problems. However, I would just like to stress four points. In the first place, we have determined the activity of the R.E. system per gramme of tissue in various animal species, starting from the mouse and going up to man. This function is a very constant one if one considers the activity per gramme of tissue. It shows that this activity is a physiological constant of remarkable fixity, regardless of the animal species involved. On the other hand, the susceptibility of these various animal species to endotoxin is extremely variable. In other words, identical functional activity of the R.E. system is associated with great differences in the response of the animal species to endotoxin. The second point I want to make is that we have shown that the activity of the R.E. cells, and especially those of the liver, i. e. the Kupffer cells, is entirely dependent on the blood supply. We have considered two types of activity — intrinsic activity and also dependent activity, i. e. the activity depending on the blood supply. In all conditions under which we have produced impairment of the blood supply, we have seen modifications in R.E. cell activity; hence, it is not surprising that in severe disturbances of the blood supply, as in shock, such modifications in R.E. activity may occur. The third point is that in adrenalectomised animals the activity of the R.E. system is absolutely normal, whereas the susceptibility to endotoxin is considerably increased. Again we have a situation in which normal activity of the R.E. system is associated with a considerable increase in sensitivity to endotoxin. The last point I would like to mention is even more striking. We have shown that injection of mycobacteria, especially BCG, considerably increases the activity of the R.E. system. The increase may amount to as much as 200% or 300%. In conditions under which the R.E.

system is markedly stimulated, the sensitivity to endotoxin is greatly increased, and one can kill an animal with a dose of endotoxin which is only $1/_{100}$ of the normal toxic dose. Here we have an exactly opposite situation, i. e. a considerable increase in the activity of the R.E. system coinciding with a decrease in tolerance to endotoxin.

FINE: I take it that Dr. HALPERN's description of the increase in activity of the R.E. system's response to BCG vaccine relates to its phagocytic function. This function and the break-down of endotoxins by this system are two different functions. We have found phagocytosis still intact when the breakdown of endotoxin was no longer taking place. Further, we have observed double the uptake of endotoxin by the injured R.E. system in response to perfusion with immune serum. Nevertheless, this system was incapable of destroying endotoxin. A normal spleen destroys endotoxin immediately. A spleen injured by endotoxin cannot do so, even after two hours are allowed for this to occur.

HALPERN: May I just say one word? We have also measured the break-down rate of denatured proteins under these conditions, and we found a good correlation between the increase in phagocytic activity and the kinetics of the break-down of proteins. This means that there is a good correlation between phagocytic and enzymatic functions.

FINE: Protein break-down is still a third function.

Hemodynamic factors in shock

By

D. E. GREGG

I should like to consider very briefly two points: first, the existing experimental data regarding the compensatory behavior of the resistance vessels during the periods of graded hemorrhage to a hypotensive level and of the decompensatory phase of irreversible or "normovolemic" shock, and secondly, our own recent experimental work on this subject.

In earlier studies summarized by WIGGERS in 1950, there appeared to be small to no significant increase in total peripheral resistance and, therefore, at best only minimal active contraction of arteriolar vessels as a compensation for hypotension induced by hemorrhage (1). During the compensatory phase of normovolemic "irreversible" shock, the systemic resistance underwent no significant change until just before the terminal phase of rapid decline in arterial pressure, when it might decrease mildly. The findings in more recent experiments were also rather moderate (2, 3). Thus, there did not appear to be any considerable increase in total peripheral resistance in simple hypotension, nor was there any clear-cut difference in the behavior of the systemic resistance between simple hypotension and the "irreversible" stage that followed a prolonged period of hypotension.

The regional resistance of the systemic circulation was studied in a number of vascular beds during the stages of hemorrhage, hypotension and cardiovascular decay that followed the blood reinfusion. For the kidney, the evidence appeared to indicate some degree of vasoconstriction during graded hemorrhage, and in the normovolemic stage of "irreversible" shock renal blood flow and resistance appeared to undergo about the same changes with declining arterial pressure as were noted during the oligemic phase (4, 5). In the skin and muscle during hemorrhage, there was a marked increase in vascular resistance, but there was insufficient data to indicate whether or not changes in flow and resistance differed in the normovolemic phase of shock (6). Splanchnic vascular resistance appeared to be mildly increased or to undergo no change during hemorrhage and the ensuing hypotensive state. Near termination of the "irreversible" shock, some hours after transfusion, hepatic artery, intestinal vascular and total splanchnic resistances were about the same as those noted in the control period (*7, 8*). In animals, in patients with various forms of "shock", and in human volunteer subjects bled until mental changes occurred, cerebral blood flow was reduced, but there was no evidence for vasoconstriction or compensatory dilatation (*9, 10*). For the irreversible phase, no adequate data are available. In the coronary system during hemorrhagic hypotension, coronary blood flow fell but coronary resistance declined. This decline also persisted in the irreversible stage and was of about the same magnitude (*11, 12, 13*).

From the preceding, it would appear that during simple hemorrhage, resistances in such regions as the kidney, skin, skeletal muscle, intestine, liver and brain may be mildly increased or unaltered, whereas resistance may decrease in the left coronary circulation. Where measured, the behavior of these regional resistances in normovolemic cardiovascular decay was not grossly different from that during simple hemorrhage. Thus, there does not appear to be evidence for a marked decrease in regional resistance as a cause of irreversibility in hemorrhagic shock.

The work just enumerated has been largely restricted to studies in experimental animals exposed to anesthesia, surgery, and varying amounts of traumatic insult. It seemed to us that a more proper approach would be in normal conscious dogs, which is now possible with methodology available in our laboratory. Accordingly, we have prepared such animals and have compared the phasic pressure-flow curves in the aorta and in various regional arteries during simple hemorrhagic hypotension, and in the same animal after reinfusion in the presence of irreversible shock resulting from spontaneous decay of the circulatory system.

Modified and improved electromagnetic flow meters of the sine wave type, constructed in our laboratory, were used to quantitate phasic and mean flows in the pulmonary artery and aorta and in the regional distribution of the latter. The flow transducers for the systemic circulation varied from 14—18 mm. in diameter and were about 1 cm. long. The flow probes for the regional arteries were from 1.5 to 4.5 mm. in diameter and were considerably shorter. For example, those used on the left coronary artery were necessarily somewhat smaller than an aspirin tablet since the space available for implantation, i. e. the maximum length of the main left coronary artery approximates 2—2.5 mm. *In vitro* calibrations of both types of probes before implantation and after subsequent removal from the animal gave linear calibrations that were within 5—10%

of each other. For the probes used to measure cardiac output, sensitivities of 1 mm. deflection per 10 cc. of flow were available; for the smaller probes, sensitivities of 1 mm. deflection per 0.1 cc. were available. However, lower sensitivities were generally used. The accuracy of the flow measurements with the electromagnetic flow meter was checked against the dye dilution technique in the case of the systemic circulation, and against the rotameter in the case of the regional circulation, and values agreed well with those obtained with these reference methods.

The studies were made on healthy mongrel dogs (15—30 kg. in weight) about one month after release from quarantine. Through a left thoracotomy, flow meters were placed on the ascending aorta (or pulmonary artery) and on the main left coronary artery or its circumflex branch, just distal to its origin. Probes were implanted by a left retroperitoneal approach on the superior mesenteric, renal and external iliac arteries, the latter being used as an index of skeletal muscle flow. For phasic arterial pressure, a nylon tube covered by a snug-fitting polyethylene tube and filled with heparin was implanted in the ascending aorta just beyond the aortic flow transducer. A plastic snare was placed around the vessel in which flow was being quantitated, and its peripheral end brought out through the skin so that zero blood flow could be determined by its temporary occlusion at any time later. In any one dog, there was implanted a pressure tube, a systemic flow transducer, and one or two regional flow transducers. The dogs, which had been previously trained, were allowed to recover for a varying number of days, during which time various physiological studies were made such as the effect of exercise, excitement, etc. Then, at the time of the shock experiment, the dog was given 2—3 mg. heparin/kg. (the dose was repeated later, if necessary), a femoral artery and vein were exposed under procaine anesthesia with clean but not sterile technique, and connected to bleeding and infusion reservoirs, respectively. The blood was kept warm and filtered before rein-fusion. Graded hemorrhage was produced by bleeding into the reservoir connected to the femoral artery. The shed blood was later reinfused into the femoral vein. Flow and pressure measurements were obtained at various blood pressure levels during the initial bleed-down, at the end of which the dog was maintained at a pressure (35 to 45 mm. Hg) and time interval ($1^1/_2$ to 3 hours) thought to be sufficient to produce irreversible shock. Blood was then reinfused, and flow and pressure measurements repeated during the spontaneous hypotension that developed, ending in death. In addition, in some dogs, as the arterial pressure in the latter period was very slowly declining, the cardiovascular system was challenged with periods of hemorrhagically induced hypotension and reinfusion.

Fig. 1 shows typical pressure and flow patterns of the resting unanesthetized dog about one week post-operatively, and obtained from the external iliac artery, superior mesenteric artery, renal artery, the main left coronary artery, ascending aorta and pulmonary artery. The horizontal line under each flow curve indicates

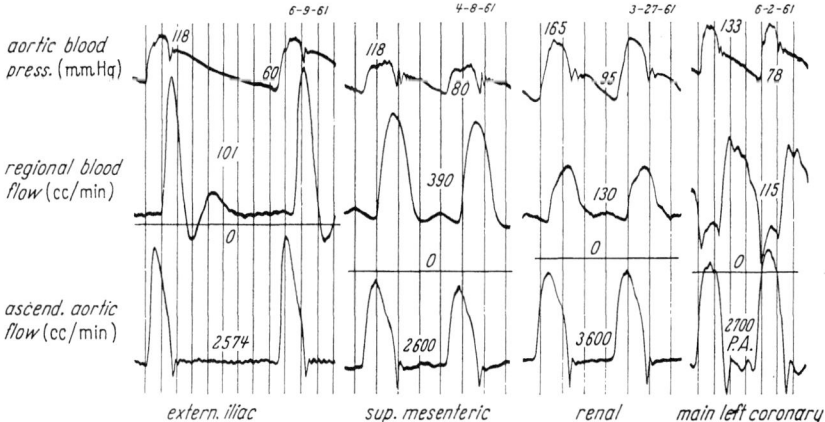

Fig. 1. Reproduction of reactions of original records of phasic aortic pressure and flow patterns taken from the ascending aorta, external iliac, superior mesenteric, renal and main left coronary artery of dogs by means of electromagnetic flow meters chronically implanted

the level of zero flow as obtained by temporary closure of the snare around the regional arteries. In the ascending aorta or pulmonary artery, zero flow occurs functionally during the latter half of diastole.

Detailed analysis of these interesting flow patterns is beyond the scope of this meeting. Attention, however, may be called to the variable relation of the flow patterns to the position of zero flow. In the renal and mesenteric arteries, the flow pattern is widely separated from the zero flow line; in the iliac artery, forward flow in late diastole is much less, and back flow occurs in early diastole. In the left coronary artery, the rate of systolic flow is less than that in diastole and it may approximate zero (*14*). It is not, however, unusual to find a sizable rate of flow during systole in both the main left coronary artery (shown here) and its major branches.

Because of time limitations, changes in phasic pressure and flow for the various vascular beds throughout an experiment cannot be shown. Fig. 2 may suffice to indicate the adequacy of the pressure and flow patterns upon which our data and calculations are based. This shows the typical patterns of pressure and flow and their values in the aorta and the renal artery during simple hemorrhagic hypotension. In this instance, by graded arterial hemorrhage of 950 cc., the mean blood pressure is reduced over a period of 31 minutes from a control mean blood pressure level of 123mm. Hg to 36 mm. Hg. The aortic flow decreases from 4,100 cc.

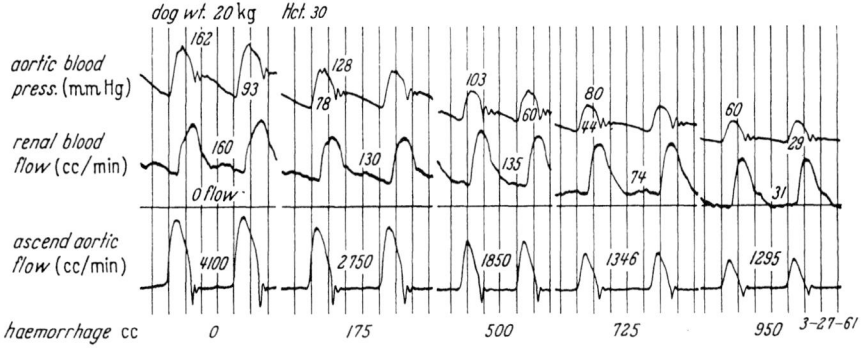

Fig. 2. Reproduction of sections of original records of phasic aortic pressure, phasic left renal flow and aortic stroke volume during hemorrhagic hypotension in the unanesthetized dog

to about 1,300 cc. The control mean renal blood flow (160 cc.) is well maintained as the blood pressure drops to 80 mm. Hg, after which it decreases to 31 cc./min. At the lowest pressure level, diastolic flow ceases and forward flow is essentially all in systole.

Fig. 3 is a chart showing in temporal fashion the typical pressure-flow relations that occur in the ascending aorta and external iliac artery during simple hemorrhagic hypotension and during the hemodynamic decay following reinfusion. During the hemorrhagic period after the removal of over 1,000 cc. of blood, the mean arterial blood pressure drops from 105 mm. Hg to approximately 35 mm. Hg for about 100 minutes. The cardiac output decreases from 1,600 cc. to 225 cc. per minute. The systemic pressure-flow ratio rises moderately throughout this period. During reinfusion, both the blood pressure and cardiac output exceed the control values and the pressure-flow ratio is moderately depressed from the level reached during the oligemic period. Terminally, as the blood pressure and cardiac output spontaneously decrease, the pressure-flow ratio rises again. During hemorrhage the external

iliac flow drops precipitously, remains quite low during the hypotensive period, and rises only mildly during the normovolemic
period. The iliac pressure-flow ratio rises considerably throughout
the experiment, roughly paralleling the resistance changes in the
aorta.

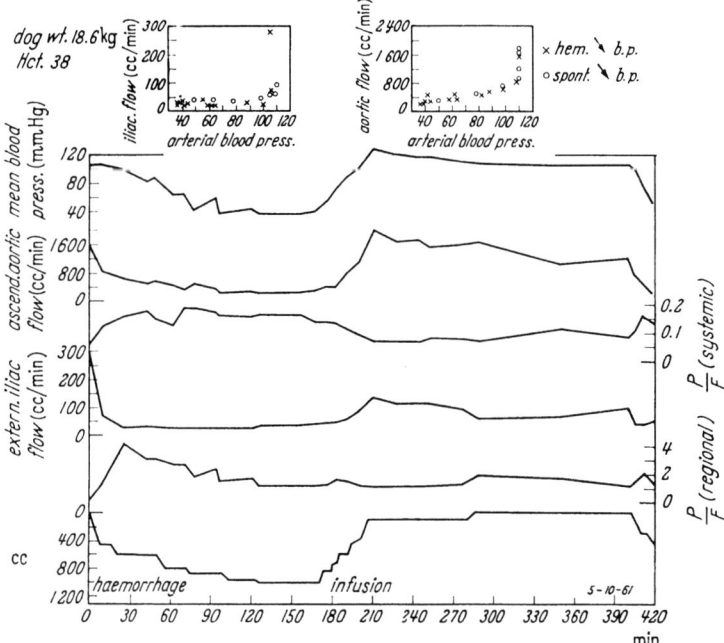

Fig. 3. Chart from representative experiment during standardized hemorrhagic shock procedure illustrating trends in mean arterial blood pressure, ascending aortic flow, total peripheral
resistance, and flow and resistance in the external iliac artery. Inserts at top are plots of
pressure-flow curves for the iliac (left) and aorta (right) during hemorrhagic hypotension and
spontaneous hypotension after reinfusion

In the top of this figure are inserted plots of the pressure-flow
curves obtained in this experiment for the aorta (top right), and
external iliac (top left), during the initial bleed-down and during
the hemodynamic decay after infusion. In each plot the position
of the points for the two periods is similar, indicating that the
resistance to flow in both the aorta and iliac artery is at least as
high during the irreversible period as during simple hypotension.

Fig. 4 is a chart similar to Fig. 3 but in which the data represent
a typical experiment showing the pressure-flow relations in the
superior mesenteric artery during the periods of oligemic and

normovolemic shock. Withdrawal of 950 cc. of blood lowers the
arterial blood pressure from 128 to about 45 mm. Hg. At the same
time, the mesenteric flow shows a precipitous drop from 420 cc./min.
to 50 cc./min. The pressure-flow ratio is considerably elevated
during the progressive hemorrhage and the following hypotensive

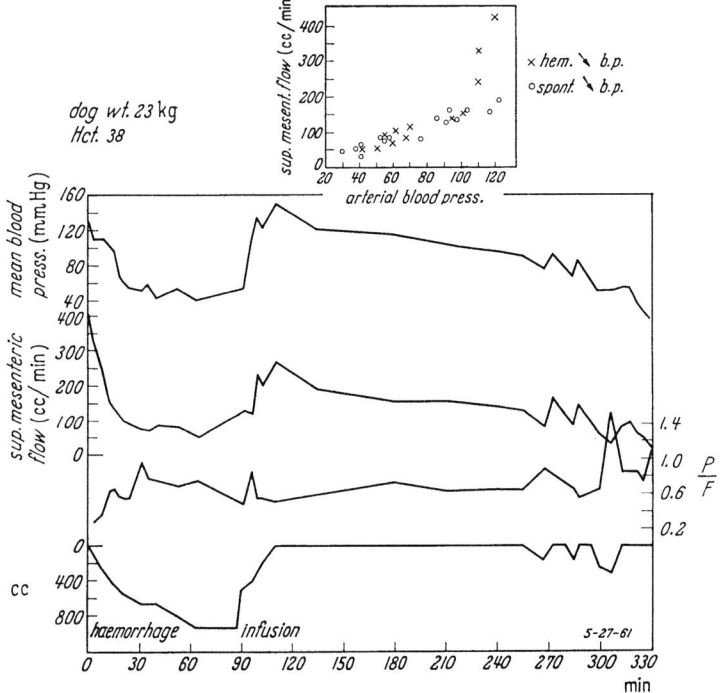

Fig. 4. Chart of data from representative experiment during standardized hemorrhagic shock
procedure showing trends in mean arterial pressure, and flow and resistance in the mesenteric
artery. Top insert is plot of pressure-flow curves

period. During reinfusion, the mesenteric flow does not return to
the control level despite an overshoot of the blood pressure. The
pressure-flow relation remains elevated. During the subsequent
gradual cardiovascular decay, which was aided somewhat by short
periods of small hemorrhage and reinfusion, the pressure-flow
relation rises still further. In the small insert at the top of this
figure, the position of points for the pressure-flow curves for the
periods of hemorrhagic hypotension and spontaneous hypotension
is similar, i.e. the flow resistance during the latter period is not less
than during the period of simple hemorrhagic hypotension.

Fig. 5 is a chart similar in design to that of Fig. 4, but in which the data represent a typical experiment for the pressure-flow relation in the left renal artery. During the hemorrhagic period, as almost 2,000 cc. of blood are removed, the arterial pressure drops from 120 to 35 mm. Hg, and the renal flow decreases from 230 to 20 cc. per minute. During the bleed-down, the pressure-flow relation in the renal artery is essentially unchanged, but throughout

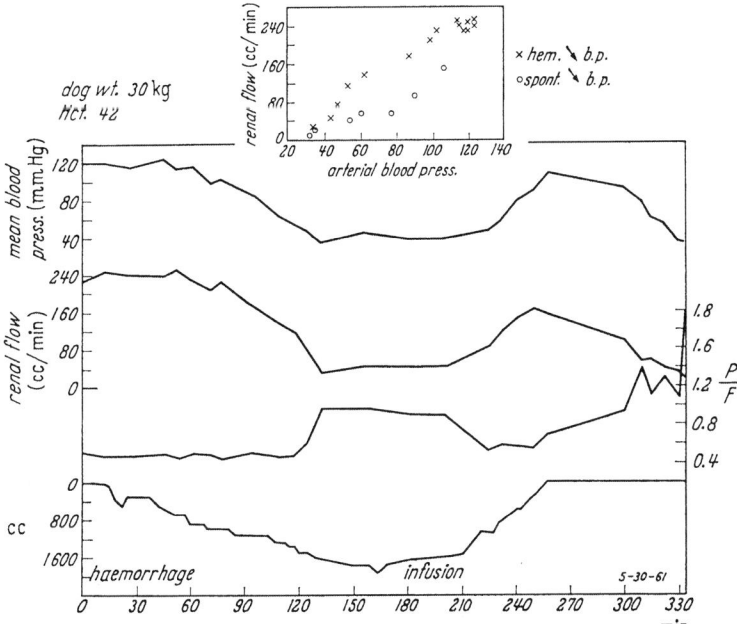

Fig. 5. Chart of data from representative experiment during standardized hemorrhagic shock procedure showing trends in mean arterial pressure, and flow and resistance in the left kidney. Top insert is plot of pressure-flow curves

the 90 minute period of maintenance of hypotension, this ratio increases considerably. During reinfusion, it returns essentially to the control level, but as the blood pressure spontaneously decreases, the pressure-flow ratio increases greatly. The insert plot at the top of the figure of the pressure-flow relation shows that the resistance is considerably higher during the period of hemodynamic decay than during the period of induced hypotension.

Fig. 6 depicts the typical trends of pressure and flow in the ascending aorta and in the circumflex branch of the left coronary artery during hemorrhagic shock. During the withdrawal of 800 cc.

of blood, the cardiac output drops from 3,600 cc. to 850 cc., as the mean blood pressure decreases from 100 to about 40 mm. Hg, where it was maintained for approximately 3 hours. The changes in aortic flow and pressure are similar to those already discussed in Fig. 3, i. e. the pressure-flow ratio rises in both the hemorrhagic and

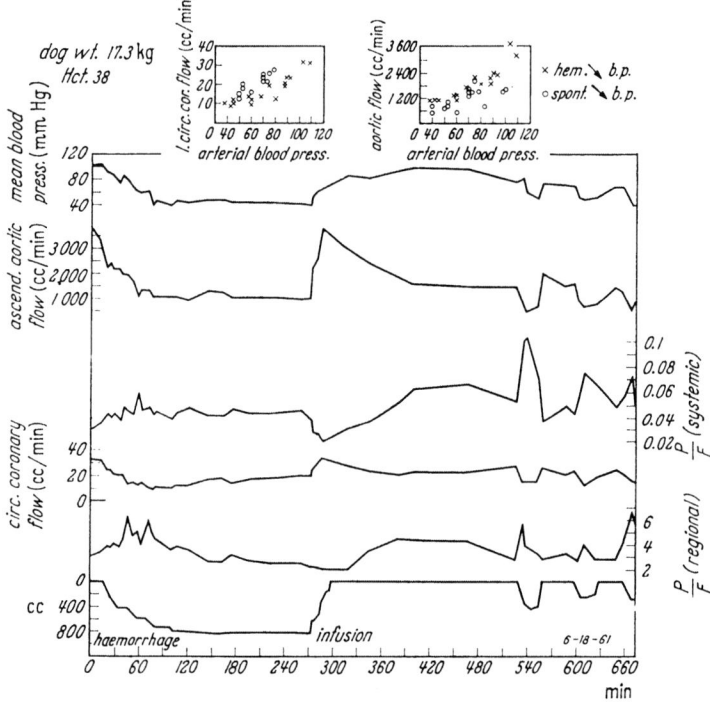

Fig. 6. Chart of data from typical experiment during standardized hemorrhagic shock procedure illustrating trends in mean arterial pressure, ascending aortic flow, total peripheral resistance, and flow and resistance in the left circumflex coronary artery. Inserts at top are pressure-flow curves for the coronary artery (left), and aorta (right) during initial hemorrhage and subsequent hemodynamic decay after reinfusion

normovolemic periods. The insert (top right) indicates that resistance to flow is at least as large during the period of spontaneous decay as during the initial hypotensive period.

During the period of bleed-down, the mean coronary flow drops from 35 to 10 cc. per minute, but during the hypotensive period it progressively rises to 20 cc. per minute, which level is fairly well maintained during the period of decay after reinfusion. These flow changes have their explanation in certain characteristic changes in the coronary flow pattern. The phasic flow pattern, initially some distance above the zero flow line throughout the cardiac cycle, moves closer to the zero flow line during hemorrhage, and back flow may appear during systole, but the magnitude of the flow pattern increases indicating increased vigor of contraction. As the hypotensive period progresses, flow is re-established in systole and increased in diastole as well. At this low level of perfusion pressure, systolic flow may now approach that during diastole for an equivalent time interval. As the coronary flow rises during reinfusion and is elevated for a short time thereafter, this type of flow pattern is exaggerated and resembles somewhat the prevailing aortic pressure pulse. During the period of spontaneous hemodynamic decay, this flow pattern with an exaggerated systolic flow reappears. As the result of these changes in flow pattern, the coronary pressure-flow ratio moderately increases during hemorrhage, progressively decreases during the hypotensive period, and is temporarily restored during the reinfusion. During the irreversible period in which the coronary flow is fairly well maintained, the pressure-flow ratio again drops. Examination of the insert of the pressure-flow curves for the coronary circulation in Fig. 6 (top left) shows that the resistance to coronary flow is somewhat less during the period of spontaneous decay than during the initial hypotensive period.

Summary

Flow-pressure relationships in different vascular beds of pre-operated, unanesthetized dogs were studied during the course of hemorrhagic hypotension and hemorrhagic shock. Blood flow was measured by electromagnetic flow meters implanted around the ascending aorta, the main left coronary artery or its circumflex branch, the mesenteric artery, renal artery and external iliac artery. Comparing the pressure-flow curves during shock to those of hemorrhagic hypotension revealed a mild increase in total peripheral resistance and in resistance in the mesenteric, renal and iliac arterial beds. Only the coronary arterial bed showed a decreased vascular resistance. It is concluded that the pathogenesis of shock in unanesthetized dogs cannot be attributed to "peripheral vascular collapse" at the arteriolar site. The hemodynamic disturbance is post-arteriolar in location.

Acknowledgements

The experiments reported here represent the collaborative efforts of Dr. D. E. GREGG, Dr. A. HUVOS, Dr. L. GRANATA and Dr. T. TSUNEKAWA.

References

1. WIGGERS, C. J.: Physiology of Shock. The Commonwealth Fund, New York 1950. — 2. REYNELL, P. D., P. A. MARKS, C. CHIDSEY, and S. E. BRADLEY: Clin. Sc. (U.S.A.) 14, 407 (1955). — 3. FOWLER, N. O. and R. FRANCH: Circulation Res. (U.S.A.) 5, 153 (1957). — 4. LAUSON, H. D., S. E. BRADLEY, and A. COURNAND: J. Clin. Invest. (U.S.A.) 23, 381 (1944). —

60   D. E. GREGG: Hemodynamic factors in shock

5. SELKURT, E. E.: Amer. J. Physiol. 145, 699 (1946). — 6. GREEN, H. D., R. N. LEWIS, N. D. NICKERSON, and A. L. HELLER: Amer. J. Physiol. 141, 518 (1944). — 7. SELKURT, E. E. and G. A. BRECHER: Circulation Res. (U.S.A.) 4, 693, 704 (1956). — 8. CULL, T. E., M. P. SCIBETTA, and E. E. SELKURT: Amer. J. Physiol. 185, 365 (1956). — 9. FAZEKAS, J. F., J. KLEH, and A. E. PARRISH: Amer. J. Med. Sc. 229, 41 (1955). — 10. KOVACH, A. G. B., P. S. ROHEIM, M. IRANYI, E. CSERHATI, G. GOSZTONYI, and E. KOVACH: Acta physiol. Acad. sc. Hungaricae 15, 217 (1959). — 11. OPDYKE, D. F. and R. C. FOREMAN: Amer. J. Physiol. 148, 726 (1947). — 12. EDWARDS, W. S.. A. SIEGEL, and R. J. BING: J. clin. Invest. (U.S.A.) 33, 1646 (1954). — 13. SIMEONE, F. A., E. A. HUSNI, and M. G. WEIDNER Jr.: Surgery (U.S.A). 44, 168 (1958). — 14. GREGG, D. E.: Coronary Circulation in Health and Disease. Philadelphia: Lea & Febiger 1950.

Nervous adjustments of the vascular bed with special reference to patterns of vasoconstrictor fibre discharge

By

B. FOLKOW

I was very interested by Dr. GREGG's findings concerning the regional blood flow changes occurring in conscious dogs upon bleeding and in the shock which subsequently develops. In many respects these data coincide with results arrived at in our laboratory in studies, performed during the last few years, concerning the patterns of vasoconstrictor fibre discharge elicited when the medullary vasomotor centre is exposed to different excitatory and inhibitory central and reflex influences (see FOLKOW 1960, 1961). It might therefore be of interest in this connection to present a brief survey of some of these results insofar as they have a bearing on the reflex cardiovascular adjustments taking place in hypotension and established shock conditions.

It has often been generally taken for granted that the sympathetic nervous system, with few exceptions, is characterised by an essentially diffuse mass activity, in which respect it contrasts with the highly differentiated somatomotor system. But on closer examination it appeared that this general assumption might after all not be correct, since previously the activity of the sympathetic nervous system had rarely been studied by methods capable of revealing regional quantitative differences in sympathetic fibre activation. A series of investigations has therefore been undertaken in our laboratory during the last ten years with the aim of obtaining more quantitative data on autonomic nervous control of the cardiovascular system, so as to permit further analysis of the functional organisation of the vasomotor centre and its subordinate cardiovascular effectors (FOLKOW 1952; CELANDER and FOLKOW 1953; CELANDER 1954; FOLKOW, LÖFVING and MELLANDER 1956; FOLKOW and HAMBERGER 1956; FOLKOW, JOHANSSON and ÖBERG 1958; MELLANDER 1960). Briefly, the results indicated (1) that the tonic vasoconstrictor fibre discharge is normally quite moderate (1—2 impulses per second or less) and that the discharge rate hardly ever exceeds some 8—10 impulses per second, even in response to extreme excitation of the vasomotor centre. Further, it was found (2)

that, for most cardiovascular effector units, the hormonal link of
the sympatho-adrenal system was of minor importance with regard
to excitatory effects; in most cases of physiological activation its
elimination resulted in hardly any weakening of the effects mediated
by direct adrenergic innervation. Lastly, an insight was gained
into the quantitative relationship between sympathetic discharge
rate and the ensuing effector response within some of the more
important "parallel-coupled" and "series-coupled" cardiovascular
sections (3). Owing to the fact that this interrelationship produced
a hyperbolic curve with a very steep initial segment, already
reaching roughly maximal values at 8—15 impulses per second, the
narrow discharge range of the autonomic fibres was nevertheless
sufficient to allow an extensive central adjustment of the cardiovascular system. When further experience had been gained, it was
also found possible to estimate approximately the average discharge
rate of the vasoconstrictor fibres in those vascular beds where the
relationship between a known discharge rate and the effector
response had been explored, as even slight shifts in fibre discharge
caused considerable adjustments of the regional flow resistance.

        With the above-mentioned data as a general background, it was
thus considered possible, by utilising suitable concomitant recordings of the effector responses, to analyse in more detail the
discharge patterns of the vasomotor centre when exposed to
graded excitatory and inhibitory influences from cardiovascular
receptors and higher autonomic structures. In this connection
certain of our recent studies which may be of special interest will
be dealt with; some related aspects have been reported elsewhere
(FOLKOW, JOHANSSON and ÖBERG 1959; FOLKOW 1960, 1961;
FOLKOW et al. 1960; LÖFVING 1960, 1961 b).

        During the last three years Dr. LÖFVING (1961 a, b) in our
department has studied the extent of the constrictor fibre adjustments taking place within some of the more important vascular
beds — the muscle vessels, the renal vessels, the intestinal vessels,
and the cutaneous vessels — under circumstances in which the
baroreceptor influence was more or less selectively eliminated, the
chemoreceptors activated, or the animals exposed to the more
complex influences resulting from bleeding or asphyxia. As partly
illustrated in Fig. 1 and Fig. 2, it was generally, though not always,
found that the muscle vessels were intensely constricted when the
baroreceptor inhibitory influence was eliminated and/or when the
chemoreceptors were activated. Under these circumstances the
renal vessels, on the other hand, were hardly affected at all and
the cutaneous vessels very little, while the intestinal vessels were

moderately constricted. It was also observed that the intense sympathetic activation induced by asphyxia influenced the muscle vessels and the intestinal vessels quite early on, whereas the renal and cutaneous vessels were not significantly affected until a fairly late stage in the progressively intensifying asphyxia.

It will be seen from Fig. 1, for instance, that the renal vessels are hardly involved at all in the reflex increase in sympathetic discharge taking place in response to carotid occlusion in the vagotomised, anaesthetised animal; the cutaneous vessels also show very little effect, whereas the muscle vessels are strongly affected. Fig. 2 illustrates how the rising phase of the blood-pressure change in the MAYER waves, which are known to emanate from rhythmic activation of the chemoreceptors (HEYMANS and NEIL 1958), is accompained by an *increase* in flow resistance within the muscles, whereas the renal vessels remain essentially unaffected as evidenced by the merely passive changes in renal blood flow. A local anaesthetic infiltrated around the carotid sinus regions eliminates the MAYER waves and the rhythmic constrictions of the muscle vessels. It is clear from the figure (D)

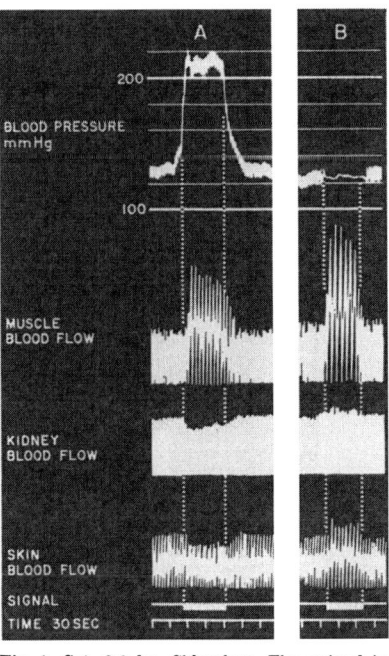

Fig. 1. Cat, 3.0 kg. Chloralose. The animal is curarised and atropinised; the vagal nerves are cut and the adrenal glands denervated. Effect of bilateral carotid occlusion on the blood pressure and blood flows in the skeletal muscles of the calf, the kidney, and the skin of the hind paw. In B the reflex blood pressure rise is compensated for by partial occlusion of the abdominal aorta just proximally to the renal arteries. Note the marked regional difference in the extent of the reflex vasoconstriction. The ordinates in the blood-flow tracings are inversely proportional to the rate of flow

that the constrictor nerves to the renal vessels were intact, as hypothalamic stimulation caused intense renal vasoconstriction.

It was possible to confirm by various means that these regional differences in reflex vasoconstriction were not due to any accidental fibre damage or simply to differences in the extent of constrictor fibre supply. As they could not be due to any counteracting local

64   B. FOLKOW:

influences on the vascular smooth muscles, they had to be ascribed
to regional differences in the average discharge rate of the constrictor fibres.

These findings thus indicate that the neuron pools supplying
the different vascular beds do not show any uniform, diffuse
activity increase when the vasomotor centre is released from the
baroreceptor inhibition and/or stimulated by the chemoreceptor
fibres. It is evident that the constrictor fibres to the skeletal

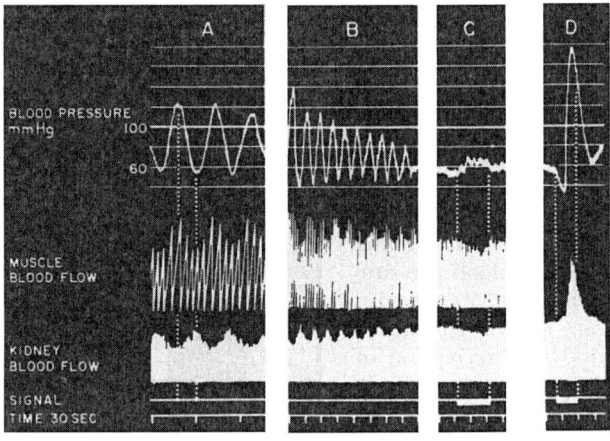

Fig. 2. Cat, 2.8 kg. Chloralose. The animal is curarised and atropinised; the vagal nerves are
cut and the adrenal glands denervated. The animal has been bled until the arterial blood
pressure reaches a level of 70—80 mm. Hg, after which the carotid arteries are clamped,
leading to the establishment of Mayer waves (A). Note that muscle blood flow *decreases* when
pressure is raised, whereas renal blood flow *increases*. — In B the carotid sinus regions have
been infiltrated with 2 ml. 2% xylocaine, which gradually depresses the rhythmic changes in
pressure and flow, until (C) carotid occlusion causes only a minor pressure increase and passive
flow increases in both tissues. — In D topical stimulation of the anterior hypothalamus is
applied, which causes an immediate, almost fourfold increase in renal flow resistance, proving
that the renal vasoconstrictor fibres were intact. — The ordinates in the blood-flow tracings
are inversely proportional to the rate of flow

muscles are markedly activated, those to the intestinal vessels
moderately so, those to the skin vessels only slightly, and those to
the renal vessels hardly at all. This means that even the basic
pattern of vasomotor fibre activity, which forms the background
to blood pressure regulation, is differentiated insofar as considerable
quantitative differences are seen between the various vascular
circuits. It is only natural, then, that central and reflex *inhibitory*
influences on the vasomotor centre will induce regional vasodilatation which is especially pronounced in those tissues where the
initial tonic vasoconstrictor fibre discharge is high, i.e. within
the skeletal muscles (LÖVFING 1961 b).

However, although the pattern of flow changes described was seen in the great majority of the animals, the results were nevertheless somewhat puzzling for several reasons. Firstly, it is well known from many studies, both in man and in animals, that under many circumstances both the renal vessels and the cutaneous vessels do constrict markedly in response to certain reflex influences. Secondly, it was occasionally observed in some of Dr. LÖVFING's experiments that only moderate constriction of the muscle vessels was induced by carotid occlusion, whereas the renal vessels could be strongly affected. It was soon realised, however, that these apparent contradictions — far from being simply due to some hidden artifact — were apparently normal variations which might be able to shed further light on the functional organisation of vasoconstrictor fibre control of the vascular bed.

Another series of studies was therefore started and so devised that the vasomotor centre could be separately or simultaneously exposed to different types of graded excitatory (or inhibitory) influences so as to induce a summation of excitatory (or inhibitory) stimuli (FOLKOW, JOHANSSON and LÖFVING 1961). Fig. 3 illustrates an experiment in which an atropinised, curarised cat was exposed to repeated carotid occlusion, while at the same time the artificial respiration was varied so as to cause moderate shifts in oxygen and carbon dioxide tension. The idea was to ascertain to what extent these environmental changes were able to affect the excitability of the different neuron pools of the medullary vasomotor centre. Blood flow in the normally innervated vascular beds of the kidney and skeletal muscles was used as an indicator because, as already mentioned, the vasoconstrictor fibres of these two vascular regions exhibited the most pronounced differences in response to increased activity during carotid occlusion. The most striking difference is seen when "D" and "E" in Fig. 3 are compared. In "D" the animal was definitely hypoventilated, and here carotid occlusion caused a considerable increase in blood pressure. Of special interest, however, is the fact that the "resting" blood flow of the two tissues was hardly affected by the hypoventilation, whereas following carotid occlusion both flow resistances increased by some 250 to 300 per cent. When hyperventilation was induced (E), this again had little effect upon the "resting" blood flow, but carotid occlusion caused only a passive flow increase within the kidney, whereas the muscle vessels were still as strongly affected as in "D", to judge from the shift in flow resistance. Cutting the regional vasoconstrictor fibres did not significantly increase renal blood flow in this experiment, whereas muscle blood flow increased

66   B. FOLKOW:

by some 60 to 70 per cent. Repetition of the carotid occlusion
under these circumstances now caused only passive flow increases.
In terms of average constrictor fibre discharge these findings
imply that the "resting" tonic discharge to the renal vessels was
negligible and only slightly enhanced in "E", whereas it must have
increased to some 3–4 impulses per second in "D". In the muscles,
on the other hand, the "resting" tonic discharge can be deduced to

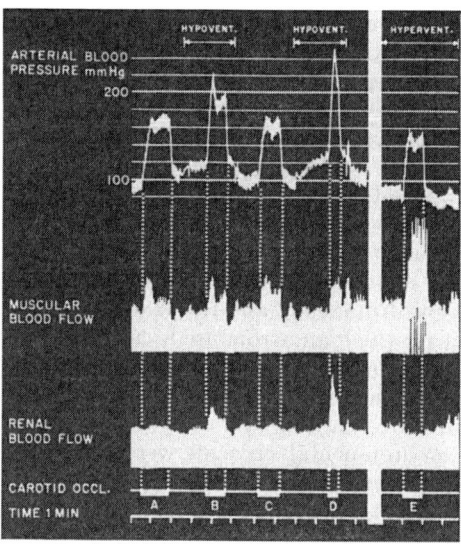

Fig. 3. Cat, 2.6 kg. Chloralose. The animal is curarised and atropinised; the vagal nerves are
cut in the neck and the adrenal glands are denervated. Effect of bilateral occlusion of the
common carotid arteries on blood pressure, muscle and renal blood flow under different
respiratory conditions. Note that the muscle vessels are considerably affected by carotid
occlusion irrespective of the respiratory state of the animal, whereas the renal vessels are
markedly affected only during periods of hypoventilation. In hyperventilation renal blood
flow is merely passively increased in connection with the reflex blood-pressure rise following
carotid occlusion. — The ordinates in the blood-flow tracings are inversely proportional to the
rate of flow

have been of the order of 1–2 impulses per second, increasing to
at least 3–4 impulses per second both in "D" and "E". In other
words, per se the environmental shift inherent in the hypoventilated
state caused hardly any intensification of the negligible resting
discharge of the renal vasoconstrictor fibres, but it did facilitate the
otherwise essentially "sub-threshold" effect of carotid occlusion
on the renal vessels, so as to cause a considerable increase in
discharge in the renal vasoconstrictor fibres.

In Fig. 4 constant artificial respiration was maintained, but
here the animal was exposed to intermittent carotid occlusion

and afferent stimulation of cutaneous "nociceptor" fibres so graded as to induce definite reflex pressor responses with only a slight effect on the constrictor fibres of the renal vessels ("A" in Fig. 4). Though carotid occlusion alone failed to exert a more significant effect on the renal vessels, when the two excitatory influences upon the vasomotor centre were superimposed on each other ("B" in Fig. 4) intense renal vasoconstriction occurred.

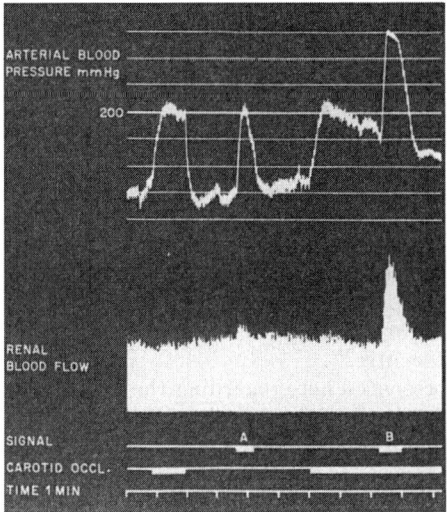

Fig. 4. Cat, 2.2 kg. Chloralose. The animal is curarised and atropinised; the vagal nerves are cut and the adrenal glands are denervated. Effects of carotid occlusions and of afferent high-voltage stimulation of a cutaneous branch of the sciatic nerve on the blood pressure and the renal blood flow. First the carotid arteries are occluded; the consequent increase in renal flow resistance is hardly any greater than that usually occurring as a result of the "autoregulation" of the renal vessels. Then (A) the afferent nerve is stimulated at 12 V, 4 msec., and 40 impulses per second; this has only a negligible effect on the renal vessels. In B the same afferent stimulation produces marked renal vasoconstriction when performed during a period of carotid occlusion which *per se* has little effect on the renal vessels. — The ordinates in the blood-flow tracings are inversely proportional to the rate of flow

The most reasonable interpretation of the data illustrated in these four figures appears to be that the different vasoconstrictor neuron pools supplying the functionally differentiated vascular beds exhibit somewhat different levels of excitability and hence different "thresholds" to excitatory influences. The fairly late involvement of the renal vasoconstrictor fibres in asphyxia, for example, seems to support this view. Such a simple difference of a mere quantitative nature, however, creates a potentiality of differentiated activation patterns, while at the same time it also implies that mass activation may occur, in which summation of *per se*

5*

subliminal excitatory influences can bring about an intense activation of "high-threshold" neuron pools, as illustrated by the
nervous effects on the renal vessels. Presumably both local chemical
changes and converging excitatory and inhibitory fibres are able to
affect the different levels of "central excitatory state" of the autonomic neuron pools. It also appears as if the potentiality of differentiated activation patterns is enhanced by differences in the extent
of convergence of the various fibre tracts, which — for example,
from central autonomic structures — establish contact with the
bulbar neuron pools. It has been observed, for instance, that slight
shifts in the electrode position within limbic autonomic structures
can considerably alter the pattern of constrictor fibre discharge to
different vascular regions (LÖFVING 1960, 1961 b; see also FOLKOW
1961).

A most dynamic and easily adjustable type of differentiation
of neurogenic cardiovascular control is thus created simply by
setting different "threshold levels" for the different neuron pools;
this is further accentuated by certain differences in the extent of
fibre convergence. This arrangement has much in common with,
for example, the organisation of central respiratory control or other
somatomotor "centres".

The data presented here regarding the organisation of constrictor fibre discharge in different situations appear to have much
in common with Dr. GREGG's interesting observation of the regional
blood-flow changes in response to bleeding. Our findings concerning
the discharge pattern after elimination of baroreceptor inhibition
and/or chemoreceptor activation are thus in agreement with
Dr. GREGG's finding that bleeding in the conscious dog causes
marked vasoconstriction in the limbs (involving mainly the muscle
vessels), whereas the renal vessels appear to be little affected. Our
findings may also explain why, in other circumstances of hypotension and shock in which, for instance, pain fibres have been
extensively activated by tissue trauma, the renal vessels and also
the cutaneous vessels can be intensely constricted.

Experiments are at present in progress in which a new technique
(MELLANDER 1960) is being utilised in order to explore whether the
constrictor fibres controlling the resistance vessels may possibly be
affected in a different manner from those controlling the capacitance
vessels (essentially identical with the veins). At present only preliminary data are available and the analysis is complex, but it would
appear that in some circumstances certain quantitative differences
exist in this respect (FOLKOW et al. 1960). Regarding the reflex
increase in constrictor fibre activity induced by elimination of the

arterial baroreceptor influence, preliminary experiments suggest that the fibres to the resistance vessels may be somewhat more affected than those to the capacitance vessels of the cat's hind quarters (Fig. 5). In "A" and "B", carotid occlusion has been performed in the vagotomised, atropinised cat; in "B" the pressure rise was compensated so as to unmask the extent of the regional neurogenic shifts in blood flow and tissue volume (blood volume).

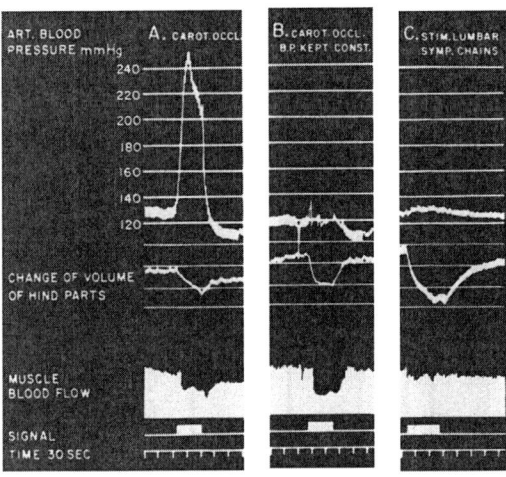

Fig. 5. Cat, 3.2 kg. Chloralose. The vagal nerves are cut and the animal is atropinised. A. Carotid occlusion. B. Carotid occlusion while blood pressure to the hind quarters is kept constant. C. Direct, low-frequency stimulation of the abdominal sympathetic trunks. Note especially the relationship between volume change and flow decrease in B and C. — The ordinates in the blood-flow recording are directly proportional to the rate of flow

Here, it is seen that the reflex decrease in blood flow was fairly marked, whereas the reflex decrease in volume was small. When, on the other hand, all the constrictor fibres supplying the hind quarters were directly stimulated at low frequency, the increase in volume was considerable, whereas the flow decrease was small. Though we are still reluctant to draw any conclusions from these data, they might be taken as suggesting that the constrictor fibres supplying the venous side participate to a somewhat lesser degree in the reflex sympathetic activation which is induced from proprioceptors situated on the arterial side of the circulation. These studies (JOHANSSON and MELLANDER 1961) will be further extended, and Fig. 5 is shown here merely to indicate that the nervous cardiovascular control may be more complex than has hitherto been assumed.

With respect to the haemodynamics of shock it is also important to know to what extent the constrictor fibres to the various
vascular sections are able to *maintain* their excitatory influence
on the vascular smooth muscles during the inevitable local ischaemia they create. The more they reduce the flow, the more the
locally produced "vasodilator metabolites" tend to relax the vessels
again. In our experience the constrictor fibres maintain their influence better on the venous side, whereas their influence on the

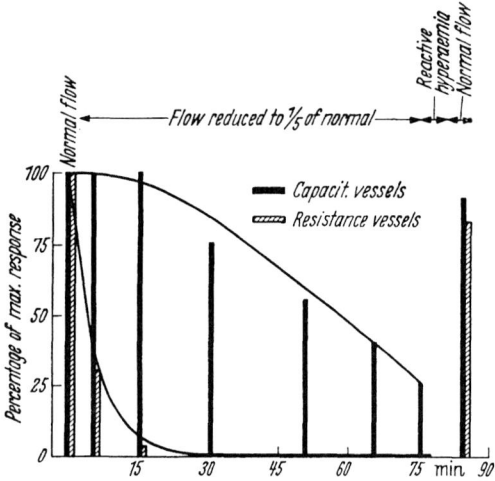

Fig. 6. Diagram illustrating how the constrictor fibre effect on the resistance vessels disappears
far more rapidly than that on the capacitance vessels in tissue exposed to prolonged relative
ischaemia. Note that the normal degree of constrictor fibre influence is restored as soon as the
relative ischaemia is eliminated

resistance vessels is more rapidly overcome by the local dilator
effect associated with the ischaemic state, in which the pre-capillary
sphincter regions in particular appear to be rapidly relaxed after
an initial vasoconstrictor response. These circumstances are illustrated in Fig. 6, showing a diagram based on the average values
obtained in about ten experiments performed by Dr. MELLANDER
with his technique for studying the separate reactions of the resistance and the capacitance vessels (MELLANDER 1960). After initial,
repeated tests to determine the influence of a graded constrictor
fibre activation upon the resistance and the capacitance vessels of
the hind quarters, a prolonged period of relative ischaemia was
produced by partial occlusion of the abdominal aorta. During the
relative ischaemia, the graded constrictor fibre activation was
repeated intermittently and its effect on the resistance to flow and

on the regional blood volume was estimated. It will be seen from the diagram that the constrictor fibre influence on the resistance vessels disappeared far more rapidly than that on the capacitance vessels. To prove that the disappearance of the constrictor fibre effects was not simply due to fibre damage resulting from stimulation, the stimulation was repeated after restitution of the normal blood supply. As is shown in the figure, the constrictor fibre stimulation again induced roughly the same effects as before the period of relative ischaemia.

With regard to the intensified constrictor fibre activity observed in shock, what probably happens is that a competitive balance is established between the released constrictor fibre transmitter and the locally produced dilator agents. The latter influence would appear to be rather more dominant with respect to the resistance vessels than to the capacitance vessels; in other words, central control of the blood depots is more persistent than that of the flow resistance. This means that post-capillary resistance is better maintained than pre-capillary resistance. However, to the neurogenic influence on the resistance vessels may soon be added other factors besides those inherent in the control of the vascular smooth muscles. If cell aggregation and sludging also occur — chiefly on the vascular side, as will be discussed by Dr. GELIN — these intravascular processes may contribute to the post-capillary flow resistance on quite a considerable scale. The net effect may even be that, after a period of constrictor discharge, mean capillary pressure can again increase while pre-capillary resistance decreases and post-capillary resistance remains high. Outward filtration will then start at the capillary level leading to haemoconcentration and to a diminishing blood volume. Thus, the immediate gain, inherent in the neurogenic mobilisation of the venous blood depots, may in some circumstances later result in part of the plasma volume being lost by outward capillary filtration.

Summary

In connection with Dr. GREGG's report concerning the regional blood-flow adjustments observed in conscious dogs following severe bleeding, the vasoconstrictor-fibre adjustments taking place in response to elimination of the baroreceptor influence and to chemoreceptor activation are discussed. Experiments are described which suggest that the various neuron pools controlling the functionally differing vascular beds exhibit somewhat different levels of excitability. This results in a constrictor-fibre discharge pattern so organised that the muscle vessels are strongly constricted, the intestinal vessels moderately so, and the cutaneous and renal vessels slightly or even insignificantly when the baroreceptor influence is eliminated and/or the chemoreceptors activated. The experimental data therefore suggest that the autonomic neuron pool controlling, for example, the renal vessels can be considered to have a higher threshold with regard to excitatory influences than, for instance, that controlling the muscle vessels. If, however, a "high-threshold" autonomic neuron pool is exposed to a very intense excitatory influence or to several concomitant, *per se* sub-threshold excitatory influences, it can be induced to discharge intensely, as is the case with the renal vaso-constrictor fibres under intense asphyxia or pain-fibre stimulation. These quantitative differences in autonomic neuron pool excitability constitute a basis for the establishment of often highly differentiated constrictor-fibre discharge patterns, but also allow for mass activation of the constrictor-fibre supply. Some implications of these findings are briefly discussed.

These studies were supported by grant No. AF 61 (052)-286 from the School of Aviation Medicine, U.S.A., and by grant No. H 5675 from the U. S. Public Health Service.

References

CELANDER, O.: Acta physiol. Scand. **32**, Suppl. **116**, 1 (1954). — CELAN-DER, O. and B. FOLKOW: Acta physiol. Scand. **29**, 241 (1953). — FOLKOW, B.: Acta physiol. Scand. **25**, 49 (1952). — Physiol. Rev. (U. S. A.) **40**, 93 (1961); — Proceedings of the Joint W. H. O.-Czechoslovak Cardiological Society Symposium on the Pathogenesis of Essential Hypertension. 247—255 (State Medical Publishing House, Prague, 1961). — FOLKOW, B. and C. A. HAMBERGER: J. Appl. Physiol. (U. S. A.) **9**, 268 (1956). — FOLKOW, B., B. JOHANSSON, and B. LÖFVING: Med. exper. (Switz.) (1961) (in press). — FOLKOW, B., B. JOHANSSON, S. MELLANDER, and B. ÖBERG: X. Physiol. Congress, Oslo 1960. Acta physiol. Scand. **50**, Suppl. 175, 51 (1960). — FOLKOW, B., B. JOHANSSON, and B. ÖBERG: Acta physiol. Scand. **44**, 146 (1958). — FOLKOW, B., B. JOHANSSON, and B. ÖBERG: Acta physiol. Scand. **47**, 262 (1959). — FOLKOW, B., B. LÖVFING, and S. MELLANDER: Acta physiol. Scand. **37**, 363 (1956). — HEYMANS, C. and E. NEIL: Reflexogenic areas of the cardiovascular system. London: Churchill 1958. — LÖFVING, B.: X. Physiol. Congress, Oslo 1960. Acta physiol. Scand. **50**, Suppl. 175, 98 (1960); — Med. exper. (Switz.) (1961 a) (in press). — Acta physiol. Scand. (1961 b) (in press). — MELLANDER, S.: Acta physiol. Scand. **50**, Suppl. 176, 1 (1960).

Discussion

RUSHMER: Does the fact that coronary flow curves reach peak flow during systole indicate that this flow is traversing arteries which are not being compressed by myocardial contraction (i. e. A-V shunts near the surface of the heart) ?

GREGG: This is a leading question. I do not know what the proper interpretation is of these changes in the coronary phasic flow curves late in the hypotensive period, in which the flow throughout the cardiac cycle rises considerably from the zero level and in which the systolic flow level may equal or exceed that in diastole. Such curves resemble those obtained in the right coronary artery under normal conditions. I do agree that the chances are good that new channels are now coming into dominance but which were not previously functional. Probably a similar mechanism is responsible for the type of response one observes in the presence of simple reactive hyperaemia in which, following release of a very temporary coronary occlusion, the coronary flow in both systole and diastole increases greatly. Experimental documentation of this view, however, is very difficult.

NICKERSON: I was impressed by the last figure shown by Dr. FOLKOW. It seems to me that his observation of the relationship between sympathetic nervous system activity and venous constriction may provide an explanation for many things that have been bothering us in the field of shock. There is considerable evidence that sympathetic overactivity may be very deleterious, reducing the effective circulating blood volume and the perfusion of tissues, and that reduction of this neurogenic vasoconstriction can be beneficial. However, the changes in total peripheral resistance often appear to be inadequate to account for the magnitude of the changes observed. I think we can conclude from the picture presented by Dr. FOLKOW that a major effect of sympathetic activity may be on the venous side, where a minor increase in resistance to the outflow from the microcirculation could alter haemodynamics so that fluid leaves the vascular system and red cells are trapped.

BACQ: As our chairman said in his introduction, questions of technique are important. If we accept the idea that the role of blood flow is primarily to maintain an adequate partial oxygen pressure in the cell, then blood flow, peripheral resistance, and so on are only some of the factors regulating the oxygen pressure in the cells. There are also other factors, e. g. the oxygen consumption of the cell and the possible short-circuits between arteries and veins. It seems to me that good progress could be expected if one could measure constantly, during all these experiments, the oxygen pressure not necessarily within the cells but in the interstitial fluid in contact with the cells; in this way, we should have a measurement that would integrate all the variations of the factors previously mentioned. This has now been done by some radiobiologists, mainly by CATER, PHILLIPS, and SILVER in MITCHELL's laboratory in Cambridge, England. They have succeeded in directly measuring the oxygen pressure in the tissues of unanaesthetised man and in animals. It seems that normally the various tissues of man do not live at the same oxygen pressure; for instance, muscles and skin have a much higher pressure (40—50 mm. Hg), while the bone marrow has a very low one (a few mm. Hg). Bone marrow normally lives practically in anoxia. If these measurements could be made and integrated with all that we have at the present time, it seems to me that many discrepancies of fact might disappear.

GREGG: The suggestion of Dr. BACQ is excellent that exploration would be profitable of tissue oxygen pressure in various regions during the shock state now that adequate methodology is available. The results should aid in resolving some of our confusion. However, when this has been accomplished, investigators will still be as unhappy as before, because it will reveal the presence of more problems, and we will not be much closer to the end of the rainbow of our desire.

FOLKOW: We plan to include also more or less continuous measurements of oxygen and carbon dioxide tension; but so far this has not been possible, because these experiments are very difficult to handle, as they involve three or four simultaneous flow recordings.

KRAMER: I would like to make a few comments on Dr. FOLKOW's experiments with regard to his findings on renal vessels. In our studies of the renal circulation, we were not interested in vasoconstrictive effects but in how to overcome constriction, in hypoxia, for example, or in asphyxia. The increase in pressure receptor activity could promote dilatation of renal vessels which were constricted, due to chemoreceptors, almost to zero in severe anoxia. I should like to ask you whether it would not be better to assume — since we don't know very much about the vasoconstrictor centre— that there may be some kind of an equilibrium between these pressor and depressor inflows and that the result finally appears as activity of the vasoconstrictor centre. Normally there is very little central constrictor influence on the renal vessels. An example of the constriction that might take place under normal conditions is that of orthostatic reactions, but this is the only one I can remember.

FOLKOW: I completely agree with you that it is a highly complex arrangement with different excitatory and inhibitory influences on the different neuron pools of the so-called vasomotor centre. By the expression "vasomotor centre" I mean here those nervous structures which are responsible for the tonic sympathetic discharge and where the most important cardiovascular receptors exert their reflex influences. It is quite possible that not only the bulbar autonomic neurons are affected by influences like carbon dioxide shifts, pain fibre stimulation, etc., but also the *spinal* autonomic neurons; however, this hardly affects the principles of differences in excitability, etc. which are under discussion. I also entirely agree with you that where one has created a situation in which there is an intense constrictor fibre discharge to the renal vessels, this discharge is promptly inhibited by, for instance, a strong activation of baroreceptors; these baroreceptors will in fact react in this way in every vascular region where there are any tonic constrictor fibres to be inhibited. This is also the case when cortical and hypothalamic sympatho-inhibitory structures are activated. All these sympatho-inhibitory effects seem to be relayed via the so-called medullary "depressor point", to judge from LÖFVING's study, which is soon to appear in Acta physiologica Scandinavica. When this area is destroyed, both the effects from the baroreceptors and the inhibitory effects from the hypothalamus and, for example, from the cingulate gyrus are eliminated. However, it cannot be said that the renal constrictor fibres are inactive in the resting animal, only because the baroreceptors keep them steadily inhibited. This was clear, for example, from the figures shown, as complete elimination of the baroreceptor influence on the bulbar vasomotor centre results in hardly any renal vasoconstrictor fibre discharge, except when these autonomic neurons are also exposed to local or reflex excitatory influences. Once there is such an activity, however, baroreceptor activation can certainly inhibit it, provided the activation is strong enough.

STRÖM: Dr. GREGG has shown us that during the hypotensive period of experimental haemorrhagic shock, a systolic peak of coronary blood flow appeared, which even persisted after the end of the hypotensive period. Dr. RUSHMER suggested that one possible explanation was that blood now flowed though channels in the heart which were not open before. An alternative explanation might be that blood instead flowed, during systole, through parts of the myocardium which were now incontractile because of myocardial damage. My question is: do you think this may be a plausible or a possible explanation, and does a similar change in the pattern of coronary circulation appear in other experimental situations in which myocardial damage has been provoked by other means?

GREGG: Yes, I agree that a possible explanation for the exaggerated left coronary flow during the prolonged period of haemorrhagic hypotension would be that regionally myocardial fibres might become "tired" or damaged, and thus intramural flow in the area surrounded by them would not be throttled or impeded during systole, with the result that they might serve in a manner as shunt channels. If such an explanation is correct, then this damage persists for a long time, for during the period of reinfusion, lasting about 30 minutes, this pattern of left coronary flow which simulates the aortic pressure pattern is still further exaggerated and is placed far above the region of zero blood flow. This picture only gradually returns to the control pattern about 30 minutes after completion of reinfusion.

I might say that coronary flow and pattern changes in other situations, such as reactive hyperaemia, might have a similar explanation. The main left coronary artery can be occluded for periods of up to 30 seconds with only a moderate systemic blood-pressure change. Following release of the occlusion, the whole flow curve is greatly elevated for 1—2 minutes, although in this instance the systolic flow does not reach the level attained in diastole. The cause of this phenomenon could be a temporary and widespread reduction in contractile power of the myocardial fibres.

Metabolic aspects of shock

By

L. MIGONE

The study of metabolism in shock involves elements of complexity inherent in the evolution of the syndrome in different successive stages — from initial circulatory disequilibrium between vascular capacity and blood content, to a phase of blood redistribution which varies from one organ to another because of vasoconstrictor reactions which are more intense in the kidneys and liver and less so in the brain and heart, and finally to a period of general decline in vasomotor reactions. The metabolic changes appear to depend not only on tissue anoxia but also on endocrine (pituitary and adrenal) and autonomic nervous (adrenergic) reactions which may appear independently of one another, producing different effects in the various organs according to the stage of shock reached and the aetiological factors involved. These variable conditions may largely explain the discrepancies between results already obtained in the experimental field and particularly in clinical practice, where circulatory disorders are often complicated by toxic and infectious factors of various kinds. For these reasons it is impossible to make a comprehensive and uniform assessment of the many contributions that have been made towards an understanding of this syndrome, since the results reported are difficult to compare with each other and are concerned with isolated phases in particular metabolic sectors, limited to a few organs or to the blood and taken from different animal species under various conditions of environment and nutrition.

Protein metabolism

In protein metabolism, hypercatabolism with loss of nitrogen, potassium, sulphates, phosphates, and uric acid has been observed (CUTHBERTSON). At first the urea in the blood increases, but later it decreases owing to insufficient formation by the anoxic liver (VAN SLYKE et al.). Accordingly, the quantity of amino-acids in the blood increases (ENGEL, RUSSEL et al.) not only because of excessive protein break-down but also because of reduced deamination (ENGEL). The catabolism also results in liberation of polypeptides from tissue protein and of hyaluronates from the mucopolysaccharide fractions (MEYER and RAPPORT) with a consequent increase in capillary permeability (CUTHBERTSON). Synthesis of peptides (ENGEL) and proteins is probably also inhibited, corresponding to a diminution in the plasma albumins, whereas the globulins (α_2 and γ) and fibrinogen may increase.

However, according to the results of experimental research by HIFT and STRAWITZ on advanced haemorrhagic shock in the dog, the hepatic mitochondria may show an increase in the protein content itself and in the functional capacity *in vitro* despite the extreme gravity of the general condition.

Lipid metabolism

As far as lipid metabolism is concerned, in haemorrhagic, tourniquet, or cold shock, hyperlipaemia seems to be frequent, with an increase in neutral fats, lipoproteins, and phospholipids in the blood (SPITZER and SPITZER, MILCH et al., JOHNSON, WADSTRÖM, etc.). In the liver, the accumulation of lipids may be parallel to the fall in glycogen (MASORO and FELTS). According to studies *in vitro* carried out by MASORO on the liver of rats exposed to cold and fasting, there is insufficient oxidation of acetate and fatty acids proportionate to the loss of glycogen and reversible to normal after the addition of glucose. It also appears that the synthesis of fatty acids is depressed owing probably to a deficiency of ATP and TPNH.

Regarding hydro-electrolytic metabolism, particularly marked changes occur in shock as a result of binding the limbs. After the limbs have been unbound there is often a conspicuous loss of water, sodium, and plasma protein in the tissue not directly traumatised, owing to the accumulation of these substances in the injured tissue. According to ROSENTHAL and MILLICAN, in tourniquet shock in rats the fluid accumulating in the injured area is equivalent to 4.6% of the body-weight, about half of this fluid coming from the blood and the rest originating from various extravascular tissues outside the traumatised area. The sodium accumulating in this area corresponds to all the sodium normally circulating in the blood and about 25% of the sodium content in the total extracellular fluid (TABOR and ROSENTHAL). At the same time, an intense liberation of potassium from the injured muscles occurs, together with an accumulation of potassium in the local oedema fluid and in all organs distant from the trauma. According to the data of MILLICAN on tourniquet-shocked mice injected with S_{35}-labelled protein, the accumulation of plasma proteins in the traumatised area may reach twice the normal content; these proteins come from uninjured tissues, which in this way are depleted of protein and lose one-third of their normal protein content. However, we did not find any significant modification of the protein content as measured by phenol group reactions in the liver and kidneys of rabbits under ischaemic shock after unbinding of the limbs.

Carbohydrate metabolism

In the field of carbohydrate metabolism, we have undertaken systematic research into the principal phases of intermediate metabolism, bearing in mind both the metabolites and the related enzymatic activities. This study has necessarily been experimental and was carried out with rabbits maintained under uniform conditions and subjected for 8 hours to tight binding of the hind limbs. The blood, homogenates, and tissue extracts were examined 8 hours after unbinding the limbs, i. e. in the stage of complete shock marked by severe plasmorrhage in the limbs freed from pressure. It is a well-known fact that, owing to the paucity of myoglobin in the muscles of rabbits, no pigmentary myoglobinuric nephrosis is found — which means that shock is not complicated by toxic causes of renal failure. Therefore ischaemic phenomena in the organs (mainly the kidneys and the liver) predominate, although one should not exclude the possibility that other products of muscular change may be released into the blood-stream.

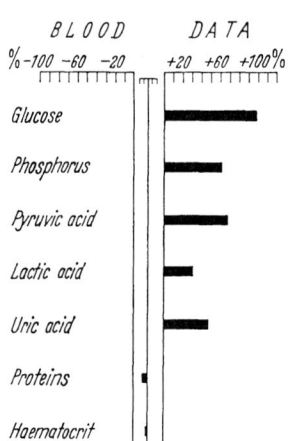

Table 1

Experiments in shocked rabbits examined 8 hours after freeing of the hind limbs, which had been subjected to tight binding for 8 hours previously. The black columns represent values for treated animals, expressed as percentage variations from the mean normal figures recorded prior to binding the limbs in the same group of animals.

The columns corresponding to the upper scale represent significant differences ($P < 0.05$). The inner columns under the smaller scale represent non-significant differences ($P > 0.05$).

Our observations have been concerned with shock in its phase of full development but not in the final stages, so that hyperglycaemia is still pronounced and the glycidic reserves are therefore not exhausted. According to recent studies by STRAWITZ et al.

on haemorrhagic shock in dogs and rats, hyperglycaemia is a physiological reaction to hypovolaemia; the rate of the decline in blood sugar is inversely proportional to the survival time, and only the beginning of hypoglycaemia indicates the transition from the reversible phase towards irreversible shock.

Table 1 shows some data on the state of the *blood* at the end of our experiment after 8 hours from the time at which the limbs were unbound; the values quoted are expressed in mean percentage variations with respect to average figures recorded before binding of the limbs in the same group of animals. There is an evident increase not only in *glycaemia* but also in *lactic acid, pyruvic acid, inorganic phosphorus*, and *uric acid*. Despite the gravity of their general condition, the animals show relative compensation of the plasmorrhage in the limbs freed from pressure, this being probably due to a shifting of fluid from interstitial to endovasal spaces. This is followed by dilution of seroproteinaemia and minimal variations in the haematocrit value.

GLYCOGEN and GLUCOSE METABOLISM

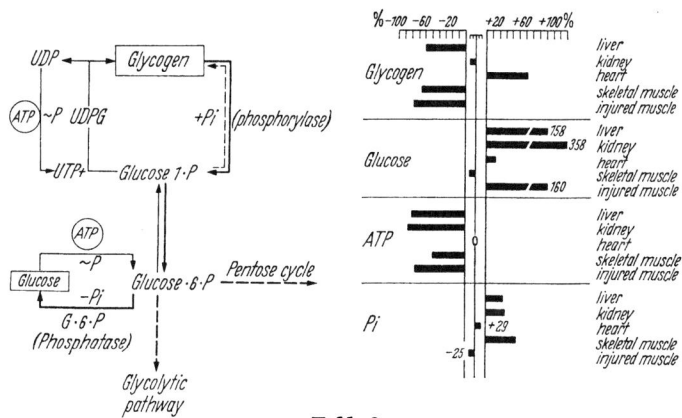

Table 2

In the diagram to the right of the table, as in all following tables (3, 4, 5, 6, 7, 8), the black columns represent mean values from the tissues of shocked animals, expressed as percentages of the mean normal values found in another group of control animals maintained under uniform conditions.

The columns under the upper scale represent significant differences ($P < 0.05$); the inner columns under the smaller scale represent non-significant differences ($P > 0.05$).

Abbreviations:

ATP = Adenosine triphosphate   UDPG = Uridin diphosphoglucose
UDP = Uridin diphosphate   Pi   = Inorganic phosphorus
UTP = Uridin triphosphate   ~ P   = Organic labile phosphorus

Table 2 shows a diagram of the metabolism of *glycogen*. The phase of glycogenolysis in shock, according to our experience and that of many other authors, is intensified. In the liver our data show a 60% loss of glycogen and an enzymatic activation of phosphorylase by 64%. It is to this enzyme that we may ascribe the prevalent influence on the break-down of glycogen *in vivo* involving the consumption of inorganic phosphate and the formation of hexose monophosphate.

We also find that the glycogen content of all the muscles, and especially the injured ones, is lowered, whereas we have observed that in the heart the opposite occurs, i. e. an increase in the glycogen reserves.

The differences in the distribution of glycogen among the various organs seem to be conditioned by the various stages of shock. According to research undertaken by STONER on rats, during the period in which the limbs are bound an increase in glycogen occurs not only in the heart but also in the liver, this being probably due to the synthesis in these organs of glycogen break-down products emanating from the skeletal muscles. But after freeing of the limbs, the glycogen diminishes in the liver but remains at a high level in the myocardium. Adrenaline exerts a determining influence on hyperglycogenolysis by activating the enzyme phosphorylase. In the liver it also (like glucagon) stimulates the formation of a mononucleotide co-factor (adenosine-3-5-cyclic phosphate) of the enzyme itself (RALL et al.). On the other hand, ACTH may promote the accumulation of this co-factor in the adrenals and the consequent stimulation of phosphorylase activity (HAYNES).

However, other different factors of adrenaline may intervene in glycogenolysis. During the later phases of shock, regulation of the glycogen content in the liver and myocardium is not apparently modified by medullectomy (STONER).

The increase in myocardial glycogen may be due to pyruvates and lactates released from the muscular lesions and from blood glucose of hepatic origin. The brain, too, except during the final stages of shock, maintains its capacity to utilise glucose, even showing an increase in hexokinase activity and a normal content of energy-rich phosphate compounds (KOVACH and FONIO). However, while the brain and the heart still retain these functional capacities, most of the other tissues show a general reduction in their utilisation of, and tolerance to, glucose. According to STONER, the muscles and liver can still synthesise glycogen, but cannot hold it, for which reason hyperglycaemia increases.

And now it is interesting to observe that the initial metabolic changes may already appear in some organs in the early or intermediate stages of shock before any marked hypoxia becomes evident; hence, these changes seem to depend on hormonal factors rather than on circulatory disorders. The observations made by STONER and THRELFALL appear to support this hypothesis. These authors noticed a reduction of temperature in the brain and liver before the appearance of ischaemia.

In the kidneys the variations we measured in the content of glycogen and phosphorylase are scarcely significant. Renal hyperglycogenolysis may perhaps develop only in stages of advanced depletion of all glycidic deposits and during hypoglycaemia.

The fall in hepatic glycogen could also be attributed to insufficient availability of ATP, as our data similarly indicate. In fact, it is well known that ATP can supply organic phosphorus for the kinasic formation of uridin triphosphate from uridin diphosphate, and that, in the synthesis of glycogen, enzymatic activity different from that operating in the break-down of glycogen is largely involved. It is a pyrophosphorylase which takes phorphorus not only from glucose-l-phosphate but also from uridin triphosphate in order to produce uridin diphosphoglucose, which, by means of a uridin diphosphoglucose-glycogen transferase gives up glucose to form glycogen. This synthetic route has not so far been examined in shock, but a deficiency of ATP might interfere with it.

I do not intend in this paper to deal with the other enzymatic activities such as amylo-1-6-glucosidase, which completes glycogenolysis hydrolytically, and amylo-1-4-1-6-transglucosidase, which instead promotes synthesis. But it is worth while bearing in mind that, according to KOVACH et al., it is actually in shock that a hydrolytic enzyme of the amylase type takes part in the intensification of glycogenolysis together with phosphorylase in the uninjured muscles and even exclusively in the injured muscles.

Finally it appears from our biochemical determinations on the liver and the kidney that the break-down of glycidic deposits extends as far as *dephosphorylation of glucose-6-phosphate* with activation of the specific enzyme *glucose-6-phosphatase*. In the kidney, an increase in this phosphatase activity can also be revealed by histochemical examination of the convoluted tubules.

Our research has also demonstrated a notable accumulation of free and true *glucose* not only in the blood but also in the traumatised muscles and the renal and hepatic tissue. The myocardium shows only a slight increase in its glucose content, while the uninjured skeletal muscles do not display any detectable variations in this metabolite. It is probable that a change in permeability permits the passage of free glucose in the injured muscles, which already definitely show some fundamental modifications in their exchanges through the cellular membranes.

In addition, the liver and the kidney, which during shock are particularly affected by ischaemia, may accumulate glucose of haematic origin owing to changes in permeability. In fact, the kidney, which shows the highest accumulation of glucose, exhibits neither hyperglycogenolysis nor loss of glycogen comparable to that encountered in the liver.

Now if we study the classical route for glycolysis, which leads from glucose-6-phosphate to the trioses, we find an increase in *glucose-6-phosphate* in the liver but not in the kidney (Table 3). It is probable that in the liver the high content of glycogen and its break-down result in an abundant quantity of metabolites belonging to the whole of the intermediate metabolism of glucides, thus revealing more readily the accumulation of glucose-6-phosphate. Other authors (THRELFALL and STONER) have also found accumulations of glucose-6-phosphate in all the muscles of rats exposed to ischaemic shock. But this finding has not been confirmed in our experience, which relates to a much more advanced stage of shock at a greater length of time following freeing of the limbs. We, in fact, have found depletion of glucose-6-phosphate in all muscles, a finding which may be explained by the general process of dephosphorylation.

We do not think that glycidic catabolism is arrested at the level of glucose-6-phosphate, since there is also an increase in other metabolites of the same glycidic cycle such as *pyruvic acid*, especially in the liver, and *lactic acid* in the kidney. From the relationship between pyruvates and lactates it is not possible to draw any conclusions as to whether the metabolism tends in an aerobic or anaerobic direction. In fact, the accumulation of these trioses could be attributable to the products of muscular break-down or to insufficient utilisation by the liver. However, it is interesting to note that the increase in the trioses involves only that part not phosphorylated, so that the triose-phosphates are normal both in the liver and in the kidney. Reduced phosphorylation of the trioses could explain the inadequate resynthesis to glucose.

Some of our experiments on homogenates, in which we studied *anaerobic glycolysis in vitro* and measured the lactic acid emanating from different metabolites, have revealed a slight glycolytic intensification of glucose-6-phosphate in the liver only, which was certainly not comparable in degree to the serious loss of hepatic glycogen. Individual enzyme activities which we measured in the same pathway appear to be unchanged; this applies to *phosphoglycomutase, isomerase, P-fructokinase, hexokinase,* and *aldolase* (Table 3).

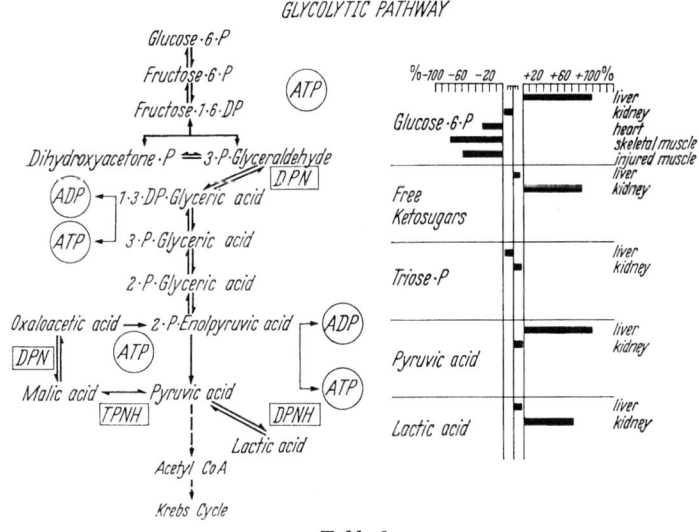

Table 3

See explanations to Table 2; for other details, see text.

To explain the loss of glycidic reserves we must therefore attribute most importance to dephosphorylation.

Similar conclusions may be arrived at by analysing the system of *glycidic interconversion* and *shunt of hexose monophosphate* (Table 4). We find that in the liver and kidney the enzymatic activities of the oxidative shunt are normal, i. e. glucose-6-phosphate dehydrogenase and 6-phosphoglunicodehydrogenase, and that the formation *in vitro* of heptose from glucose-6-phosphate takes place normally. Besides this, in the homogenates of the liver and kidney, the addition of ribose-5-phosphate as an exogenous substrate gives rise — both in shock and in control animals — to equal formation of the various metabolites of the *pentose cycle,* namely ribulose-5-phosphate, xylulose-5-phosphate, sedopeptulose, tetrose, fructose-6-phosphate, and triose-phosphate. We can therefore assume that the enzymes related to these transformations are normally preserved.

On the other hand, we note in the kidney, and even more so in the liver, an accumulation of *ketopentoses* and especially of fractions which are not phosphorylated (Table 4). Again, an accumulation of non-phosphorylated pentoses could be interpreted along lines similar to the arguments that have just been applied to the

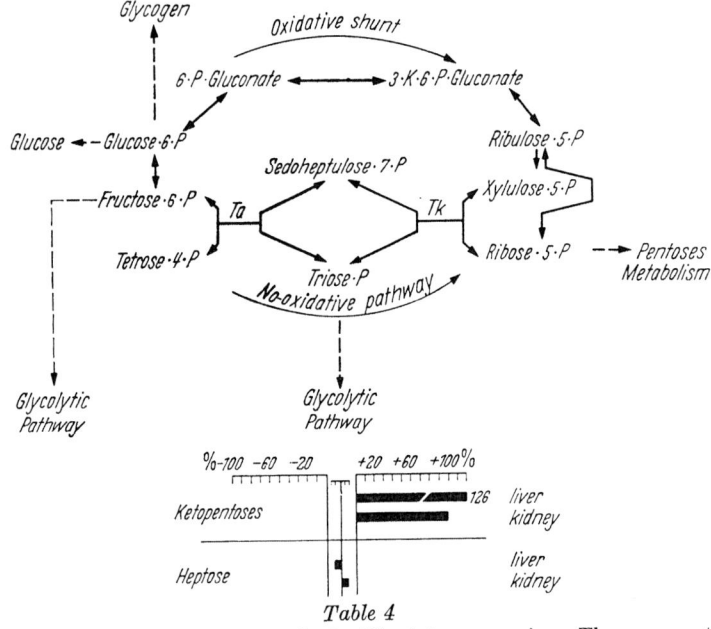

Table 4

Diagram of the system of glycidic interconversion. The enzymatic activities referred to here are:

glucose-6-P dehydrogenase, involved in the oxidation of G-6-P to 6-P-gluconate; 6-phosphogluconic-dehydrogenase, involved in the oxidation of 6-P-gluconate to 3-keto-6-P-gluconate; non-oxidative hepto-formation from glucose-6-P, and the pentose cycle. Among the main transformations occurring in this latter cycle, and the related enzymatic activities, are the following: ribulose → ribose (isomerase); ribulose → xylulose (epimerase); ribose + xylulose → sedoheptulose + triose (transketolase) = Tk; sedoheptulose + triose → tetrose + fructose (transaldolase = Ta).

At the bottom of the figure, the percentage variations of the ketopentoses and heptose are indicated as in the preceding tables

other metabolites freed from phosphoric bonds and so excluded from utilisation. But the possible passage into the circulation of pentoses either free or bound to radical nucleotides emanating from the traumatised muscles should also be borne in mind.

Nucleotides

Following ischaemia of the limbs, some authors have in fact reported an accumulation of plasma pentoses (in rats: MCSHAN et al. 1945, Green et al. 1949) and an increase in the equivalent adenosine of the blood (in rabbits: Billings and Maegraith 1937, Stoner and Gray 1947). In the injured muscles we find a substantial fall in the *nucleotides*, whereas the pentose free from phosphate is almost unchanged (Table 5). It is probable that changes in the permeability of the ischaemic muscles allow the release and passage into the blood-stream of pentoses both before and after their

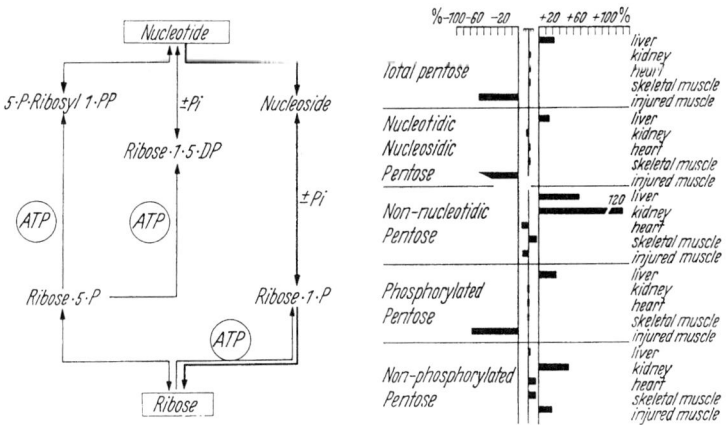

Table 5

See explanations to Table 2.

Note the fall in total, nucleotidic, nucleosidic, and phosphorylated pentose in injured muscles and the accumulation of nucleotidic pentose in the liver and kidney. The latter pentose fraction is "non-phosphorylated", as indicated by our findings on the accumulation of free ketopentose in the same organs.

separation from the bonds of the nucleotides. According to Threlfall and Stoner, the latter leave the injured muscles after transformation into inosinemonophosphate.

The loss of nucleotides also affects ATP, not only in the injured muscles but also in important organs like the liver and kidney, which thus reveal an effect of ischaemia pertaining to the advanced state of shock upon which we have been experimenting (Table 6).

In this way we have been able to confirm the findings of other authors (Lepage, Kovach), in contrast to those of Goramson et al. and of Threlfall and Stoner. According to the latter authors, the fall in ATP and other phosphorated organic compounds, such as phosphocreatine, is limited to the traumatised muscles and appears only during the phase of ischaemia together with the increase in inorganic phosphates. But after revascularisation of the muscles, these latter compounds are also diminished and the values of the entire acidosoluble phosphorus are lowered by a kind of washing of the phosphorate compounds (TRÉMOLIERES and DERACHE). The resynthesis of phosphocreatine and of ATP also appears to be inhibited.

However, the findings of STONER and co-workers concerning the normality of the content of labile organic phosphorus referable to the ATP in non-traumatised tissue are based on experiments in which both the ischaemia and the subsequent period were of short duration. Only in the most advanced stages, when circulatory insufficiency becomes apparent in the various organs, is there (as in our cases) a more extensive decrease in energy-rich phosphorus reserves. These facts have also been noted in the researches of KOVACH and FONIO on the brain of the dog in the most advanced stages of haemorrhagic or ischaemic shock. According to these authors, an increase in inorganic phosphates in the brain occurs again before the fall in the ATP, with lowering of acidosoluble organic phosphorus from a different source.

Phosphorus fractions

According to our observations on the liver and the kidney, the fall in ATP (measured by specific enzymatic methods) appears, on the other hand, to be connected with an increase in inorganic phosphorus in the blood and in the same organs, and is not always revealed by fractionated measurements of organic phosphorus according to the time of hydrolysis. Such measurements do not permit precise evaluations, because of the interference of other compounds of labile organic phosphorus derived from its initial break-down or at any rate different from ATP and probably less sensitive to metabolic lesions at the stage we have examined (Table 6). In the injured muscles, where the lesions directly due to the trauma and to the general effects of shock are concentrated, both ATP and labile phosphorus of 10' are reduced.

On the other hand, the fractions we determined of phosphorus bound to lipids, proteins, nucleic acids, and ribonucleic compounds show no modification, at least in the liver and kidney (Table 7).

These latter data, integrated with the finding of a normal content of glycolipids and glycoprotein in some carbohydrates (hexoses and heptoses) and of a normal content of protein and ribonucleic acid, show us that shock — while still determining the important alterations in glycidic and phosphorus metabolism which we have noted — can still leave the proteic cellular structure unchanged.

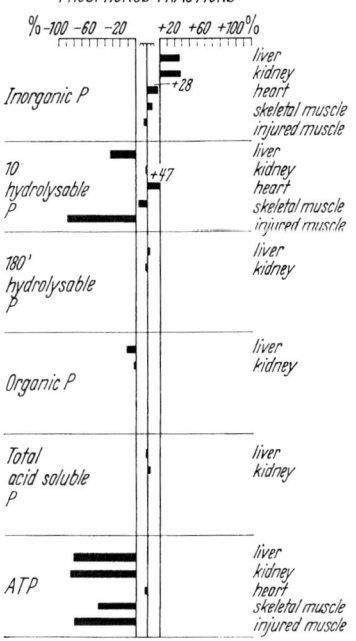

Table 6
See explanations to Table 2.
Note the fall in ATP in the liver, kidney, and muscles (especially the injured muscles) and the greater decrease in labile phosphorus of 10′ seen in the injured muscles. Significant increase in inorganic phosphorus is limited to the liver and kidney.

Table 7
See explanations to Table 2.
The lack of significant variations in phosphorus bound to lipids, proteins and nucleic acid, in the carbohydrate content of lipids and proteins, and in ribonucleic acid (RNA), and the normal protein content in the main organs indicate preservation of proteic cellular structure under our experimental conditions.

Pyridine co-enzymes

It has already been observed that total measurement of the nucleotides shows lowered values only in the traumatised muscles; but detailed examination of the *pyridine co-enzymes* reveals a lowering of their concentration which is particularly distinct in the injured muscles but which is also evident, though to a lesser extent, in other tissues examined (Table 8). In particular, diphosphopyridine nucleotide showed a fall in values in the kidney, in the heart, and in the traumatised muscles. A prevalent diminution in the oxidised fraction (as revealed by an increasing DPNH/DPN ratio) appears in the liver and in all the muscles. It is now well known that DPN, in the various tissue preparations usually obtained, appears in greater quantities in oxidised form owing to the continuous effect of the respiratory enzymes. And, on the other hand, the oxidised form of DPN may act in important stages of glycidic metabolism, namely: in the dehydrogenation of triose-phosphate with formation of phosphoglyceric acid, in the dehydrogenation of lactic acid with formation of pyruvic acid, and in the KREBS cycle via the oxidative chain with dehydrogenation of isocitric, alphaketoglutaric and malic acid.

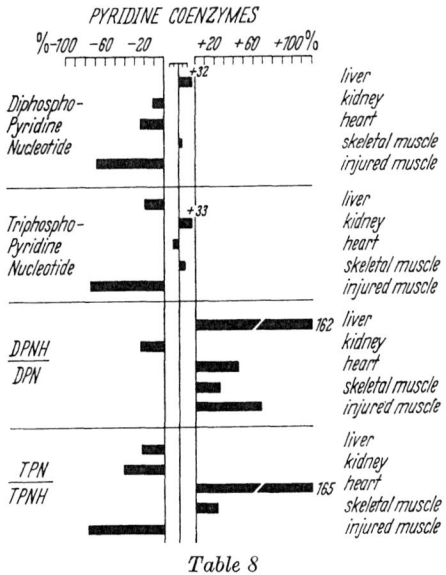

PYRIDINE COENZYMES

Table 8

See explanations to the diagram accompanying Table 2.

For an interpretation of the main variations in the pyridine co-enzymes, see text.

A decrease in triose-phosphate dehydrogenase depending on DPN might account for the accumulation of particular metabolites, as postulated by STONER for fructose-diphosphate, according to KREBS and KORNBERG.

Turning now to the behaviour of the total triphosphopyridine nucleotide, one observes that it decreases in the liver and in the traumatised muscle (Table 8). In the myocardium and in the nontraumatised muscle (as revealed by the increasing TPN/TPNH ratio) it is the reduced form which is mainly diminished, i. e. that form which is always prevalent in all normal cells owing to the special importance of this co-enzyme in the functions of biosynthesis (carboxylation and reduction from pyruvic to malic acid, and from ketoglutaric to isocitric acid). In the other organs, by contrast, such as the liver, the kidney, and the injured muscle, the diminution affects chiefly the oxidised form, whose importance in the dehydrogenating processes of the oxidative shunt and KREBS cycle (from isocitric acid to oxalsuccinic acid) is well known. However, our limited physiological knowledge makes quantitative evaluations of these data rather uncertain.

Oxygen consumption

A more direct study of metabolism, involving measurement of the *consumption of oxygen* in the Warburg apparatus, has yielded normal values with respect to the homogenates of various organs, using pyruvate, glutamate, and fumarate as substrates. These *in vitro* findings cannot be applied with certainty to conditions in living organs, but they do at least show that, in separate tissues not directly affected by a trauma, some enzyme structures maintain their respiratory capacity in the presence of the related substrates. Moreover, these normal findings agree with others reported in the literature, provided that the values of consumed oxygen are referred not to the fresh weight of the organ but to the same quantity of glycogen and protein both in the shock and in the control animals. According to HANNON and COOK, it is only in the most advanced stages of depletion of the glycogen reserves, even where anaerobic glycolysis is still normal, that depression of oxygen consumption may occur.

During the ischaemic period and in the first few hours following release of the tourniquet from the limbs, KOVACH and FONIO and CATER et al. found an increase in the oxygen consumption of the brain. There was also a rise in the oxygen tension in the brain, as well as in the liver and uninjured muscle. But as the shock increases in severity the oxygen uptake diminishes until the terminal stages.

With regard to measurements *in vivo*, not carried out by us but reported by other authors, it may be recalled that the transformation of acetate in various metabolites of the KREBS cycle is slowed down in rats under drum-shock, whereas oxidation *in vitro* is normal reckoning from the substrates of the same metabolites of the cycle (malic acid, succinic acid, and citric acid: KOLTURN and GRAY). According to STONER, during the first hour following ischaemia of the limbs, the oxygen consumption of rats *in vivo* is lowered, despite the fact that the oxidation values of the liver mitochondria *in vitro* remain normal under the same experimental conditions (ALDRIDGE).

Some measurements *in vivo*, relating to the liver (MYERS) and the brain (KOVACH and FONIO) in haemorrhagic or ischaemic shock, indicate a decrease in blood flow parallel with an increase in the arteriovenous oxygen difference. But the $a-v$ O_2 difference does not rise to compensate for the decrease in blood flow when the saturation of venous blood is markedly decreased. It is therefore probable that the increased oxygen uptake, together with the slowing of the circulation, causes a reduction in the oxygen tension. Thus the stagnant anoxia has an adverse effect although the oxygen uptake is increased.

In other organs, such as the heart and kidney, the oxygen consumption varies directly with the blood flow, the $a-v$ O_2 difference tends to remain almost constant with a normal venous and capillary O_2 saturation, and O_2 extraction is maintained at relative uniformity, at least in levels of ischaemia equivalent to a quarter of the normal blood flow (DOLE). According to MUNK, LASSEN et al., in several cases of acute anuria in humans the renal oxygen uptake was reduced to about the same basal or resting level as found experimentally *in vivo* and *in vitro* under conditions where sodium reabsorption is arrested. These clinical observations, combined with experimental findings on haemorrhagic shock, have cast some doubt on the importance or the frequency of protracted renal anoxia.

Oxidative phosphorylation

We also carried out research *in vitro* on *oxidative phosphorylation*, using distinct homogenates of kidney, liver, diaphragmatic muscle, and myocardium in saccharose and Versene under conditions arranged so as to maintain the integrity of the mitochondria. In none of the tissues examined did we notice any significant difference in the P/O ratio as between animals under shock and the control animals, either by using a substrate of sodium succinate in the presence of a cytochromic system or by adding flavine-adenine-dinucleotide to this medium of incubation.

This unexpected normality of the *in vitro* findings, despite the reduction in the content of ATP already seen, could lead to the assumption that phosphorylation coupled with oxidation are compromised only *in vivo*, i. e. owing to altered relationships or exchanges between the mitochondria and the cytoplasm structures.

Modification of the structures and relationships of the cytoplasm during preparation of the homogenates might perhaps permit greater activity of the mitochondria *in vitro*; alternatively, and more probably, the addition of co-enzymes *in vitro* might reveal a normal phosphorylating capacity which was unable to manifest itself fully *in vivo* owing to co-enzyme insufficiency. But these explanations are of course merely hypothetical. At all events, it is certain that the fall in ATP does not depend on activation of the ATP-ase enzyme, since the latter does not appear to be hyperactive but if anything depressed (at least in the liver and the kidney) under our experimental conditions.

On the other hand, a decrease in oxidative phosphorylation seems to have been demonstrated *in vitro* in the case of isolated myocardial mitochondria during haemorrhagic shock in the dog (STRAWITZ and HIFT), as well as in isolated mitochondria of the heart and brain during the irreversible stage of haemorrhage, tourniquet, and drum-shock (PACKER et al.), and also in homogenates or isolated mitochondria of the liver of rats exposed to cold and fasting (MASORO and FELTS, HANNON, LIAMIDES and BEYER).

But according to STRAWITZ et al., in irreversible shock in the dog, the liver may still present normal oxidative phosphorylation (from media containing succinate and co-enzyme A) and even respiratory hyperactivity, despite exhaustion of glycogen reserves. The discrepancy between this normality of behaviour *in vitro* and the insufficiency of glycogen synthesis *in vivo* would seem to suggest that some organs, as long as they remain exposed to humoral pathological factors of shock in the living organism, maintain their metabolic changes, but that the latter become reversible when the tissue is removed from these general factors and subjected to *in vitro* conditions which produce normal functioning.

No conclusions regarding oxidative or phosphorylating metabolism can be reached until *in vitro* research has been completed with the various substrates of the KREBS cycle, from which the different findings can be compared with each other in the various phases of shock and in the individual organs.

At present, some metabolic changes of the cytoplasm occurring in the intermediate and advanced stages of shock are already known. In the soluble part of the cytoplasm a break-down of the glycogen reserves takes place owing to hyperglycogenolysis and dephosphorylation of glucose through activation of the specific phosphatase enzyme. In the mitochondria the production of ATP is lowered. Hence, the syntheses are limited, free and inert sugars and inorganic phosphates accumulate, and the various metabolites and co-enzymes are eliminated from their cycles of utilisation.

It is probable that, in addition, changes in the permeability of the membranes between the nuclei, mitochondria, cytoplasm, and interstitial surroundings are influential in producing the effects we have noted. Many points remain obscure as regards the localisation of the metabolic processes occurring during the evolution of shock from the initial to the terminal stages. The furtherance of our knowledge will depend upon a more precise definition of the aetiological and pathogenetic factors involved, upon constant reference to the relevant stage of the vast syndrome of shock, and finally upon progress made in the acquisition of physiological knowledge in the field of biochemistry.

Summary

After a brief survey of the principal discoveries relating to protein, lipid, and hydro-electrolytic metabolism during shock, the present paper deals in particular with experimental research undertaken by the author and his staff on several metabolic and enzymatic activities of tissue during the shock syndrome of the rabbit in the stage following release of the hind limbs from pressure by tight binding. The blood data reveal an increase in lactic, pyruvic, and uric acid, inorganic phosphorus, and hyperglycaemia. The glycogen content is decreased in the liver and skeletal muscles, increased in the myocardium, and unchanged in the kidney. There is a notable increase in the dephosphorylation of glucose-6-phosphate and an activation of the specific enzyme glucose-6-phosphatase. Evidence is presented of a corresponding accumulation of free and true glucose not only in the blood but also in injured muscles and renal and hepatic tissue. The content of many dephosphorylated trioses is increased in various organs, too, while glycolysis *in vitro* does not display intensification comparable to the glycogen loss. Single metabolic steps of glycidic interconversion, oxidative shunt, and the pentose cycle appear to be unchanged. On the other hand, the content of ATP is appreciably reduced, as is also that of pyridinic co-enzymes. Certain measurements of oxidated and reduced fractions of pyridinic co-enzymes are illustrated. However, when the tissue is removed from the humoral factors of the living shocked organism and placed *in vitro* in artificial selected media, respiration and phosphorylation capacities appear to be normal.

The shock syndrome is dependent on circulatory or ischaemic factors as well as on hormonal (i. e. pituitary and adrenal) and autonomic nervous (i. e. adrenergic) factors. The main metabolic disturbances resulting from these factors are the break-down of glycogen and dephosphorylation of glucose in the cytoplasm and lowered production of ATP in the mitochondria. Biosynthesis is hence impaired, and there is an accumulation of free and inert sugars and inorganic phosphates; thus, the various metabolites and co-enzymes are eliminated from their cycles of utilisation.

Acknowledgements

The following members the staff of the Institute of Medical Pathology of the University of Parma (Head: Prof. L. MIGONE) have contributed to the experimental research referred to in this paper: S. AMBROSOLI, G. AZZOLINI, A. BORGHETTI, G. COCCONI, F. DELINDATI, V. FERIOLI, F. FIACCADORI, G. LA GRECA, R. MAIORCA, G. MISSALE, F. PISANO, L. SCARPIONI, L. VITALI-MAZZA. The original publications of these authors are quoted in the papers of L. MIGONE et al. (1957) and L. MIGONE (1960) (see References).

References

1. ALDRIDGE, W. N.: Biochem. J. (U.S.A.) **67**, 423 (1957). — 2. BIL-LINGS, F. T. and B. G. MAEGRAITH: Quart. J. Exper. Physiol. (G.B.) **27**, 249 (1937). — 3. CATER, D. B., A. F. PHILLIPS, and I. A. SILVER: Proc. Roy. Soc., Biol. Sc. (G.B.) **146**, 289 (1957). — 4. CUTHBERTSON, D. P.: In: The Biochemical Response to Injury. A Symposium. 193. Oxford: Blackwell; Paris: Masson. 1960. — 5. DOLE, V. P., K. EMERSON Jr., R. A. PHILLIPS, P. HAMILTON, and D. D. VAN SLYKE: Amer. J. Physiol. **145**, 337 (1945—1946). — 6. ENGEL, F. L.: In: Shock Syndrome. Ann. N. Y. Acad. Sc. (U.S.A.) **55**, 381 (1952). — 7. ENGEL, F. L., M. G. WINTON, and C. N. H. LONG: J. Exper. Med. (U.S.A.) **77**, 397 (1943). — 8. GORANSON, E. S., J. E. HAMILTON, and R. E. HAIST: J. Biol. Chem. (U.S.A.) **174**, 1 (1948). — 9. GREEN, H. N., H. B. STONER, and M. BIELSCHOWSKY: J. Path. Bact. (U.S.A.) **61**, 101 (1949). — 10. HANNON, J. P.: Amer. J. Physiol. **196**, 890 (1959). — 11. HANNON, J. P. and S. F. COOK: Amer. J. Physiol. **180**, 580 (1955). — 12. HAYNES, R. C. Jr.: J. Biol. Chem. (U.S.A.) **233**, 1220 (1958). — 13. HIFT, H. and J. G. STRAWITZ: Amer. J. Physiol. **200**, 264 (1961). — 14. KOLTURN, W. L. and I. GRAY: Amer. J. Physiol. **190**, 183 (1957). — 15. KOVACH, A. G. B., I. BAGDY, R. BALAZS, F. ANTONI, J. GERGELY, J. MENYHART, M. IRANYI, and E. KOVACH: Acta physiol. Acad. sc. Hungaricae **3**, 331 (1952a). — 16. KOVACH, A. G. B. and A. FONYO: In: The Biochemical Response to Injury. A Symposium. 129. Oxford: Blackwell; Paris: Masson. 1960. — 17. KOVACH, A. G. B., L. TAKACS, S. KISS, and J. ANTAL: Acta physiol. Acad. sc. Hungaricae **10**, 291 (1956). — 18. KREBS, H. A.: In: Lectures on the Scientific Bases of Medicine. **5**, 126 (1956). — 19. KREBS, H. A. and H. L. KORNBERG: Erg. Physiol. (G.) **49**, 212 (1957). — 20. JOHNSON, S. R. and L. B. WADSTRÖM: Scand. J. Clin. Laborat. Invest. **8**, 323 (1956). — 21. LASSEN, N. A.: Minerva cardioangiol. (It). **9**, 433 (1961). — 22. LE PAGE, G. A.: Amer. J. Physiol. **146**, 267 (1946). — 23. LIANIDES, S. P. and R. E. BEYER: Amer. J. Physiol. **199**, 836 (1960). — 24. MASORO, E. J.: In: The Biochemical Response to Injury. A Symposium. 175. Oxford: Blackwell; Paris: Masson. 1960. — 25. MASORO, E. J. and J. M. FELTS: J. Biol. Chem. (U.S.A.) **231**, 347 (1958). — 26. MASORO, E. J. and J. M. FELTS: J. Biol. Chem. (U.S.A.) **234**, 198 (1959). — 27. MEYER, K. and M. M. RAPPORT: Advances Enzymol. (U.S.A.) **13**, 199 (1952). — 28. MIGONE, L.: Renal Metabolic Disturbances During Shock. Proceedings of the Ist Int. Cong. of Nephrology. Basle-New York: Karger 1961. — 28a. MILCH, L. J., R. F. REDMOND, and W. CALHOUN: J. Laborat. Clin. Med. (U.S.A.) **43**, 603 (1954). — 29. MIGONE, L., S. AMBROSOLI, G. AZZOLINI, A. BORGHETTI, R. MAIORCA, and L. SCARPIONI: Medicina (Parma) **7**, 141 (1957). — 29a. MILLICAN, R. C.: In: The Biochemical Response to Injury. A Symposium. 269. Oxford: Blackwell; Paris: Masson. 1960. — 30. MUNK, O. et al.: quoted by LASSEN. — 31. MYERS, J. D.: In: Shock and Circulatory Homeostasis. 121. New York: Josiah Macy Jr. Foundation 1955. — 32. PACKER, L., M. MICHAELIS, and W. R. MARTIN: Proc. Soc. Exper. Biol. Med. (U.S.A.) **98**, 164 (1958). — 33. RALL, T. W. and E. W. SUTHERLAND: J. Biol. Chem. (U.S.A.) **232**, 1065 (1958). — 34. RUSSELL, J. A., C. N. H. LONG, and F. L. ENGEL: J. Exper. Med. (U.S.A.) **79**, 1 (1944). — 35. MC SHAN, W. H., V. R. POTTER, A. GOLDMAN, E. G. SHIPLEY, and R. E. MEYER: Amer. J. Physiol. **145**, 93 (1945). — 36. SPITZER, J. J. and J. A. SPITZER: J. Laborat. Clin. Med. (U.S.A.) **46**, 461 (1955). — 37. STONER, H. B.: Brit. J. Exper. Path. **39**, 251 (1958). — 38. STONER, H. B.: Brit. J. Exper. Path. **39**, 635 (1958). — 39. STONER, H. B. and H. N. GREEN: J. Path. Bact. (U.S.A.)

57, 337 (1954). — 40. Stoner, H. B. and C. J. Threlfall: Biochem. J. (U.S.A.) **58**, 115 (1954). — 41. Stoner, H. B. and C. J. Threlfall: In: The Biochemical Response to Injury. A Symposium. 105. Oxford: Blackwell; Paris: Masson. 1960. — 42. Stoner, H. B., C. J. Threlfall, and H. N. Green: Brit. J. Exper. Path. **33**, 131 (1952). — 43. Strawitz, J. G. and H. Hift: Proc. Soc. Exper. Biol. Med. (U.S.A.) **91**, 641 (1956). — 44. Strawitz, J. G., H. Hift, A. Ehrhardt, and D.-W. Cline: Amer. J. Physiol. **200**, 261 (1961). — 45. Tabor, H. and S. M. Rosenthal: Publ. Health Rep. (U.S.A.) **60**, 373 (1945 a). — 46. Tabor, H. and S. M. Rosenthal: Publ. Health. Rep. (U.S.A.) **60**, 401 (1945 b). — 47. Threlfall, C. J. and H. B. Stoner: Quart. J. Exper. Physiol. (G.B.) **39**, 1 (1954). — 48. Threlfall, C. J. and H. B. Stoner: Brit. J. Exper. Path. **38**, 339 (1957). — 49. Trémolieres, J. and R. Derache: In: The Biochemical Response to Injury. A Symposium. 23. Oxford: Blackwell; Paris: Masson. 1960. — 50. Van Slyke, D. D., R. A. Phillips, P. B. Hamilton, R. M. Archibald, V. P. Dole, and K. Emerson Jr.: Transact. Ass. Amer. Physicians **58**, 119 (1944).

Discussion

KRAMER: I shall limit my question to the kidney. It consists of two different structures, cortex and medulla, and they have very different functions. Did you differentiate between these two types of tissue in your investigations?

We believe that cortical tissue does not consume glucose but actually makes it, and since it does not store glycogen, this new glucose must be constantly removed by the blood. If blood flow after tourniquet shock is markedly decreased, but if some gluconeogenesis continues, is it not possible that this could account for your finding a 360% increase in the glucose content of renal tissue?

MIGONE: All our metabolic measurements involving renal tissue were limited to the cortical region. Here, the high increase in true glucose during shock to over 350% of the control values could not be accounted for in terms of hyperglycogenolysis, because the normal content of cortical glycogen was very low and did not show any significant modification in our shocked animals. The increase in renal cortical glucose was actually double that measured in the liver, which, by way of contrast, showed intense hyperglycogenolysis. It might be supposed that the increased renal glucose is of haematic origin, i. e. brought about by an alteration in cellular permeability. But we cannot exclude the possibility that the ischaemia causes a stagnating accumulation of glucose produced in the kidney from other metabolic sources, although quantitative data on this relationship are still lacking at present.

BACQ: The adrenal cortical hormones are known to affect oxidative phosphorilations, and I would like to ask if there is any evidence of their participating in the biochemical disorders you have observed, Dr. MIGONE.

MIGONE: Our normal findings on oxidative phosphorilation obtained *in vitro* do not afford any evidence that hormonal pathological factors are involved. But this biochemical problem does not seem to have been solved yet — nor is it likely to be until research is extended to other substrates and different preparations of mitochondria and possibly to investigations *in vivo* using labelled P^{32}. Regarding other metabolic data, I am particularly interested in the increase in glucose-6-phosphatase found in the liver and kidneys of our shocked animals. Research undertaken by other authors seems to indicate that such enzymatic activity is enhanced by cortisone.

Microscopic observations of the mesenteric circulation in rabbits subjected to reversible and irreversible haemorrhagic shock

By

S. Bellman, P. B. Lambert, and J. Fine

The changes occurring in the peripheral circulation in severe shock have been described by Chambers and Zweifach and their associates in terms of a progressive loss of tone in the peripheral vessels, especially of the splanchnic area, beginning with a reduction in "vasomotion" and eventually terminating in paralysis affecting most intensely the precapillary sphincters and venules. This description is based mainly on microscopic observations *in vivo* of the exteriorised mesentery of dogs and rats subjected to haemorrhagic shock (*1—2*). We report here similar experiments performed on rabbits put into shock by the elevated reservoir technique.

Material and methods

Animals: 25 adult rabbits, male and female, were observed. The standard procedure for inducing shock was used. After heparinisation of the rabbit, a femoral artery was cannulated under local anaesthesia and connected to a mobile reservoir. The animal was allowed to bleed freely into the reservoir, which was adjusted so that the level of the exsanguinated blood corresponded to a hydrostatic pressure of 40 mm. Hg throughout the experiment. The animal remained at this level of pressure until death or transfusion.

Vital microscopy: A specially built unit was used. The laboratory microscope objectives were $\times 10$ and $\times 30$ and the oculars $\times 5$ and $\times 10$. The light source was an Orthophot illumination unit with 300 watt incandescent lamp and a 5 cm. thick heat filter of water with a small amount of copper sulphate. A large movable metal stage carried the whole animal. On this stage was placed a chamber of plexi-glass to be used as a stage under the optical system of the microscope. It was arranged so that it would fit smoothly against the mid-line of the belly of a rabbit lying on its side. By moving the large animal-carrying stage, the microscopic field could be changed without causing traction upon the tissue under study.

The observations were performed upon the mesentery of the small gut, a short loop of which was taken out as gently as possible through a small mid-line incision made under local anaesthesia. This loop was placed in the plexi-glass chamber filled with Ringer-gelatin solution as used by CHAMBERS and ZWEIFACH. The loop was covered with a sheet of clear plastic to prevent evaporation and improve insulation. The immersion fluid was kept at 39° C by an electric heater with a thermo-regulator. Measurements on the surface of the loop of gut showed the temperature to be 38.5 to 39° C. The observation stage was tilted forward by 10°; this made even very short exteriorised loops of small bowel remain on the observation stage by gravity, instead of falling back in the abdominal cavity as they would have done with the stage in a horizontal position.

In each experiment the mesentery was exteriorised and the microcirculation watched during the second hour of a 2-hour exposure to shock or during the fifth hour of a 5-hour exposure to shock at an arterial blood pressure of 40 mm. Hg. At the end of this period of time, the blood still remaining in the reservoir was infused, and the mesenteric microcirculation observed for some time thereafter.

Results

The microscopic observations showed the well-known pattern of the mesenteric microcirculation with a flow that was active and free of stagnation. This was the case for rabbits in shock for 5 hours as well as for 2. There was nothing in the pattern of the microcirculation to distinguish the first group of rabbits in the reversible state from the second group in the irreversible state of shock.

A moderate degree of sludging was observed. As a field of the mesentery was watched for 5 to 10 minutes, occlusion by red-cell aggregates of small vessels, particularly veins, gradually took place. This, however, was quite clearly an artifact caused by the examination technique, since newly exposed parts of the mesentery did not show this. The artifact may have been partly caused by heat from the illumination; but even with very short periods of weak illumination this change was seen to take place in the part of the mesentery that was kept on the observation stage. In normal, i. e. unshocked control rabbits, with the mesentery exteriorised under local anaesthesia, the same change was seen. When it appeared, a new part of the mesentery was selected for examination.

Under the conditions obtained here "vasomotion", i.e. rhythmic narrowing and widening of small vessels, was not seen in normal or shocked rabbits. Opening and closing of capillary sphincters was seen in all animals, but the capillaries appeared to close less frequently in the shocked animals than in normal animals. The rate of blood flow in the vessels of the shocked animals appeared to be normal.

Three animals died on the stage while the mesenteric circulation was being watched. In all three, the blood flow stopped in a second or two without any preceding signs of disturbances in flow. The mesenteric circulation, which appeared to proceed at a normal speed as far as this could be judged by observation through the microscope, contrasted sharply with the poor general condition of the irreversibly shocked animals and with the pale bluish colour of their noses and ears. There was barely perceptible blood flow in the ears, and the cut ear hardly bled.

In some of these animals the femoral artery and vein on the uncannulated side were exposed under local anaesthesia. These were very narrow and the artery did not pulsate. Division of the femoral vein produced only a few drops of blood.

In some instances the vessels were hypersensitive, i. e. moving the loop of gut caused a complete arrest of the microcirculation for one to two minutes, an event which we did not see in normal animals. Cooling the perfusion fluid by three degrees also increased this kind of hypersensitivity.

Crowding of white cells along the walls of the small vessels, which did not occur in normal rabbits, gave the impression of an increased number as compared to normal, but repeated white-cell counts showed no change.

Thus we found an almost normal microcirculation in the mesentery during reversible and irreversible shock, apart from the sticking of white cells, and apart from the sludging which we consider artifactual. Pooling of blood was not observed. We are therefore obliged to conclude that there is marked dissociation between the good flow in the small vessels in the mesentery and the obviously poor flow in the ears and extremities.

References

1. ZWEIFACH, B. W.: In: Methods in Med. Res., The Year Book Publishers, Vol. 1, page 131, 1948. — 2. ZWEIFACH, B. W.: In: Shock and Circulatory Homeostasis. Transactions of the first conference, October, 1951, New York, N. Y.

Discussion

SPINK: I wonder if I can ask a question just for information. My understanding is that the original observations of DELAUNEY and RILEY almost 20 years ago showed a rhythmic alteration of vasoconstriction and dilation in the mesenteric vessels of animals when subjected to endotoxin, and this is also what ALGIRE showed at the National Institute with bacterial polysaccharide. In our experiments using the dog's mesentery under direct observation, the typical rhythmic vasoconstriction and dilation were seen. Why do your results differ from these findings?

BELLMAN: We were looking for this from the beginning and were quite concerned at not seeing it. After trying for a whole year, we were convinced that it did not occur in rabbit mesenteries which were kept at a normal temperature and were subjected to little trauma by the method of investigation. If we lowered the temperature of the immersion fluid, vascular constrictions occurred; in our set-up, these were clearly artefacts.

SPINK: But it may be a different type of shock that you were employing. You induced shock with haemorrhage. We have used endotoxin. May not your observations tend to show that endotoxin is not always involved in the irreversibility of haemorrhagic shock?

FINE: You are right in saying that endotoxin produces both vasoconstriction and vasodilatation. We have observed in the cheek pouch of the hamster vasoconstriction alternating with vasodilatation following the induction of a peritonitis. But the conditions of this experiment and of your experiment in which you inject endotoxin intravenously are not comparable to those of Dr. BELLMAN's experiment. You flood the circulation in a manner that is not at all comparable to what might be going on in haemorrhagic shock or in spontaneous infection. In the latter circumstances, the amount of endotoxin present at any one time in the circulation, and its rate of accumulation, is certainly very much less and the vascular responses, too, might very well be different.

GELIN: I would like especially to stress the difference between haemorrhagic shock and traumatic shock in accordance with the original title of this subject. May I show a couple of slides with data from a contused animal in answer to the query regarding the difference between haemorrhagic shock and traumatic shock? The first figure (Fig. 1) shows variations in the viscosity of blood and plasma at different time intervals after a severe contusion injury. The first curve, marked a and A, represents the viscosity of plasma and whole blood at 37° C and at different rates of shear before contusion. The viscosity was determined in a Brookfield viscosimeter permitting estimation of the viscosity at different rates of shear. Curve B is taken 2 hours after contusion; viscosity is now very elevated, the increase being significant at all rates of shear, but most marked at low shear rates. The haematocrit is also elevated at this time, which may account for part of the increase in viscosity. The viscosity curve 16 hours after the injury is represented by curve C; viscosity has now dropped towards the normal value, while at the same time the haematocrit has dropped to 32. (A lowering of the haematocrit results

7*

in a decreased viscosity of the whole blood. An unchanged viscosity despite a lowered haematocrit must indicate an alteration of the viscous properties of the whole blood.) The viscosity curve 96 hours after contusion, i.e. curve D, shows that the viscosity of the whole blood has decreased as compared to the pre-experimental values. This is due to the very low haematocrit — 24. The viscosity of plasma is slightly increased 2 hours and 16 hours after contusion; 96 hours after contusion, the viscosity of plasma (curve d) is significantly increased at any rate of shear. These changes indicate an altered distribution of the protein molecules in the plasma. The last curve represents distilled water under the same conditions.

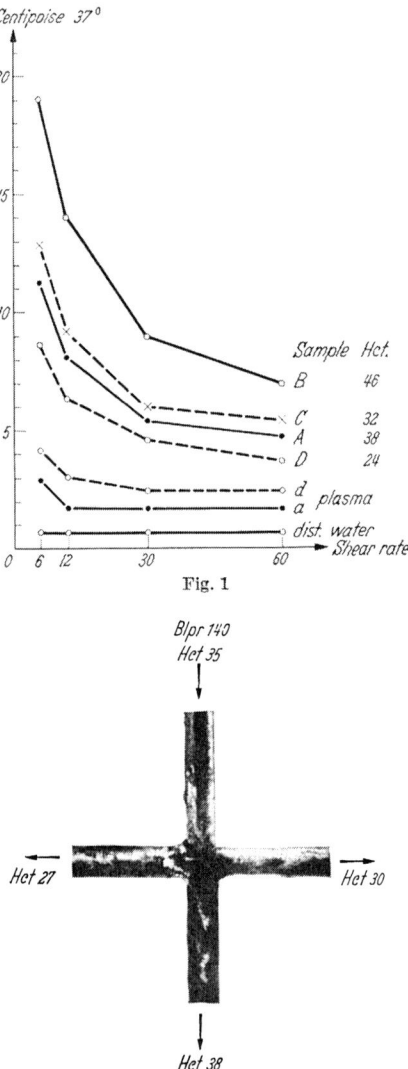

Fig. 1

Sample	Hct.
B	46
C	32
A	38
D	24

Centipoise 37°

Shear rate

Fig. 2

Thus, tissue injury is followed by significant alterations in the rheological properties of blood. These alterations must influence the flow of blood, especially at low flow rates. Determinations of viscosity can, however, only give information on the properties of blood as such, but not, of course, on the behaviour of blood in different parts of the vascular system. To clarify this influence on flow, besides the vascular reactions and vascular tone responses, we have tried to analyse these flow disturbances in a model.

We know from earlier studies that the viscosity of blood streaming through capillary tubes less than 300 μ in diameter is changed by the orientation of the cells towards the axis, resulting in a broader plasma layer at the margin of the tube. In this way, viscosity is decreased by decreasing the haematocrit. This orientation is in turn dependent on the viscous properties of blood, its haematocrit, and its emulsion and suspension stability. These have been clarified in the case of blood streaming through rigid linear tubes; such studies, however, merely imitate arteriolar flow, but not venular flow. Since stasis of cells and occlusion by aggregated cells in the venules are such a dominant finding in the microcirculatory flow pattern of blood after tissue injury, it is essential to study these flow characteristics of blood in models with branching and post-capillary tubes. This is what has been done in the following experiment illustrated in Fig. 2.

When blood with decreased suspension stability is perfused through a branched capillary device, as shown in Fig. 2, orientation of the cells occurs in the central inlet tube. In the cross area, there will be turbulence; there is increased skimming of plasma in the lateral outlets, but no central orientation of the cells in the central outlet tube. The haematocrit in the central *inlet* tube is 35, and the perfusion pressure 140 mm. Hg. The haematocrit in the *lateral* tubes is lower (27, 30), but higher in the *central outlet* tube.

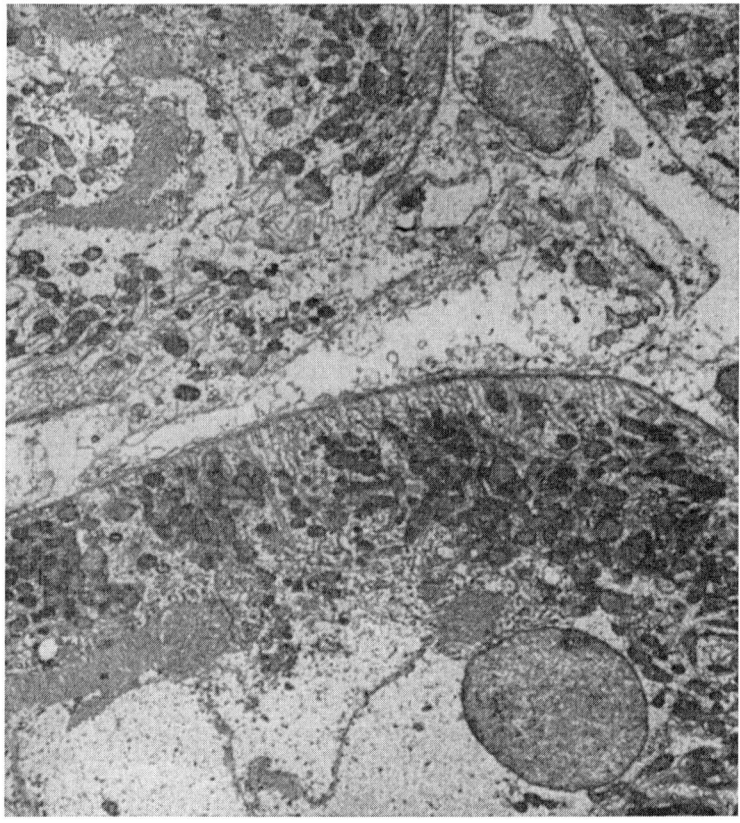

Fig. 1 (see Discussion MIGONE)

The post-capillary flow seen in prolonged tubes from this model shows stasis of cells relative to the plasma which flows ahead of the cells. This separation of plasma flow and cell flow in the presence of decreased suspension stability of blood will also be apparent in some clinical conditions, especially in so-called "red shock", where hypostasis of cells may be demonstrated by very persisting pale pressure marks in the skin.

Thus, this perfusion of blood through narrow branched capillary tubes, and the aggregation of blood cells observed, clearly demonstrate the separa-

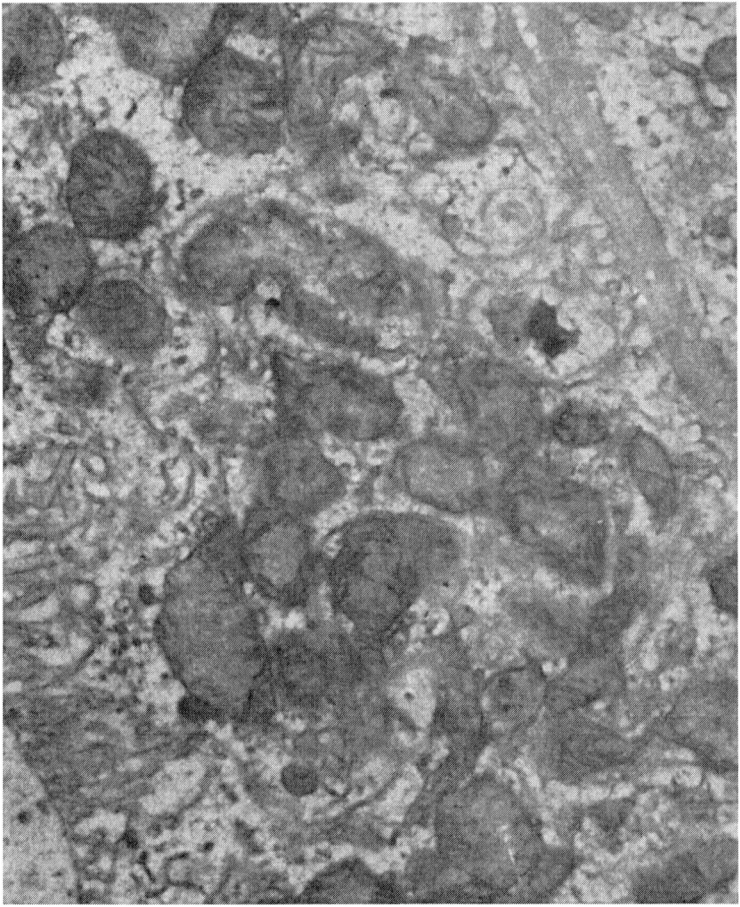

Fig. 2 (see Discussion MIGONE)

tion of plasma flow and cell flow which takes place. This separation may occur independently of the vascular tone and results in skimming of plasma and in post-capillary stasis of red cells. The degree of separation and stasis increases as the suspension stability of the blood decreases; this phenomenon is encountered in traumatic shock but not in acute haemorrhagic shock.

MIGONE: Regarding the biophysical factors involved, I should like to stress the importance of changes in cellular permeability occurring during shock. I have some electron-microscopic pictures showing aspects of the

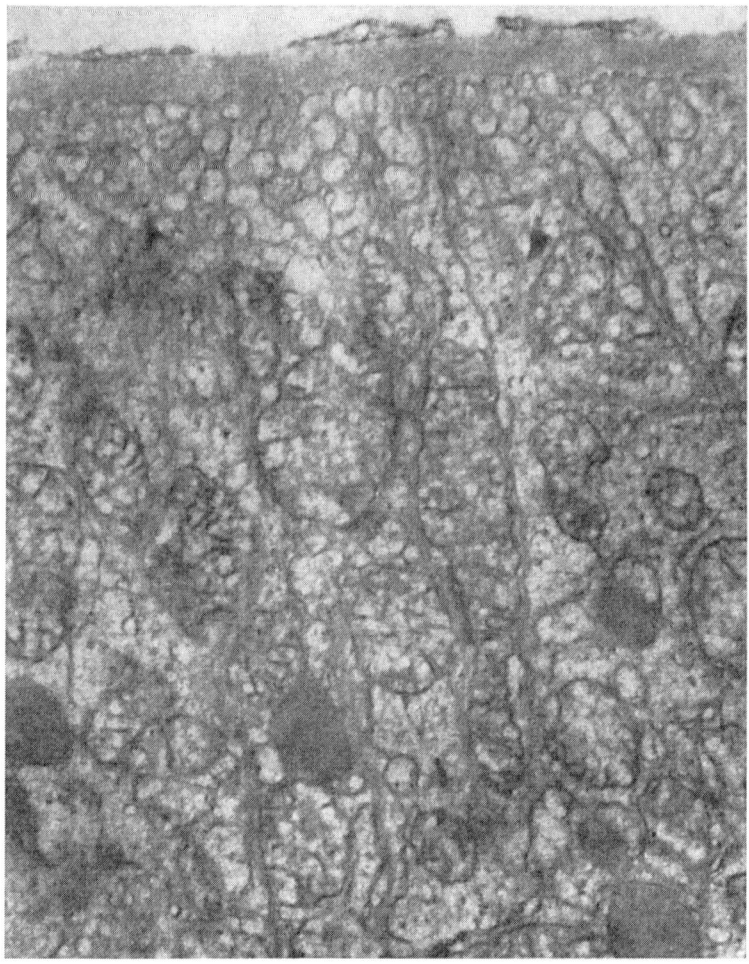

Fig. 3

renal tubular cells, which not only indicate a morphological basis for the enzymatic alterations, but which also suggest probable shifts of co-enzymes and metabolites between nuclei, mitochondria, cytoplasm, and the interstitial surroundings.

Fig. 1 shows a partial section of three proximal tubules of the kidney. In the lower half of the picture, a tubule has been transected obliquely. The mitochondria appear irregular in their distribution, shape, and volume. On the luminal side of the cell, swelling and clearing of the ultrastructures is visible; the hyaloplasma is clear and fibrillar. The brush border is broken and thin in several points.

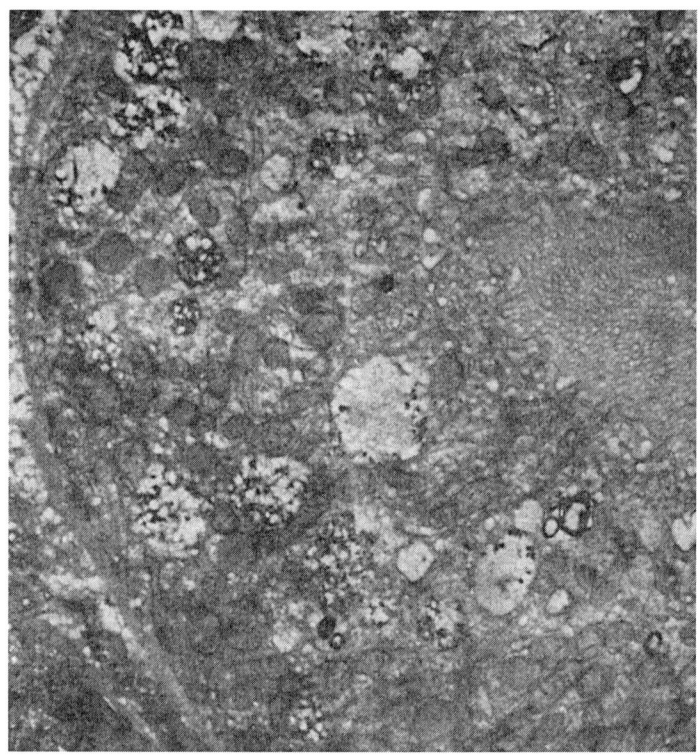

Fig. 4

In the middle, to the left of the photo, there is also a rupture of the basal and cellular membrane, the mitochondria and other cellular materials pouring out into the interstitial spaces ($\times$ 8,000).

Fig. 2 shows alterations in the mitochondria at a higher magnification, i.e. swelling and fragmentation of the cristae and clearing of the ground substance. The β-cytomembranes are indistinct, ruptured, and irregular ($\times$ 30,000).

Fig. 3 shows intense vacuolation and swelling of the mitochondria and of the hyaloplasm ($\times$ 42,500).

In addition to the alterations already described, Fig. 4 shows an increased number of large vacuoles with electron-dense granules ($\times$ 17,000).

IMHOF: With respect to Dr. BELLMAN's paper, I should like to draw your attention to a clinical condition which demonstrates impressively the importance of splanchnic vasomotor control in maintaining a normal blood pressure. Paraplegics with high traumatic lesions of the spinal cord all exhibit postural hypotension to a greater or lesser degree, whereas paraplegics with low lesions do not. The critical level which separates normal from abnormal reaction seems to be around the 5th thoracic vertebra, and this is just the level where the splanchnic nerves originate.

BEIN: To revert to Dr. MIGONE's slides, I wonder whether these changes in the electron-microscopic picture are specific for shock or whether they can be seen in all states of hypoxaemia or anoxia.

MIGONE: I do not think these alterations are specific. They appear very frequently in shock and in other experimental conditions of toxic hypoxia.

GROSS: I should like to ask Dr. BELLMAN if he has done any studies on the response of the microcirculation to various vasoactive drugs during the shock stage.

BELLMAN: No, we have not. It was obvious that there must be a reduction in vascular tonus, but this could not be quantitated with the technique employed and formed no reliable basis for the evaluation of therapeutic measures.

HALPERN: To emphasise once again that we are dealing with different forms of shock, I want to add that we have also studied microcirculation under the microscope in the anaphylactic type of shock (Slides). Here you have the same preparation at 11.05 and at 11.06, i. e. after an interval of only one minute. In this case, you can see that dramatic changes are brought about within a very short space of time. Again it would probably be unwise to generalise about what happens in one type of shock and what can happen in another type of shock.

NICKERSON: Did you make an attempt to reproduce the results of CHAMBERS and ZWEIFACH in the rat ? In our hands, and I think in the hands of several other workers, the rabbit is a peculiar animal. I wonder if the species rather than the experimental conditions may account for the different results.

FINE: May I reply to Dr. NICKERSON, because his remark involves me. The preparation that CHAMBERS and ZWEIFACH used, i. e. the rat's exteriorised appendiceal mesentery, was not intended to depict the state of shock. It was used for assaying sensitivity of the microscopic circulation to topically applied adrenaline. Their model for study of the microscopic circulation of the dog was the mesentery or omentum. We know that the portal circulation of the dog is so different from that of other mammals that this model cannot be relevant for other species.

The nature of irreversible shock:
its relationship to intestinal changes

By

R. C. Lillehei, J. K. Longerbeam, and J. C. Rosenberg

What has been is what shall be,
What has gone on is what shall go on,
And there is nothing new under the sun.
Men may say of something, "Ah, this is new!"
But it existed long ago before our time.
The men of that old time are now forgotten,
As men to come shall be forgotten,
By those who follow them.

Ecclesiastes 1, 9—11

The numerous theories conceived over the years to explain the nature of irreversible shock can perhaps be grouped under one or the other of three major headings. First, that prolonged vasoconstriction accompanying shock causes enough cellular damage alone, due to mechanical limitation of blood flow and attendant ischemia, to result in the irreversible state. MALCOLM 1905 (*1*), BAINBRIDGE and TREVAN 1917 (*2*), ERLANGER and GASSER 1919 (*3*), and CANNON 1923 (*4*) deserve mention as early votaries of this theory, along with FREEMAN 1933 (*5*) who gave it new life. Or secondly, that toxic products and/or bacteria are released from tissues such as liver or muscle during shock, and these products and/or bacteria are responsible for the irreversible state. AUB 1944 (*6*) and SHORR 1945 (*7*) were early proponents of this idea. More recently, FINE 1954 (*8*) has revivified this theory with 15 years of continuous research — which points to bacteria and their products (endotoxins) as being responsible for the development of the irreversible state — anchoring his findings by stating that the irreversible state can be prevented by appropriate antibiotic treatment. Finally, there is the most recent theory that sludged blood [KNISELY 1945 (*9*)], combined with resulting intravascular aggregation, agglutination and thrombosis [HEIMBECKER and BIGELOW 1950 (*10*), McKAY 1956 (*11*), GELIN 1956 (*12*)] is the basic factor responsible for the development of the irreversible state.

Over the past 7 years, the authors have systematically examined much of the evidence for each of these theories in an attempt to establish the basis for the development of the irreversible state. This investigation has developed in the following manner. Initially, a reliable, valid method to induce irreversible hemorrhagic

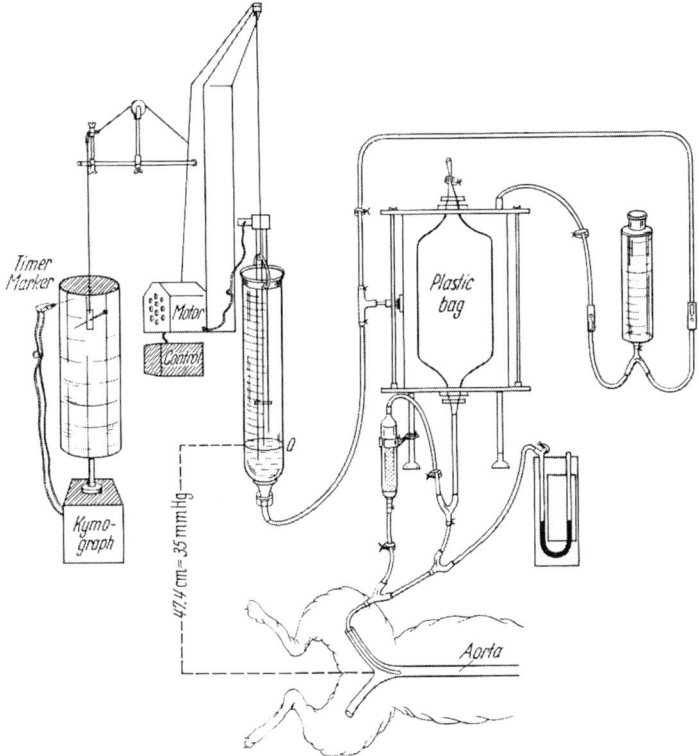

Fig. 1. New electronic device and blood reservoir used in this study to produce irreversible hemorrhagic shock. The dog bleeds into a limp plastic bag enclosed in a water-filled tank. The blood displaces an equal amount of water into the open cylinder. Sensing electrodes connected to an electronic control maintain the water surface in the cylinder at 47.4 cm. (equals 35 mm.Hg) above the aorta of the dog, regardless of the bleed-out or uptake volume, by means of a reversible motor which can raise or lower the cylinder. Changes in bleeding volume are recorded on a moving kymograph by means of a pulley system connected to the cylinder. By adjustment of clamps at the end of the experiment, water can be pumped back into the tank at any desired speed with the syringe. This forces blood back into the dog through the filter. A mercury manometer provides a constant reading of the dog's systemic arterial pressure, or pressures can be continuously recorded with transducers and a Sanborn Polyviso Recorder

shock was established in the dog. Then the pathological changes occurring in the various organ systems as a result of the irreversible state were indexed. Finally, the effect on the irreversible state of altering or preventing such pathological changes was observed, not only in the irreversible state following hemorrhage but also in that due to endotoxins of gram-negative bacteria, to epinephrine, or to occlusion of the superior mesenteric artery. These observations have revealed a unity in the nature of the irreversible state by implicating hemorrhagic necrosis of the intestinal mucosa as the common denominator in the etiology of irreversible shock.

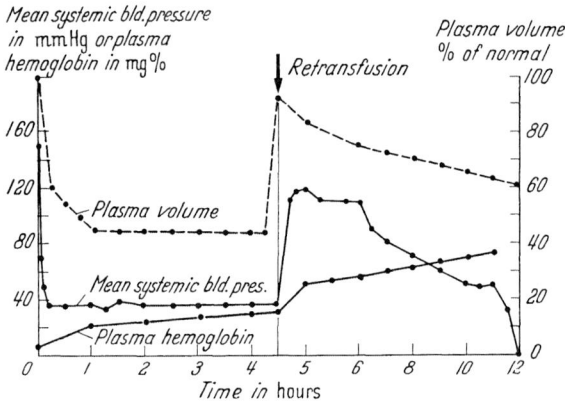

Fig. 2. Typical course of irreversible hemorrhagic shock in the dog. Bleeding begins at time 0

In encompassing such a thesis in a single paper it has not been possible to give credit to all those whose work has formed the basis for the present report; nor has space been available to trace the historical evolution of our knowledge of shock to the present day. On both scores, the authors can perhaps partially repay their debt to those who have preceded them by providing some small aid to those who will surely succeed them in this field.

Establishment of a method

Our initial task was to establish a reliable and valid method for the production of irreversible hemorrhagic shock. With the use of a new electronic device and blood reservoir (Fig. 1), we modified the Lamson-Fine technic to produce a standardized type of irreversible hemorrhagic shock in sedated dogs (13). This apparatus enabled us to overcome many of the vagaries associated with this type of experiment. We found that 4.5 to 5 hours of oligemia at 35 or 40 mm. Hg mean arterial pressure followed by retransfusion resulted in typical irreversible hemorrhagic shock with subsequent death of over 90 per cent of dogs in 12 hours or less (Table 1).

Table 1. *Standardization of irreversible hemorrhagic shock*[1]

Level of hypotension. Mean in mm. Hg	End point for retransfusion	No. dog	Pre-hemorrhage				Maximal bleeding volume (MBV)		Retransfusion		No.[2] survivors	Fatalities. Time to death in hours	Mean plasma loss in % 2 hours following retransfusion
			Body weight kg.	MABP mm. Hg	Blood volume (BV) ml./kg.	Hematocrit %	ml./kg.	% B. V.	% uptake	Time in hours			
30	Cardiorespiratory failure (CRF)	15	19.5 ± 6.8	117 ± 12	92.0 ± 12	52 ± 4	56.9 ± 11	59.3 ± 7.0	31.5 ± 17	3.95 ± 1.5	3	9.50 ± 7.9	22.6 ± 7.3
30	CRF or[3] 40% uptake	10	16.7 ± 1.8	131 ± 19	94.6 ± 13	49 ± 4	58.8 ± 5.2	61.5 ± 6.3	29.0 ± 12	3.47 ± 1.6	1	8.03 ± 6.3	26.2 ± 5.6
35	CRF	10	17.0 ± 5.0	111 ± 9.3	93.0 ± 8.5	49 ± 6	59.0 ± 5.6	57.6 ± 4.7	51.6 ± 28	5.38 ± 1.8	1	5.83 ± 7.4	27.4 ± 15
35	CRF or[3] 40% uptake	16	19.1 ± 3.2	124 ± 12	91.5 ± 9.8	51 ± 4.5	57.7 ± 4.3	57.5 ± 7.2	34.3 ± 10	4.68 ± 1.6	1	7.49 ± 9.3	29.1 ± 10
35	4.5 hours	15	20.0 ± 5.1	133 ± 15	99.0 ± 15	50 ± 5	57.3 ± 5.5	53.5 ± 4.6	25.7 ± 5.9	4.40 ± 0.40	1	6.39 ± 3.9	26.5 ± 13
40	CRF or[3] 40% uptake	10	21.0 ± 3.7	120 ± 12	93.0 ± 9.4	46 ± 6	58.6 ± 4.7	59.0 ± 5.5	35.3 ± 8.0	5.10 ± 2.2	2	8.21 ± 7.2	25.6 ± 9.1

[1] Mean values with standard deviations
[2] Alive 72 hours following an experiment
[3] Dogs were retransfused at whichever end point was first attained

Following retransfusion and prior to death, a characteristic triad of findings, harbingers of the irreversible state, were noted. These were a progressive increase in hematocrit and plasma hemoglobin and a concomitant progressive loss of circulating plasma volume as measured with the T-1824 method (Fig. 2). At autopsy, there were some pathological changes in all the visceral organs, but the striking finding was hemorrhagic necrosis of the intestinal mucosa, most marked in the small intestine. Subsequent studies showed that the hemoconcentration, plasma hemoglobin increase and plasma volume loss were all related to the appearance of hemorrhagic necrosis of the intestinal mucosa (14).

Differential organ perfusion

Having catalogued the pathological findings in individual organs associated with irreversible shock, attempts were begun to prevent such changes from occurring by differential organ perfusion, the method used for such experiments having been described in more detail elsewhere (13). These studies (Table 2) pointed inescapably to the importance of the intestinal damage in the genesis of irreversible shock. When the integrity of the intestinal mucosa was preserved by maintaining its circulation during shock, almost all dogs survived. These dogs did not show the hemoconcentration, plasma hemoglobin increase and plasma volume loss characteristic of irreversible shock, and at sacrifice their intestinal mucosa was normal. Perfusion of other organs, including the liver or a section of the body, did not prevent the harbingers of the irreversible state from appearing and death inevitably occurred, although brain perfusion via the carotid artery during shock did significantly prolong the survival of dogs before they died. It should be noted that the same salutary results of "bowel" perfusion were obtained in chronic Eck fistula dogs, all portal blood being diverted into the inferior vena cava, as in normal dogs. This indicated that indirect liver perfusion by increasing portal flow as a result of superior mesenteric arterial perfusion was not a factor in promoting survival.

The role of bacteria within the intestinal lumen

One's first impression when interpreting the perfusion results was to indict the bacteria within the bowel lumen, which were presumed to escape into the systemic circulation as a result of the destruction of the intestinal mucosal barrier. Yet in our experience bacteremia was not a concomitant of irreversible shock. Moreover, pre-treatment of dogs with oral neomycin, sulfasuxidine and

Table 2. Results in perfusion studies[1, 2]

Group	Type of perfusion	No. dogs	No.[3] survivors	Maximal bleeding volume ml./kg.	% Blood volume	Start in hours after hemorrhage	Flow ml./kg./min	Hours in shock	Blood volume change immediately after retransfusion in %	Mean plasma loss 2 hours after retransfusion in %	Hours to death after retransfusion
1	Superior mesenteric arterial	30	27	60.0 ±9.4	58.6 ±7.6	1.48 ±0.38	8.84 ±2.2	4.90 ±0.23	6.21 ±4.2	18.6 ±10.7	
2	Superior mesenteric-arterial-Eck fistula	10	9	50.9 ±3.9	51.5 ±3.9	1.01 ±0.28	9.52 ±2.3	5.0 ±0.2	7.33 ±6.3	9.79 ±3.2	6.39 ±3.9
3	None—Normal dogs	15	1	57.3 ±5.5	53.5 ±4.6			4.40 ±.40	7.21 ±3.3	28.8 ±9.1	18.5 ±9.1
4	None—Eck fistula	8	0	56.0 ±8.6	53.0 ±5.3			4.92 ±.06	9.10 ±3.9	22.7 ±6.8	5.86 ±3.1
5	Inferior vena caval	10	2	60.4 ±9.3	56.0 ±4.5	1.30 ±0.07	9.0 ±.92	4.94 ±0.29	6.87 ±4.0	23.1 ±13	17.5 ±6.7
6	Inferior vena caval-Eck fistula	3	0	61.5 ±6.0	56.4 ±2.1	1.33 ±0.30	8.41 ±1.1	4.98 ±0.10	9.53 ±3.1	22.6 ±6.4	7.03 ±6.1
7	Lower abdominal aortic (hind-quarters)	10	2	57.8 ±6.4	57.3 ±5.6	1.32 ±0.19	10.9	4.64 ±0.2	7.60 ±4.6	25.6 ±9.1	12.5 ±6.8
8	Celiac axial	10	4	63.7 ±9.0	57.8 ±7.3	1.37 ±0.23	9.86 ±0.72	4.97 ±0.14	4.98 ±5.1	15.4 ±10	9.64 ±4.5
9	Portal	10	3	43.9 ±14	51.2 ±7.3	1.44 ±0.36	10.9 ±2.2	4.95 ±0.10	8.34 ±3.4	19.3 ±9.5	26.2 ±4.0
10	Carotid	10	2	51.3 ±7.9	53.9 ±8.0	1.25 ±0.19	8.72 ±0.83	4.92 ±0.06	7.81 ±6.9	21.1 ±10	

1 Mean values with standard deviations
2 Hemorrhagic shock at 35 mm. Hg mean arterial blood pressure for all groups
3 Alive 72 hours following experiment

Table 2a. *Plasma hemoglobin in hemorrhagic shock*[1]

Group	Type of perfusion	No. of dogs	No. survivors[2]	Hours to death after retransfusion	No. dogs studied	Plasma hemoglobin in mg.%					
						Pre-hemorrhage	Post-retransfusion (hours)				
							$1/2$	3	7	24	
1	Superior mesenteric	30	27	—	15	5.53 ±3.5	20.5 ±13	16.8 ±5.8	9.0 ±5.3	7.0 ±6.7	
2	Superior mesenteric Eck fistula	10	9	—	2	5.75 ±4.2	17.3 ±13	—	—	5.89 ±5.4	
3	None	15	1	6.39 ±3.9	7	3.43 ±2.4	41.3 ±13	67.2 ±24	74.2 ±40	Dead	
4	None—Eck fistula	8	0	18.5 ±9.1	6	Normal[3]	18.7 ±8.7	35.8 ±11	61.9 ±14	Dead	
5	Inferior vena caval	10	2	5.86 ±3.1	1	Normal[3]	17.5	43	Dead	—	
6	Inferior vena caval Eck fistula	3	0	17.5 ±6.7	3	1.66 ±1.7	17.7 ±10	33.3 ±10	44.3 ±28	Dead	
7	Lower aortic (hind-quarter)	10	2	7.03 ±6.1	5	5.10 ±3.7	20.8 ±15	34.7 ±13	Dead	—	
8	Celiac	10	4	12.5 ±6.8	5	4.38 ±3.4	20.7 ±2.7	25.1 ±11	42.0 ±6.5	Dead	
9	Portal	10	3	9.64 ±4.5	8	Normal[3]	23.2 ±9.5	27.6 ±15	35.5 ±12	Dead	
10	Carotid	10	2	26.2 ±4.0	6	2.55 ±1.5	28.5 ±9.1	41.8 ±19	42.5 ±22	59.3 ±22	

[1] Mean values with standard deviations
[2] Survived 72 hours
[3] In some instances the pre-hemorrhagic plasma specimen was noted to be colorless, indicating a normal plasma hemoglobin and the quantitative determination was therefore omitted

streptomycin for several days, so that stool cultures on the day of an experiment were sterile for both aerobic and anaerobic organisms, did not influence the results of hemorrhagic shock experiments in our hands (Table 3). The course prior to death and the hemorrhagic necrosis of the intestinal mucosa at autopsy did not differ in these dogs from other dogs not receiving oral antibiotics. Heparin was also administered in large doses, 30 mg./kg. intravenously, and also failed to alter the outcome of these experiments (15). Rather, the importance of the intestine apparently lay in the susceptibility of its arterioles and venules to the profound vasoconstriction occurring during shock, the massive amounts of tissue destruction alone evidently being enough to cause the death of the animals. Such a conclusion is supported by the results of shock experiments in germ-free animals carried out by others (16).

Gram-negative septicemia and shock

In mathematics, things equal to the same things

Table 3. Evaluation of heparin and oral antibiotics in preventing irreversible hemorrhagic shock[1,2]

Group	No. dogs	Pre-hemorrhage Body weight kg.	MABP mm.Hg.	Blood vol. ml./kg.	Hemato-crit %	Maximal bleeding volume (MBV) ml./kg.	% BV	Retransfusion % Uptake	Time in hours	No. survivors	Fatalities Time to death in hours	Mean plasma loss 2 hours following retransfusion in %
Control	16	19.1 ±3.2	124 ±12	99.5 ±9.8	51 ±5	57.7 ±4.3	57.5 ±7.2	34.3 ±10	4.63 ±1.6	1	7.49 ±6.3	27.4 ±15
Heparin 30 mg./kg. i.v.	10	17.9 ±2.3	121 ±12	97.3 ±16	48 ±5	55.8 ±9.6	59.3 ±6.3	36.4 ±7.4	4.88 ±0.98	0	4.18 ±2.4	29.1 ±10
Neomycin-sulfasuxidine 7 days prior to shock	10	17.4 ±2.6	130 ±15	94.8 ±12	47 ±7	55.2 ±7.3	58.7 ±5.4	32.9 ±6.9	4.90 ±1.0	0	8.1 ±4.7	28.3 ±7.9

[1] Hemorrhagic shock at 35 mm. Hg mean arterial blood pressure (MABP) with retransfusion at end point of cardiorespiratory failure or 40 per cent uptake of maximal bleeding volume, whichever occurred first

[2] Mean values with standard deviations

8

are equal to each other. Similar reasoning is of aid in studying the genesis of irreversible shock. Gram-negative septicema is probably the most common cause of clinical irreversible shock in the hospital. It is well known that the deleterious effects of these bacteria are due to the endotoxins contained within their cell wall. It is not so well appreciated, however, that these endotoxins either directly or indirectly act upon the arterioles and venules of the viscera to cause the shock which is characteristically seen (17).

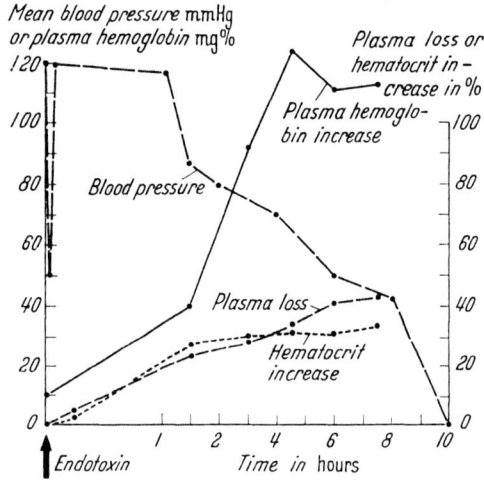

Fig. 3. Typical course of irreversible endotoxin shock in the dog

The clinical counterpart of gram-negative bacteremic shock can be reproduced in the dog by the injection of crude or purified endotoxin taken from any of the gram-negative bacteria, although the endotoxins of *Escherichia coli* are more frequently used in the experimental situation. Such experiments can be standardized on the dog to produce the typical type of endotoxin shock shown in Fig. 3 (18).

Again we found in these experiments on dogs that the bowel proved the most susceptible organ to the vasoactive effects of the endotoxins. Before death the triumvirate, the harbingers of the irreversible state, appeared, i.e. hemoconcentration, plasma hemoglobin increase and plasma volume loss (Table 4). All were also again related to the hemorrhagic necrosis of the intestinal mucosa found at autopsy in these dogs. So, the hypotension resulting from gram-negative endotoxins was not an occult affair (so-called "normovolemic shock") but was due, as in hemorrhagic shock, to an intravascular hypovolemia. What can be done to prevent these intestinal changes from occurring? Merely replacing plasma volume losses is of only temporary benefit, again as in irreversible hemorrhagic shock, because the administered blood or plasma continues to leak from the damaged intestine. A number of

Table 4. *Shock following injection of endotoxin of Escherichia coli*[1]

Group	No. dogs	No. permanent survivors[2]	Duration survival in hours	Hematocrit increase %[3]	Plasma volume loss %[3]	Increase plasma hemoglobin in mg.%[3]
1. Controls	90	6	10.3 ± 5.5	36.1 ± 14	34.8 ± 13	91.0 ± 49
2. Enterectomy	10	1	21.8 ± 5.1			
3. Hypothermia	10	1	10.5 ± 5.6	28.9 ± 10	33.4 ± 9.4	82.6 ± 16
4. Exchange transfusion . . .	5	0	13.0 ± 4.2			
5. Levophed (norepinephrine) .	10	0	10.2 ± 5.2	29.7 ± 12	34.7 ± 14	144 ± 58
6. Aramine (metaraminol) . .	10	0	5.10 ± 2.8	31.5 ± 9.1	40.4 ± 8.5	193 ± 83
7. Sublethal endotoxin and Aramine .	5	0	15.8 ± 6.1	27.0 ± 7.7	34.9 ± 13.1	113 ± 34
8. Chlorpromazine 25—50 mg./kg.	10	6		12.1 ± 5.0	10.3 ± 6.1	28.0 ± 4.0
9. Dibenzyline	10	9		6.70 ± 3.8	6.72 ± 8.2	28.2 ± 15
10. Hydrocortisone	10	9		7.91 ± 3.5	4.06 ± 3.7	33.2 ± 13

[1] Mean values with standard deviations
[2] Survived 72 hours or more
[3] Maximums measured in first 8 hours

procedures and technics have been used in an attempt to ameliorate or to prevent the intestinal damage caused by endotoxins from occurring in order to observe the effects of such procedures on the irreversible state.

Enterectomy, hypothermia, exchange transfusion

Two facts prevented us from differentially perfusing separate organs *in vivo* as was the case in the hemorrhagic shock experiments. First, the extremely high resistances encountered in endotoxin shock, higher even than those found in hemorrhagic shock, and second, the bleeding diathesis resulting from endotoxin administration which precluded the dissection required for the perfusion type of experiment. Nevertheless, merely excising the entire intestine did increase survival of dogs given lethal doses of endotoxins, although obviously prolonged survival could not be obtained with such an animal (Table 4). Dextran infusion (high molecular weight), hypothermia or exchange transfusion had no advantage over doing nothing. All such dogs died in the usual period of time and had hemorrhagic necrosis of the intestinal mucosa at autopsy (Table 4).

Drug treatment of endotoxin shock

In this phase of the study we compared the effects of drugs [chlorpromazine and phenoxybenzamine hydrochloride (Dibenzyline)] which would counteract a vasospastic effect of endotoxin with the effect of drugs [norepinephrine (Levophed), metaraminol (Aramine), and hydrocortisone] which currently form the basis for the clinical treatment of shock due to gram-negative bacteria (19). The results of these experiments are seen in Table 4. It is apparent that those drugs which have a vasoconstrictive effect of their own did not influence the outcome of endotoxin shock or in some cases actually intensified the pathological changes seen in the intestine at autopsy besides worsening the ischemic changes in all the other viscera and the brain as well. Indeed, sublethal doses of endotoxin are potentiated by metaraminol, causing death in all dogs in which this combination was used (Table 4).

In contrast are the results with the antiadrenergic agents. Both chlorpromazine and dibenzyline favorably influenced the outcome of these experiments. The more potent of the two agents, Dibenzyline, prevented death in almost all dogs. Moreover, the usual hemoconcentration, plasma hemoglobin increase and plasma volume loss did not occur (Table 4). This could be correlated with a normal intestine on sacrifice of the survivors. Again, there was no difference in the findings in the liver between survivors and fatalities. Both groups showed hepatic congestion at sacrifice or autopsy.

The beneficial effects of hydrocortisone were obtained only with intravenous doses of 15 mg./kg. or larger (Table 4), indicating that the effect was primarily a pharmacological rather than a physiological one. Hydrocortisone in this dosage in some way protected the dogs against the excessive vasoactivity induced by the endotoxin. This theory for its action is strengthened by the ability of hydrocortisone also to protect dogs against lethal doses of epinephrine (19) (see below). The intestines of dogs

pre-treated with hydrocortisone and surviving usually lethal endotoxin shock have appeared normal at sacrifice, and this has correlated closely with the absence of the plasma findings of the impending
irreversible state.

Other drug treatment

In Table 5 are the results of other experiments in which still
other drugs were used to ameliorate or prevent the intestinal
changes resulting from the injection of lethal doses of endotoxins.

Table 5. *Shock following injection of endotoxin of Escherichia coli*[1]

Group	No. dogs	No. sur-vivors[2]	Dur-ation sur-vival in hours	Hemat-ocrit[3] increase %	Plasma loss %	Plasma hemo-globin[3] increase mg.%
1. Antibiotic sterilization of gut .	11	1	12.3 ± 6.0	37.2 ± 19	38.4 ± 9.1	84.7 ± 44
2. Heparin 30 mg./kg. i. v. . . .	10	1	12.1 ± 7.6	28.9 ± 14	35.0 ± 5	66.5 ± 26
3. Phenergan 25 mg./kg. i. m. . .	10	3	7.6 ± 13	24.6 ± 10	33.1 ± 8.6	73.2 ± 2.1
4. Reserpine 0.25—0.50 mg. orally X 7—10 days	10	0	11.9 ± 11	25.4 ± 9.9	32.5 ± 12	45.4 ± 17
5. Iproniazid (Marsilid)	5	0	5.8 ± 3.4	—	—	—

[1] Mean values with standard deviations
[2] Alive 72 hours following an experiment
[3] Maximum values measured in the first 8 hours following administration
of endotoxin

Antibiotics were again used to sterilize the intestinal lumen and,
as in hemorrhagic shock, were without effect. Heparin in large
doses, 30 mg./kg. intravenously, was also used prior to induction of
endotoxin shock, since, again as in hemorrhagic shock, it has been
postulated that the irreversible state results from a "Swartzman-
type" reaction following absorption of endogenous endotoxin from
the gut damaged by the injection of the exogenous endotoxin. A prime
characteristic of such a reaction is that it can be prevented by
pre-treatment of the experimental animal with heparin (*20*). In
our studies (Table 5) heparin did not alter the outcome of the
irreversible state in any way, indicating that widespread small
vessel thrombosis as a result of a "Shwartzman-type" reaction
was apparently not a factor in the etiology of the irreversible
state.

118   R. C. LILLEHEI, J. K. LONGERBEAM, and J. C. ROSENBERG:

Phenergan and reserpine were used in the endotoxin experiments for two reasons. First, both chlorpromazine and dibenzyline have some antagonistic effect toward histamine and serotonin as well as being adrenergic blocking agents (21). Both these latter substances have been suspect as agents which may mediate or be the actual cause of irreversible shock. It is conceivable then that the beneficial results obtained with chlorpromazine and dibenzyline might be due to their antagonism toward histamine and serotonin rather than toward adrenergic substances. Again, however, neither Phenergan nor reserpine influenced the outcome of the endotoxin experiments (Table 5). The ability of reserpine to deplete vessel walls of catecholamines as well as serotonin (22) may leave such vessels still more reactive to circulating vasoactive substances present in endotoxin shock and explain the lack of beneficial effect of this drug. Iproniazid (Marsilid), a drug interfering with the metabolism of catecholamines and serotonin (23), was also found to be without beneficial effect and seemed to accentuate the physiological disturbances caused by endotoxin injection.

Finally, serotonin itself was administered, since determinations in our laboratory indicated that this substance was invariably decreased in shock induced by endotoxin (24). Again, however, this vasoactive substance, similar to the vasopressor agents previously cited, potentiated rather than ameliorated the shock.

The analysis of both irreversible hemorrhagic and endotoxin shock has suggested the importance of excessive vasoactivity in the genesis of irreversible shock. It is but a short step then to compare these forms of shock with another type of shock which they so closely resemble in many respects — shock due to the intravenous injection of epinephrine.

Epinephrine shock

The physiological disturbances caused by epinephrine are strikingly similar to those already seen in hemorrhagic or endo-

Table 6. *Epinephrine shock* (16—17 μg./kg./min. × 120 min.)[1]

Group	No. dogs	No. survivors	Duration survival in hours	Hematocrit increase %	Plasma loss %	Plasma hemoglobin increase mg.%
Controls	10	1	19.9 ± 16	29.7 ± 9.3	40.4 ± 9.9	161 ± 64
Hydrocortisone	10	8		25.3 ± 12	29.7 ± 11	119 ± 56

[1] Mean values with standard deviations

toxin shock: large plasma deficits and hemorrhagic necrosis of the intestinal mucosa (Fig. 4). The pathological sequence of events leading to death caused by epinephrine can, of course, be blunted or blocked completely by the use of adrenergic blocking agents. Hydrocortisone in pharmacological doses will also provide almost

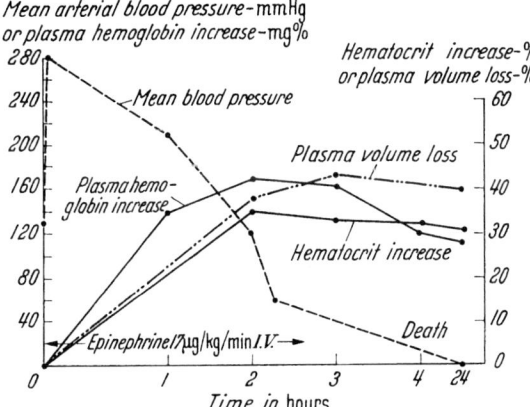

Fig. 4. Typical course of irreversible epinephrine shock in the dog

complete protection against the deleterious effects of the epinephrine (19). This result is provocative and perhaps gives a hint why such large doses are also useful in preventing death from usually lethal doses of endotoxins (Table 6).

Tolerance to shock

It occurred to us that if profound vasoconstriction is intimately related to the development of intestinal ischemia and subsequently to the occurrence of irreversible shock, whether due to prolonged hemorrhage, endotoxins or epinephrine, then it might be possible to make animals resistant to the deleterious effects of vasoconstriction by gradually building up their tolerance to epinephrine. We did find that dogs could be made tolerant to the usually lethal dose of epinephrine (2 mg./kg. intravenously) if this dose was gradually arrived at over a period of several weeks. And such dogs were then able to survive both usually lethal periods of hemorrhagic shock and usually lethal injections of endotoxins. The same interrelationships were found when dogs were gradually made tolerant to lethal doses of endotoxins over a period of weeks and then subjected to usually lethal hemorrhagic shock or injections of epinephrine (Table 7).

Table 7. *Interrelationship between shock due to epinephrine, endotoxin and hemorrhage*

Group	No. dogs	No. survivors[1]
Hemorrhagic shock "controls"	41	2
Hemorrhagic shock in endotoxin tolerant dogs . . .	10	9
Hemorrhagic shock in epinephrine tolerant dogs . .	10	8
Endotoxin shock "controls"	90	6
Endotoxin shock in epinephrine tolerant dogs . . .	10	7
Epinephrine shock "controls"	10	1
Epinephrine shock in endotoxin tolerant dogs . . .	10	9

[1] Survived 72 hours or more.

Electromagnetic measurements of blood flow

The observation that procedures or drugs which preserve the integrity of the bowel during shock also usually prevent the onset

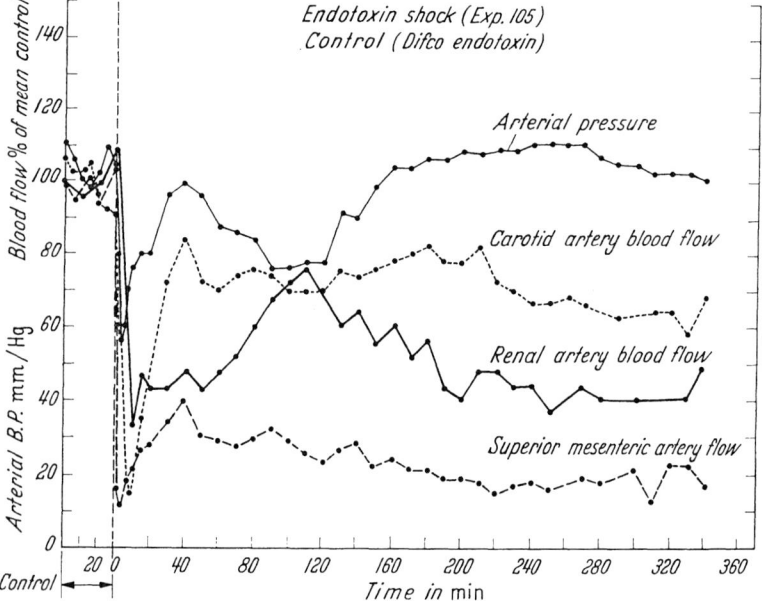

Fig. 5. Measurements of blood flow to various organs made with the Electromagnetic Flow Meter during endotoxin shock

of the irreversible state spurred our desire to make quantitative measurements of blood flow to the bowel as well as to other organs during various types of shock. By means of the electromagnetic flow meter, it has been possible to obtain such flows without cannulation of the vessels and with little disturbance to the dog (25). These studies have shown us that the blood flow to the bowel via the superior mesenteric artery falls almost to zero within one hour after profound shock has been induced by hemorrhage, endotoxins, or epinephrine. This reduction in flow through the superior mesenteric artery is of a greater magnitude than the reduction in cardiac output or the reduction in arterial flow to other organ systems measured (Fig. 5). This minute blood flow to the bowel during shock, usually averaging less than 1 ml./kg./min. (normal, 10—12 ml./kg./min.) is almost exactly the same as the collateral blood flow through the bowel after experimental occlusion of the superior mesenteric artery of the dog.

In general, those drugs which have been shown to increase the number of survivors from the various types of shock have also increased the amount of blood flowing to the bowel. Perhaps the most important finding is that those vasopressor substances (e. g. metaraminol, norepinephrine) which are commonly used to raise systemic blood pressure in clinical shock result in even further lowerings of blood flow to the bowel as well as to other visceral organs even though the systemic arterial pressure is raised to normal levels (Fig. 6).

Shock due to occlusion of the superior mesenteric artery

The similarities in the dog between the findings in superior mesenteric arterial occlusion, irreversible hemorrhagic shock, irreversible gram-negative endotoxic shock, and epinephrine shock are many. In all these conditions the characteristic findings in the irreversible state are an increasing hematocrit, a progressive plasma loss and a rising plasma hemoglobin. In all, we have found that intestinal antibiotics per se will not prevent the development of the irreversible state. Again in all, although plasma volume losses are large, mere replacement of such losses is of only temporary benefit and the animals proceed inexorably to death because of the underlying bowel pathology which is responsible for these plasma losses. These bowel findings are intimately related to the development of the irreversible state and are not only responsible for marked fluid losses but also for the rise in plasma hemoglobin which is the harbinger of impending death in these conditions. The elevated plasma hemoglobin, like the plasma volume loss, is not apparently lethal in itself but indicates that the integrity of the intestinal mucosa has been lost and that blood is accumulating within the intestinal lumen. There it is hemolyzed

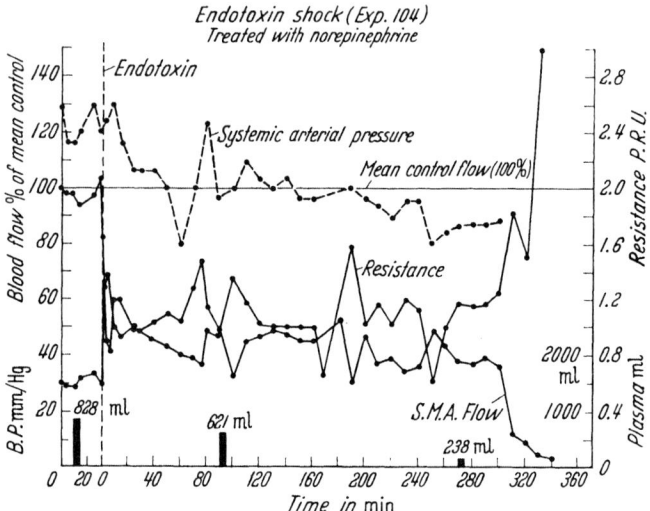

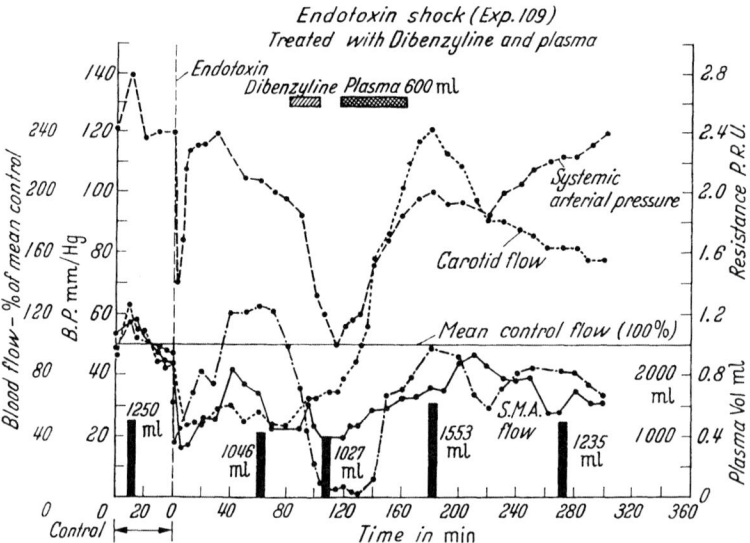

Fig. 6. Measurements of blood flow to the intestine with the Electromagnetic Flow Meter
and adrenergic blocking

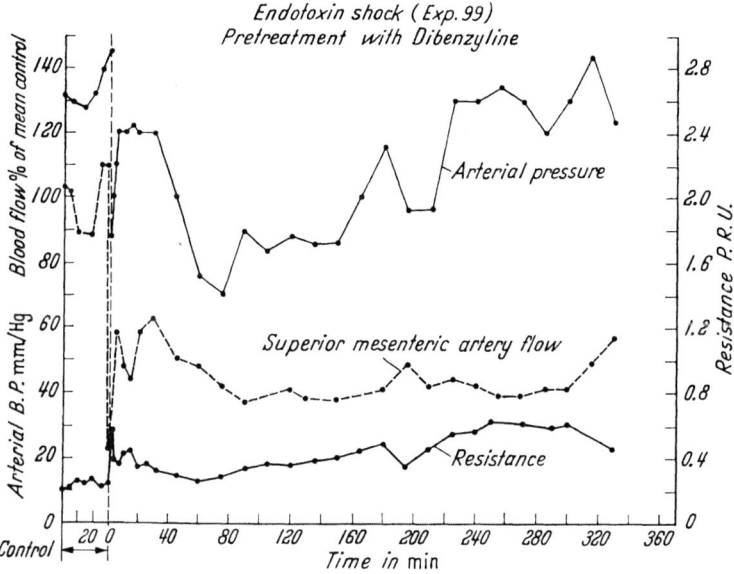

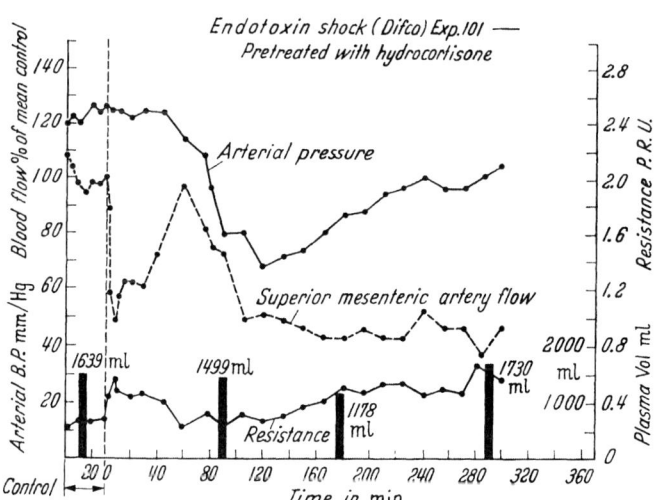

during varying types of shock treated with vasopressors, adrenergic blocking agents, or plasma
agents, and hydrocortisone

and then reabsorbed again into the circulation through the necrotic mucosa, doubtless along with other toxic products resulting from mucosal necrosis (26).

It is interesting that irreversible hemorrhagic shock with its inevitable hemorrhagic bowel necrosis occurs only after 4 to 5 hours of profound oligemic hypotension followed by retransfusion. So, also, the characteristic bowel finding in superior mesenteric arterial occlusion occurs only after four to five hours of occlusion followed by release of the occlusion (Fig. 7, Table 8). If the superior mesenteric occlusion is maintained permanently, however, along with division of collaterals, the characteristic plasma findings do not occur until much later and survival is also prolonged although eventual death occurs. This is because fluid losses are minimized and the break-down products of intestinal necrosis are not washed

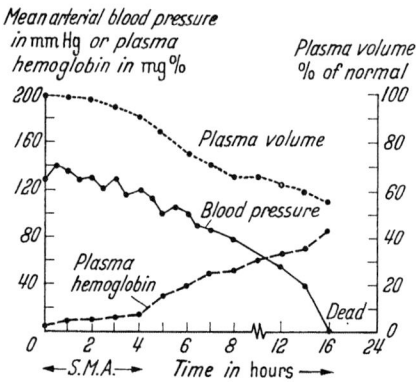

Fig. 7. Typical course of shock following occlusion of the superior mesenteric artery (S.M.A.) in the dog

Table 8. *Superior mesenteric arterial (S.M.A.) occlusion*[1]

No. dogs	Group	Duration of occlusion (hours)	Maximum values within 8 hours following release of occlusion			No. survivors 48 hours or more
			Plasma volume loss (%)	Hematocrit increase (%)	Plasma hemoglobin increase (mg.%)	
10	S.M.A. occlusion	5	44.9 ± 12	30.9 ± 6.9	108 ± 49	1
10	S.M.A. occlusion following 5—7 days pre-treatment with neomycin-sulfasuxidine	5	37.8 ± 11	35.4 ± 7.8	90.7 ± 12	0

[1] Mean values with standard deviations.

directly into the general circulation by release of the occlusion but are denied access to the circulation until they have permeated through the bowel wall and then been reabsorbed from the peritoneal cavity.

Determination of plasma catecholamine and serum serotonin levels

Finally, to put all the results described above on a more quantitative basis, chemical determinations of plasma catecholamines

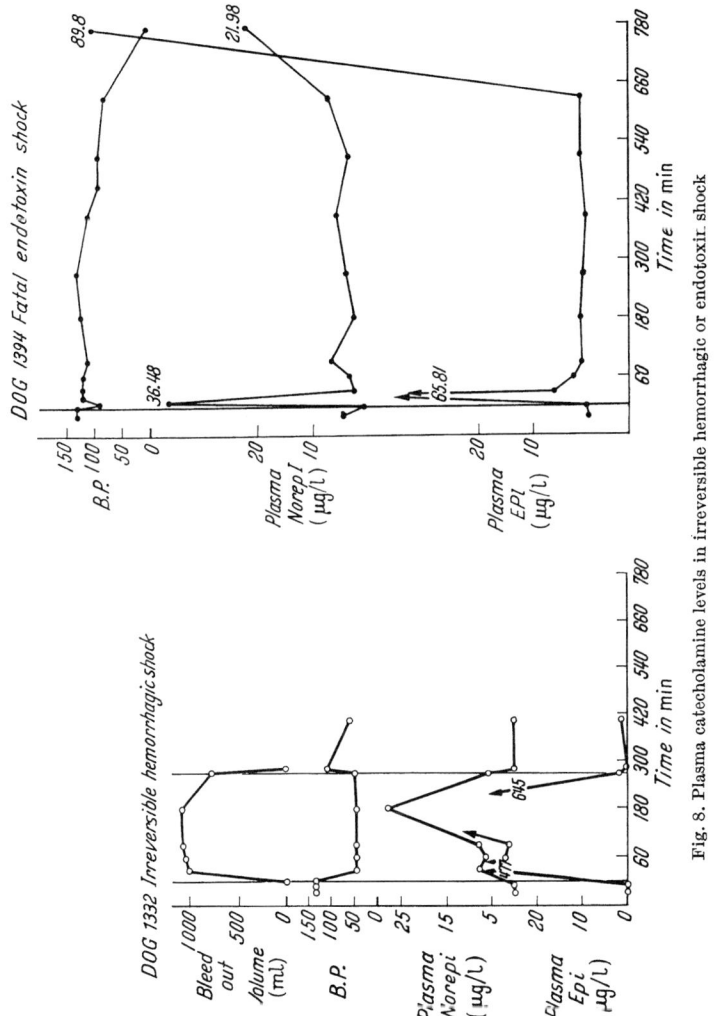

Fig. 8. Plasma catecholamine levels in irreversible hemorrhagic or endotoxic shock

and serum serotonin have been and are being made in dogs subjected to the various procedures outlined above. The work in this field has been dealt with in more detail elsewhere (24, 27), but in summary we have found that, in both prolonged hemorrhagic and endotoxin shock, the catecholamine levels increase from 30 to 100 times or greater, more than sufficient to provide the mechanical limitation of blood flow necessary to cause the visceral changes so characteristic of irreversible shock (Fig. 8). The changes in serotonin have not been so striking, although they are depressed more in irreversible endotoxin shock than in hemorrhagic shock. In our experience, however, restoring this deficit with intravenous injections of exogenous serotonin did not favorably influence endotoxin shock experiments.

The application of experimental concepts to clinical thinking

It is evident from these studies that the vasculature of the bowel of the dog is unusually sensitive to circulating vasoactive substances, whether endogenous or exogenous in origin. The metabolic rate of the bowel, which is greater than that of almost any other tissue, emphasizes the effects of the resulting mechanical limitation of blood flow (28). Moreover, SPANNER 1934 (29) has shown that there are innumerable arteriovenous shunts in the submucosal layer of the bowel of the dog. With a low arterial perfusion pressure and a high resistance in the rich vascular network of the mucosa, almost all blood by-passes the mucosa via these shunts. Similar shunts are found in the human intestine, but in this case they are in the mucosa. Therefore, under the conditions of low perfusion pressure and high resistance occurring in shock in the human, it is the submucosa of the human intestine which is by-passed. This anatomical difference between the dog and human intestine may perhaps account for the fact that the intestinal changes associated with shock in the human are submucosal in location and easily overlooked (30—35) compared with the mucosal lesions in the dog which are readily apparent. The formation of pseudomembrane in the intestine of humans is actually a manifestation of severe shock, corresponding to the intestinal changes in the dog.

While studies in this field are continuing, it appears that enough evidence is available to suggest that one should turn one's thinking back to that early theory which indicated excessive vasoconstriction, with its resulting mechanical limitation of blood flow to vital organs, as the primordial factor in irreversible shock. This concept when applied to clinical thinking and judgment is of urgent concern, for it would mean the virtual elimination of the use of vasopressor agents in the treatment of traumatic or bacterial shock, and the substitution in their place of agents designed to overcome excessive vasoactivity. Indeed, on the surgical services at the University of Minnesota Hospitals, the use of vasopressor agents has been all but eliminated in the treatment of shock. In place of the vasopressors, massive doses of hydrocortisone and plasma (or blood when indicated) have usually restored systemic blood pressure while also restoring vitally needed blood flow to the viscera. Agents such as chlorpromazine and Dibenzyline are also being used in selected patients.

This long overdue disenchantment with the vasopressors can be best expressed in the words of SHAKESPEARE's King Henry IV: "they surfeited with honey and began to loathe the taste of sweetness, whereof a little more than a little is by much too much".

Summary

A standardized method to produce irreversible hemorrhagic shock based upon a modification of the LAMSON-FINE technic has been developed. This method utilizes an electronically controlled leveling device to maintain a constant counterpressure and includes a closed plastic blood reservoir which prevents bacterial contamination and facilitates carrying out the mechanics of the hemorrhagic shock experiments. Using this method, we found that 80 per cent or more of unanesthetized, sedated, adult mongrel dogs, bled to 30, 35, or 40 mm. Hg mean systemic arterial blood pressure, died following the retransfusion of all shed blood when the retransfusion was carried out either at the end-point of 40 per cent uptake of the maximal bleeding volume (acute respiratory failure) or after 4.5 hours of elapsed time from the onset of hemorrhage. Following retransfusion, the period before the death of these dogs was characterized by a progressive fall in the plasma volume and a progressive rise in the hematocrit and plasma hemoglobin. At autopsy, the striking finding was hemorrhagic necrosis of the mucosa of the bowel, most pronounced in the small bowel. Irreversible hemorrhagic shock was not prevented or altered in any way by pre-treating dogs with intravenous heparin or by sterilizing the gut of dogs with intestinal antibiotics prior to the hemorrhage. In contrast, irreversible hemorrhagic shock was prevented in 90 per cent of normal and chronic ECK-fistula dogs by perfusing the superior mesenteric artery at normal pressure and flow with arterial blood from a donor dog during a 5 hour period of hemorrhagic shock at 35 mm. Hg mean pressure. The irreversible state was not prevented by perfusing the liver or lower systemic arterial or venous systems of dogs similarly shocked. Brain perfusion during hemorrhagic shock increased the duration of survival of shocked dogs but did not prevent the irreversible state from ultimately occurring. In the dog, apparently the intestine is the organ most sensitive to the ischemia attendant upon prolonged hemorrhagic shock.

Plasma loss, hematocrit increase, plasma hemoglobin increase, and hemorrhagic necrosis of the bowel, all of which characterize irreversible shock following prolonged hemorrhage, also characterize shock due to the endotoxins of gram-negative bacteria. These findings in endotoxin shock are apparently due to the sympathomimetic action of endotoxin on the vasculature of the bowel, resulting in mechanical limitation of blood flow and subsequent irreversible ischemia of the bowel. Agents which have an adren-

128   R. C. LILLEHEI, J. K. LONGERBEAM, and J. C. ROSENBERG:

ergic blocking effect prevent these deleterious effects of endotoxin and prevent death of the animal, while the vasopressor drugs which are commonly
used to treat this type of shock either are without effect or else, by increasing
visceral ischemia, potentiate the shock caused by endotoxin. Evidence has
also been presented that the cause of the visceral ischemia which characterizes
the response of experimental animals to endotoxin and leads to the irreversible
state is neither a result of bacterial invasion from the damaged gut nor a result
of the release by the tissues of histamine or serotonin. While part of the
sympathomimetic effect of endotoxin may be direct, plasma catecholamine
levels of dogs given endotoxin have increased 50 to 100 times, and this may
account for the critical visceral ischemia which occurs. The same high "toxic"
levels of plasma catecholamines were also found in the dog during prolonged
hemorrhagic shock.

Hemorrhagic shock and endotoxin shock closely resemble shock which
follows the injection of epinephrine both in the hemodynamic effects on the
circulatory system as well as in the visceral changes seen at autopsy. This
similarity has led to experiments in which dogs were made tolerant to the
vasospastic effects of endotoxins or epinephrine by gradually injecting increasing amounts of these substances. Such tolerant dogs are then also able to
survive usually lethal periods of hemorrhagic shock as well as lethal amounts
of endotoxin or epinephrine. Latterly, measurements of blood flow to the
viscera during varying types of shock have been made with the electromagnetic flow-meter, and blood flow to the gut has consistently fallen to lower levels
than seen in any other organ. This finding perhaps explains why the bowel
suffers such severe damage during shock whether it be due to hemorrhage,
endotoxins, or epinephrine and why these forms of irreversible shock so
closely resemble a similar condition induced by a 4.5—5 hour period of occlusion of the superior mesenteric artery.

Thus these studies give further evidence that there is a unity in the nature
of the organism's response to shock as well as a unity in the nature of irreversible shock itself. In the light of such findings, the authors feel that our
usual methods of treating clinical shock in patients with vasopressor substances need a drastic revision.

Supported by U. S. P. H. S. Grant No. 2941 and a grant from the Minnesota Heart Association.

References

1. MALCOLM, J. D.: Lancet (G. B.) **1905/II**, 573. — 2. BAINBRIDGE, F. A.,
and J. W. TREVAN: J. Physiol. (G. B.) **51**, 460 (1917). — 3. ERLANGER, J., and
H. S. GASSER: Amer. J. Physiol. **49**, 345 (1919). — 4. CANNON, W. B.:
Traumatic Shock. New York: D. Appleton & Co. 1923. — 5. FREEMAN, N. E.:
Amer. J. Physiol. **103**, 185 (1933). — 6. AUB, J. C.: N. England J. Med.
231, 71 (1944). — 7. SHORR., E., B. W. ZWEIFACH and R. F. FURCHGOTT:
Science (U. S. A.) **102**, 490 (1945). — 8. FINE, J.: The Bacterial Factor in
Traumatic Shock. p. 43. Springfield: Charles C. Thomas Co. 1954. —
9. KNISELY, M. H., T. S. ELIOT and E. H. BLOCH: Arch. Surg. (U. S. A.) **51**,
220 (1945). — 10. HEIMBECKER, R. D., and W. G. BIGELOW: Surgery
(U. S. A.) **28**, 461 (1950). — 11. McKAY, D. G., and G. H. WOHLE Jr.:
Arch. Path. (U. S. A.) **60**, 679 (1955). — 12. GELIN, L. E.: Acta chir.
Scand. Suppl. 210 (1956). — 13. LILLEHEI, R. C.: Surgery (U. S. A.)
42, 1043 (1957). — 14. LILLEHEI, R. C.: Circulation Res. (U. S. A.) **6**, 438
(1958). — 15. LILLEHEI, R. C., and A. EINHEBER: Amer. J. Physiol. **183**, 611
(1955). — 16. ZWEIFACH, B. W., H. A. GORDON, M. WAGNER and J. A.

REYNIERS: J. Exper. Med. (U. S. A.) **107**, 437 (1958). — 17. DELAUNAY, A., P. BOQUET, J. LEBRUN, Y. LEHOULT and M. DELAUNAY: J. physiol. (Fr.) **40**, 89 (1948). — 18. LILLEHEI, R. C., and L. D. MACLEAN: Ann. Surg. (U.S.A.) **148**, 513 (1958). — 19. LILLEHEI, R. C., and L. D. MACLEAN: Arch. Surg. (U. S. A.) **78**, 464 (1959). — 20. GOOD, R. P., and L. T. THOMAS: J. Exper. Med. (U. S. A.) **97**, 871 (1953). — 21. GADDUM, J. H., and M. VOGT: Brit. J. Pharmacol. **12**, 323 (1957). — 22. BURN, J. H., and M. J. RAND: Brit. Med. J. 1958/I, 903. — 23. FOUTS, J. R., and B. B. BRODIE: J. Pharmacol. Exper. Therap. (U. S. A.) **116**, 480 (1956). — 24. ROSENBERG, J. C., R. C. LILLEHEI, W. H. MORAN and B. ZIMMERMANN: Proc. Soc. Exper. Biol. Med. (U. S. A.) **102**, 335 (1959). — 25. LONGERBEAM, J. K., and R. C. LILLE-HEI: Fed. Proc. (U. S. A.) **21**, 116 (1961). — 26. LILLEHEI, R. C., B. GOOTT and F. A. MILLER: Ann. Surg. (U. S. A.) **150**, 543 (1959). — 27. ROSENBERG, J. C., R. C. LILLEHEI, J. K. LONGERBEAM and B. ZIMMERMANN: Ann. Surg. (U. S. A.) (to be published October, 1961.). — 28. SPECTOR, W. S. (Editor): Handbook of Biological Data, p. 260. Philadelphia: W. B. Saunders Co. 1956. — 29. SPANNER, R.: J. Morph. Mikr. Anat. 1. Abt. **89**, 394 (1932) — 30. PENNER, A., and A. I. BERNHEIM: Arch. Path. (U. S. A.) **28**, 129 (1939). — 31. PENNER, A.: J. Exper. Med. (U. S. A.) **10**, 453 (1939). — 32. PENNER, A.: Arch. Path. (U. S. A.) **27**, 966 (1939). — 33. KLEMPERER, P., A. PENNER and A. I. BERNHEIM: Amer. J. Digest. Dis. (U. S. A.) **7**, 410 (1940). — 34. PENNER, A., and L. J. DRUCKERMAN: Gastroenterology (U. S. A.) **11**, 478 (1948). — 35. WEIL, M.: J. Clin. Invest. (U. S. A.) **31**, 940 (1958).

Discussion

NICKERSON: I should like to begin by complimenting Dr. LILLEHEI, not only on his beautiful experiments, but also on an excellent preview of the last section of this symposium, on the drug treatment of shock. I find very little to disagree with him on this point. I would like to ask two questions. First, does he have evidence on the effectiveness of massive doses of adrenal steroids in shock due to procedures other than the administration of endo-toxin? My second question has to do with the longer survival of animals with permanent than of those with temporary occlusion of the superior mesenteric artery. Is it possible that the difference is due to loss of fluid into the viscera rather than to release of toxic material?

RUSHMER: Does the use of survival as an end-point in such experiments imply the assumption that the cause of death is the same in all the animals? Secondly, do the patterns of change in blood pressure and gross pathology indicate functional similarity in the various kinds of shock that have been described?

LILLEHEI: Let me first answer Dr. NICKERSON's question on the effective-ness of adrenal steroids. In general we have used hydrocortisone in massive doses (10—15 mg./kg.) intravenously in any patient suffering from shock who has not responded to replacement of actual or estimated blood losses. In this connection, I would emphasise again that losses are usually greater than anticipated, and many cases of profound shock occur merely because losses of red cells and/or plasma have not been adequately replaced. The patients whom we see suffering from shock are usually post-operative, so that the causes of shock are manifold. That is, there is the general trauma of the surgery with plasma loss, especially from the traumatised bowel. There is actual blood loss from the surgery as well as following surgery, and there is gram-negative septicaemia with its attendant "endotoxin" shock, or gram-positive (staphylococcal) septicaemia with its attendant "exotoxin" shock. In such patients, we have found that blood and/or plasma replacement, combined with the intravenous use of 500 to 1,000 mg. of hydrocortisone, is an effective means of returning blood pressure toward normal levels without the further visceral ischaemia inevitably occurring when vasopressors, such as l-norepinephrine or metaraminol, are used to raise blood pressure. Latterly, we have been using adrenergic blocking agents, such as chlor-promazine or phenoxybenzamine (Dibenzyline), given intravenously and accompanied by blood or plasma to "fill up" the enlarged vascular space resulting from the use of such agents. With this regimen, we have rarely failed to restore blood pressure. It is of course then imperative to find any source of blood or plasma loss and to drain any abscess or anastomotic breakdown in the viscera causing the shock. We have reduced the hydrocortisone dosage gradually and then eliminated it entirely in 4—5 days. In the laboratory, we find that such a regimen restores flow to the brain, heart, and viscera as well as restoring blood pressure. We are now engaged in quantitating such findings in the human as well.

The question has been asked whether all our findings could not be explained simply by plasma loss from the bowel. Certainly the large amounts of plasma lost in these experiments (30—50% of plasma volume) are important, but replacing such losses only temporises or delays the eventual death if nothing is done to correct the ultimate cause of the losses, which is critical ischaemia and eventual necrosis of the bowel. At the present time, we have worked out techniques to remove the entire bowel, small and large, and later replace it as an autograft with indefinite survival of the dog. If refrigerated *in vitro* to 5° C the bowel need not be replaced and circulation restored for up to 6 hours. Having established the technique, we are now removing the bowel of dogs and cooling it to 5° C *in vitro*, while the dog is subjected to one of the types of shock described in this presentation. Following the end of the shock experiment, the bowel is replaced. Similar experiments are being done with the stomach and kidneys in order to further clarify the "intestinal" factor in irreversible shock.

Dr. RUSHMER has asked whether gross and microscopic examination of tissues at post mortem should be used to establish the cause of irreversible shock before death. I might add here that we have much other data available, such as continuous pressure and flow recordings, electrocardiograms, respiration tracings, chemical analysis of blood, etc., which correlate with the more significant data presented here. We have by no means solved the problem of irreversible shock, but I think we have established some general concepts which are of value in clinical thinking. JOHN HUNTER summed up more succinctly what I am trying to say in the folllowing way: "We should never reason on general principles only, much less practise upon them when we are, or can be, master of all the facts; but where we have nothing else but the general principle, then we must take it for our guide."

GREGERSEN: It seems, Dr. LILLEHEI, that the term stagnant anoxia could well be used as designating the central feature and common denominator in all forms of shock.

With reference to the effects of tying off vessels, no one so far has mentioned the possible damage done by leaving the blood in the tissues instead of first expelling the blood as with an Esmarch bandage. Some years ago, a surgeon came to me with this problem. In dogs he succeeded in demonstrating to me a few times that if he first flushed out the blood in the brain with saline, he could stop the heart for 30—40 minutes and still bring back spontaneous breathing and some reflexes when the heart was started and cerebral circulation re-established. I suggested the test be done on other tissues presenting less formidable technical difficulties.

BACQ: How do you explain on the basis of your general idea the failure of reserpine to have a favourable effect, whereas you do have a favourable effect with Dibenzyline?

LILLEHEI: Dr. GREGERSEN's suggestion of a revival of the term "stagnant anoxia" is a good one. I like the term, as does Dr. GREGERSEN, because it aptly describes the end result occurring following a number of varied types of stress. It is the common denominator resulting from prolonged haemorrhage, injection of endotoxins, gram-negative septicaemia, trauma, and the injection of vasopressor agents. What I am suggesting is that "stagnant anoxia" is most pronounced in the bowel of the dog, and the resultant ischaemic necrosis of the bowel causes the death of the animal.

Dr. GREGERSEN also asked another question concerning the possible detrimental effects of stagnant blood itself within an organ. We have done a number of transplantation experiments as described above, in which the entire bowel or stomach has been removed and kept *in vitro* for periods up to 6 hours before such organs have been replaced as an autograft. While the organ was held *in vitro*, we found no advantage in washing the blood from the bowel or stomach or in giving the animals heparin before removing the organ in question.

After the organ is removed from the dog, the blood within the organ does not clot, similar to cadaver blood, and dogs receiving autotransplants of the entire bowel or stomach have survived indefinitely.

Dr. BACQ has asked about the effects of reserpine in these experiments. The failure of reserpine to protect dogs also surprised us, but I think there is probably a logical explanation for this. BURN and others have shown that reserpine depletes the blood-vessel walls of both serotonin and catecholamines. This leaves the vessels sensitised to vasopressor agents similar to the sensitisation following sympathectomy. When dogs, pre-treated with reserpine, are subjected to the sympathomimetic effects of endotoxins or the increased catecholamine levels in prolonged haemorrhagic shock, then these sensitised vessels perhaps go into an even more profound spasm than usual, thus resulting in severe stagnant anoxia and an accelerated decline to death. More data are of course required before this theory can be considered fact.

MIGONE: According to your clinical experience, has hydrocortisone good effects in preventing advanced shock and during the full development of the syndrome as well ? It would be interesting to know the relations between the therapeutic effect of hydrocortisone and the reactions caused by endogenous catecholamines.

LILLEHEI: Dr. MIGONE has asked about the mode of action or the beneficial effects of hydrocortisone when given either after the onset of shock or as pre-treatment. At present, we are trying to get more quantitative data to explain this observation of protection with hydrocortisone. With the use of the electromagnetic flow-meter and with measurements of pressures across the capillary beds in varying types of experiments we have obtained some evidence to explain this beneficial effect of hydrocortisone. Hydrocortisone possibly works in at least two ways in these experiments. First of all, it may blunt the full sympathomimetic effect of endotoxin acting on the blood vessels, and perhaps it also allows cells to survive ischaemic or "stagnant" conditions which ordinarily would result in the death of the cell. The problem is complex because of the rapidity with which events occur in shock, especially in shock due to gram-negative bacteria. Dr. SPINK has written that if one could explain what occurred in the first 30 seconds after the injection of endotoxin, the remainder of the problem could easily be solved. The ability of hydrocortisone to protect dogs against lethal doses of epinephrine suggests from a clinical point of view that it may be wise to include massive doses of hydrocortisone in any situation in which the physician feels that a vasopressor agent is necessary to raise the blood pressure of a patient. This may enable one to derive some beneficial effect from the vasopressor agent on blood pressure without causing added damage to the viscera due to further reduction in blood flow to these organs. From our own clinical experience, however, we feel that the use of vasopressor agents is rarely indicated and that the blood pressure can be supported by much more physiological means, such as described above.

BEIN: Dr. LILLEHEI, how long have you been treating your dogs with reserpine ? I think that you can get a complete loss of the stored catecholamines only after prolonged pre-treatment with reserpine. Secondly, I do not think that one can call endotoxin a sympathomimetic. I shall probably come back to this in my own paper. Thirdly, you have pre-treated dogs with endotoxin and found that they could tolerate haemorrhagic shock. I do not know whether in your experiments you have observed a pharmacological type of action of endotoxin, because if you pre-treat guinea-pigs with endotoxin you can also protect them against anaphylactic shock or other allergic phenomena[1].

GILBERT: I would like to compliment Dr. LILLEHEI for this stimulating talk, though there are some things with which I disagree. The first point: The blood volume in man with bacteraemic shock is, as far as I know, normal, barring complications such as dehydration. Studies in monkeys by other people have shown no reduction in blood volume after endotoxin. The haematocrit does not rise. Point two: I have been waiting for comments, but the fact that this was pre-treatment should be emphasised. The data which were obtained by Dr. SPINK's group showed that post-treatment of endotoxin shock with steroids is more effective when combined with a pressor drug such as metaraminol.

LILLEHEI: To Dr. BEIN: It is difficult to pre-treat dogs with reserpine for much more than a week to 10 days. With dogs of 10—15 kg. body-weight, reserpine, in 0.5—1 mg. doses daily, usually produces profound lethargy by the end of a one-week period of pre-treatment. When pre-treatment with reserpine is carried past two weeks, many of the dogs die spontaneously with severely congested livers. I believe that a week's pre-treatment is probably sufficient to deplete tissue serotonin and catecholamine stores.

I think that endotoxin can truly be called sympathomimetic in action in the viscera of the dog for the following reason. If one measures pressure in the superior mesenteric artery and portal vein along with flow in the superior mesenteric artery, resistance in the portal system is seen to increase progressively during the course of shock caused by the injection of endotoxin (see Fig. 5). The same is true for shock induced by prolonged haemorrhage or injection of epinephrine (see Fig. 5). Dr. BEIN has also asked about the significance of the tolerance experiments. We are currently trying to establish the basis for such tolerance. In preliminary experiments we have found that flow to the viscera and especially to the bowel of tolerant dogs is not depressed to the usual low level seen during shock in control dogs.

Many investigators, as well as Dr. GILBERT, have commented on the fact that shock due to septicaemia is not accompanied by any blood-volume loss. The study of EBERT and STEAD in 1941[2] is usually cited to support such a statement. Actually, the patients studied by these investigators were all suffering from septicaemia with gram-positive organisms, which do not possess endotoxin within their cell wall. We are currently measuring blood volumes in patients suffering from shock due to gram-negative organisms in hopes of resolving this controversy.

Dr. GILBERT has also asked about the combined post-treatment of shock with hydrocortisone along with vasopressor agents. As mentioned above, the use of hydrocortisone with vasopressor agents may protect the animal or patient from the deleterious effects of the vasopressor agent. I would re-emphasise my own thoughts that even better results are obtained with hydrocortisone when no vasopressor agents at all are used; instead, the hydrocortisone is given along with blood plasma or low molecular weight dextran and an adrenergic blocking agent.

---

[1] MEIER, R., H. J. BEIN, and R. JAQUES: Int. Arch. Allergy (Switz.) 11, 101 (1957); JAQUES, R., H. J. BEIN, and R. MEIER: Int. Arch. Allergy (Switz.) 14, 144 (1959).

[2] J. Clin. Invest. (U. S. A.) 20, 671 (1941).

Renal failure in shock

By

K. KRAMER

As a consequence of acute circulatory failure due to hemor-rhagic, traumatic or toxic shock, renal failure develops. After the peripheral signs of shock have disappeared and blood pressure is restored, urine flow declines to such low values that solute ex-cretion is almost completely suppressed. The serum urea level climbs day by day to values which may reach 600 mg.% or more. In patients who recover, a polyuric phase sets in after a week of oliguria. However, the concentrating power of the kidney is by no means regained. Creatinine U/P's show values as low as 5, and urine tonicity — as revealed by a specific gravity of 1012 — is equal to that of serum. The state of uraemia shows very little change until the concentrating function of the kidney has been restored (Fig. 1).

MUNCK's (9) measurements of RBF (radioactive krypton) during oliguric and polyuric phases have revealed that the reduc-tion is not of such a degree that hypoxia could be held responsible for what occurs. MUNCK has found that on an average 30% of the normal blood flow is still maintained during renal failure in man. However, the GFR, as measured by endogenous creatinine-clearance in daily urine collections, decreases to extremely low values (such as 1—2% of normal). It remains low even during the polyuric phase. After a period of 3 weeks or more, about 30% of normal is regained. Even after months the GFR does not yet return to normal levels.

It has long been recognised that the GFR becomes zero at arterial pressure levels lower than 60 mm. Hg. At this level the blood flow per gramme tissue is still above that of any other organ, since renal vascular resistance is very low. However, during haemorrhagic shock, as SELKURT (13) has shown in anaesthetised dogs, reflex vasoconstriction also takes place in the renal vessels leading to an increase in vascular resistance of about 100% (Fig. 2). Dr. THURAU, using Gregg's electromagnetic flow-meter, has performed a few experiments inducing haemorrhagic shock in conscious dogs. At 60 mm. Hg the RBF has fallen to 30% of the control value — a disproportion which indicates vasoconstriction. This increase in resistance in shock persists in the post-infusion period except in a few instances. Even after 24 hours a slight

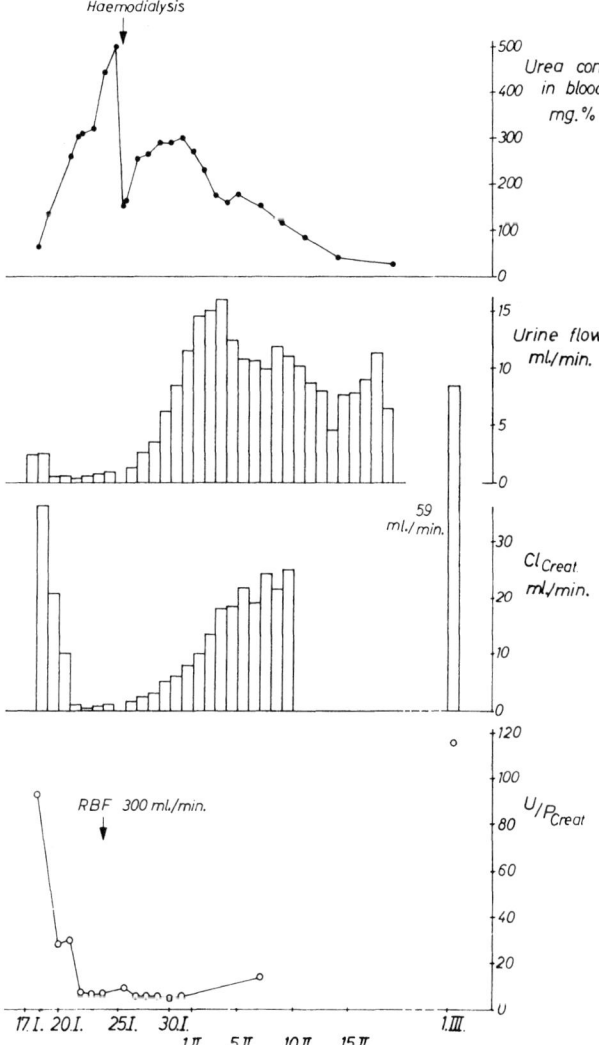

Fig. 1. Data obtained during the course of acute renal failure following 36 hours of shock due to barbiturate poisoning. The change in creatinine clearance and U/P serum urea levels and urine volume are plotted against time in days. Note that the return of concentrating power (U/P creatinine) corresponds to the recovery of GFR (Cl creatinine). (From MUNCK, O.)

increase in resistance is still found in animals which go on to complete recovery.

This finding of protracted renal vasoconstriction even in cases which recover is in good agreement with the results in humans in

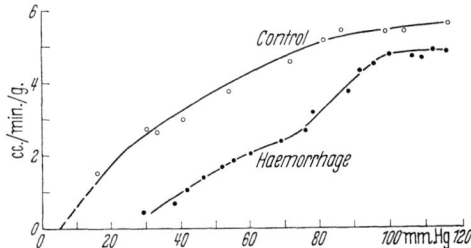

Fig. 2. Effect of haemorrhage on the pressure-flow relationship. Variation in arterial pressure was obtained by graded clamping of the renal artery. (From E. SELKURT)

shock. This increase in vascular resistance, however, is not enough to reduce the blood supply to the kidney to such a degree that hypoxia of renal tissue occurs. The O_2 saturation of venous blood is found to be not lower than 80 % with a normal arterial saturation. It has been objected that in spite of highly oxygenated venous

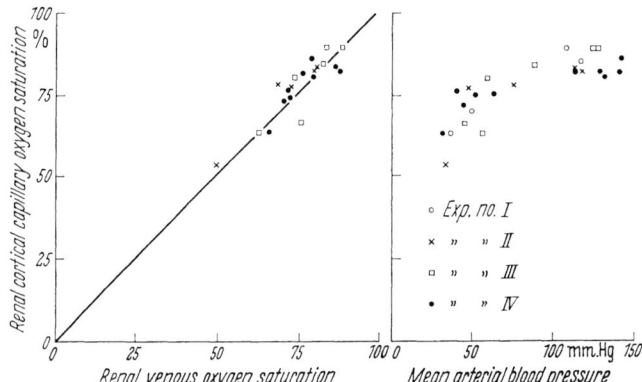

Fig. 3. Cortical capillary O_2 saturation in relation to renal venous O_2 saturation (a) and mean arterial blood pressure (b) during haemorrhagic shock. (From MUNCK, O., N. LASSEN, P. DEETJEN and K. KRAMER, Lancet, in press)

blood the renal tissue suffers under hypoxia because of a low O_2 saturation in the capillaries due to a shunt mechanism such as described by TRUETA (14) or PAPPENHEIMER (12).

By the photo-electric technique of KRAMER and ULLRICH (3), MUNCK et al. (10) have shown that this objection is not valid.

Capillary O_2 saturation was never lower than renal venous O_2 (Fig. 3) in haemorrhagic shock of 2 hours' duration. Even at an arterial pressure of 50 mm. Hg, capillary saturation was found to average not less than 70%.

WIGGERS (17) in his book, the "Physiology of Shock" (1950), sums up current ideas of renal oxygen consumption by saying:

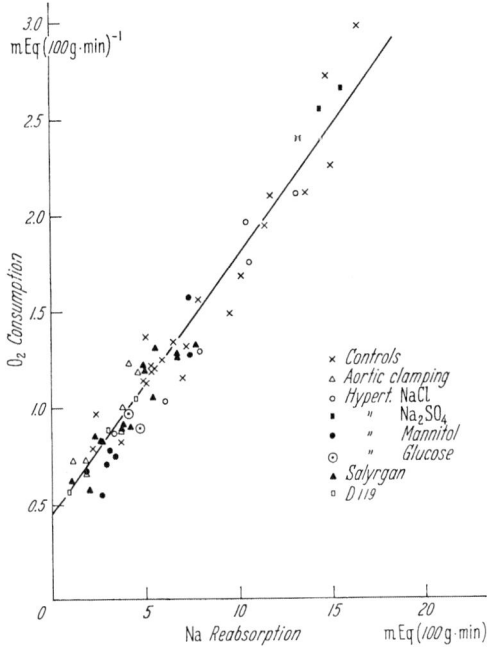

Fig. 4. Renal O_2 consumption as a function of sodium reabsorption. The sodium load was changed by either aortic clamping, spontaneous renal vasoconstriction, osmotic diuresis or mercury poisoning (Salyrgan). (From DEETJEN, P., and K. KRAMER)

"Contrary to most other tissues studied renal cells appear to have the ability of reducing their oxygen consumption in proportion to that supplied." Since we now know that renal O_2 consumption depends mainly on the sodium load and its reabsorption, we interpret this observation in a different light (2, 8). Oxygen is the price paid for active transport of sodium in the renal tubules (Fig. 4). This explains the proportionality of O_2 consumption to blood flow, since the latter is closely related to the GFR and consequently to the sodium load. The proportionality ends when levels of 50 to 60 mm. Hg and about 30% of normal blood flow are reached. At lower pressures O_2 consumption is exponentially related to further reduction of blood flow (Fig. 5). This exponential relationship (5) is found in most other organs and indicates that with decreasing pressure the number of open capillaries decreases and the diffusion distances increase to such an extent that O_2 supply is no longer

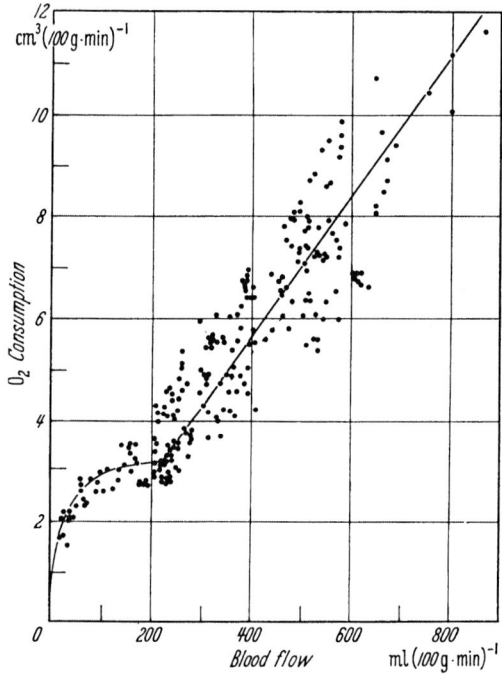

Fig. 5. Renal O_2 consumption in relation to blood flow. Note that in the range of blood flow from 0—200 ml./min. O_2 consumption increases exponentially. Above 200 ml./min., when glomerular filtration sets in, a linear relationship obtains. (From KRAMER, K., and P. DEETJEN, 1960)

adequate. This, however, does not happen until very low blood flow values are reached (less than 10% of normal). It is here that the ischaemic changes described by OLIVER (11) in fatal cases must occur.

We may conclude from these findings in humans and dogs in circulatory shock that, in cases which survive, renal hypoxia is very unlikely to occur.

Acute renal failure following haemorrhagic shock in dogs has not been described. DEETJEN and I have carried out experiments on dogs in which a 3-hour period of shock was induced by haemorrhage. Transient renal insufficiency was observed for 5 hours following the reinfusion of blood. After this period the animals were sacrificed and their kidneys subjected to histological examination. During the post-infusion period vasoconstriction persists in varying

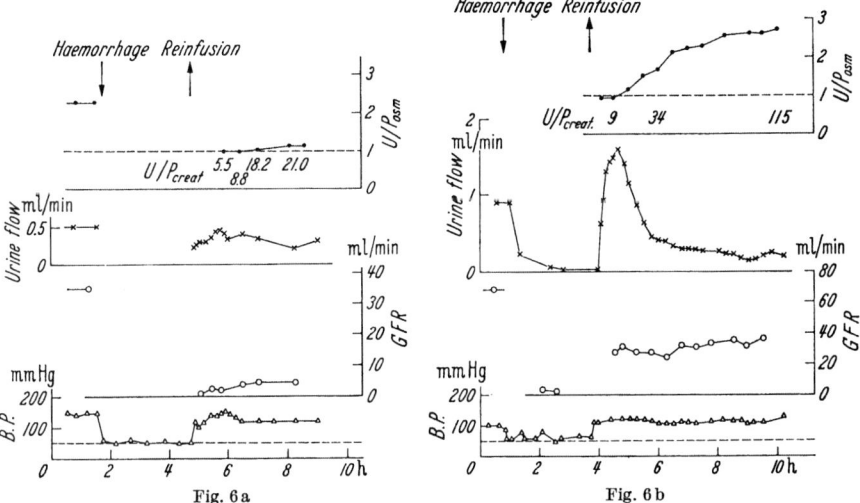

Fig. 6a   Fig. 6b

Fig. 6a and b. Renal function in anaesthetised dogs following (a) severe and (b) moderate haemorrhagic shock. Note that in (a) GFR reaches only 10% of the normal and no concentrating power is restored during the post-infusion period. In (b) a return to 50% of normal GFR is associated with a return of concentrating ability. (From KRAMER, K., and P. DEETJEN, 1961)

degree depending on the severity of shock. Animals in which the arterial pressure dropped to values lower than 40−45 mm. Hg showed longer vasoconstriction periods than those in which the pressure fluctuated around 60 mm. Hg. Typical records of these two different events obtained from dogs of similar size are shown in Fig. 6a and b. In severe shock the GFR does not recover to more than 12% of normal. U/P osmols are around 1, indicating that no concentration of urine has taken place. U/P creatinines show values of 5.5−21.0. In mild shock the GFR recovers to about 50% of normal. This is followed by an increasing concentration of urine

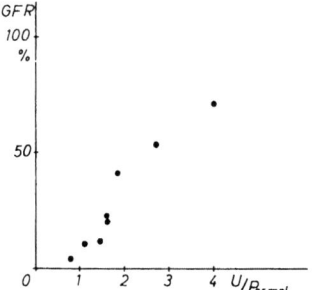

Fig. 7. U/P osmols as a function of GFR in per cent of normal. Data obtained in steady states of the post-infusion period of haemorrhagic shock in 8 dogs. (From KRAMER, K., and P. DEETJEN, 1961)

after a short period of polyuria, during which isotonic urine is excreted. These results have been confirmed in 8 experiments. When steady state values of U/P osmols in progressive states of recovery are plotted against the GFR a good proportionality is found (Fig. 7).

The sequence of events so far may be pictured in the following way:

1. Persisting vasoconstriction prevents the development of a proper GFR in varying degrees related to the severity of shock in circulatory failure.

2. The recovery of the kidney's urine concentrating power is closely related to the restoration of the GFR.

Our first problem, as to what causes the persistent renal vaso-constriction, has long been recognised and is still obscure. The assumption that pressor agents, such as renin or other types of substance, are produced during circulatory shock has often been discussed. I do not have any new results to add. It seems necessary to reinvestigate the matter since more reliable assays have been developed by many authors.

But the second problem – the cause of failure to concentrate the urine – can now be tackled with more success. The concentrat-ing mechanism is found in the countercurrent system of Henle's loops and much has been learned in recent years about this system.

I should like to give you a brief outline of what we know about the countercurrent system in the renal medulla. The primary treatment of a loop system by WERNER KUHN (7) presupposes that sodium in the fluid of the ascending limb of Henle's loop is transported out into the descending limb at a constant rate (Fig. 8a). This would lead, by virtue of the so-called "single effect", to an increase in sodium concentration from base to tip of the papilla. The process by which the final urine is concentrated is brought about by water reabsorption from the collecting duct into the loops (Fig. 8b). This hypothesis involves a few rather perplexing assumptions, i. e. one part of Henle's loop must be water-permeable and another not. We must also suppose that volume flow increases in the loop system since fluid from the collecting duct is added. The increase of inulin U/P ratios from 3 to 11 at the tip of the papilla, however, indicates that water has left the loops.

This fact points to the function of the medullary blood vessels, which carry away about 25% of the glomerular filtrate (16). They, like Henle's loops, are also formed as hairpin loops and should function as a countercurrent system. This, however, would conflict

with their obvious task of carrying away 25% of the GF including solutes. By mathematical means it can be shown that
solutes entering the interstitial space, and also the blood vessels,
at a constant rate will be concentrated
from the base to the tip of the papilla
(Fig. 9). But this concentration process
is diminshed by the rate of blood flow.
This diminishing effect is of great im-

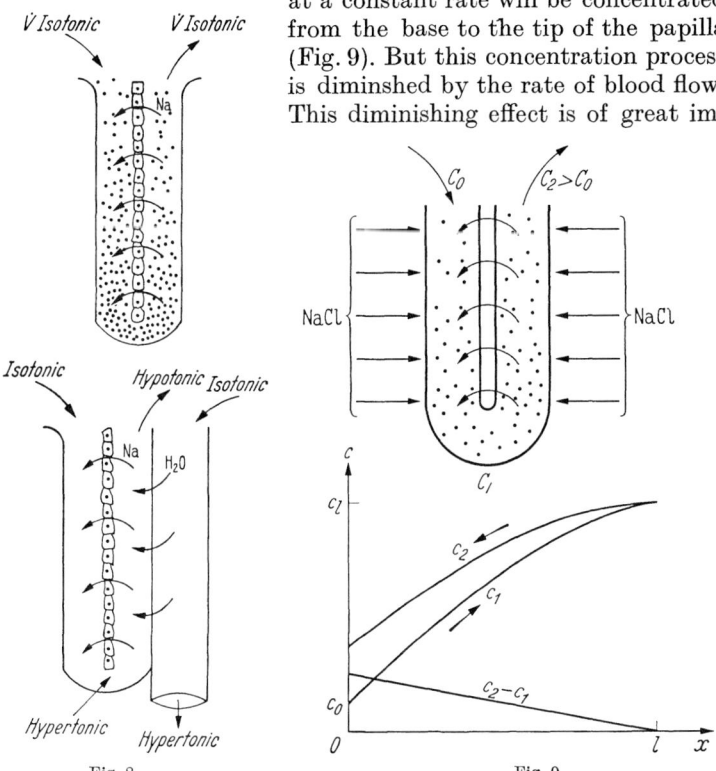

Fig. 8

Fig. 9

Fig. 8. Model of the countercurrent system according to W. KUHN, applied to the renal
medullary structures (see text)

Fig. 9. Model to illustrate countercurrent exchange of NaCl entering by diffusion throughout
the length of a loop comparable to a vasa recta hairpin. Diagram describes the course of
NaCl concentration entering along the length (1). The concentration rises along curve c_1 and
returns along the curve c_2 corresponding to the in-going and out-going vessel. (From
ULLRICH, K., K. KRAMER and J. W. BOYLAN)

portance, since it is related to the square of the blood flow. Therefore we have to consider several functions of the blood vessels, and
of Henle's loops as well, which cooperate in such a way that an
osmotic gradient in the medulla is built up and maintained. The
osmolar gradient will be greater as the volume flow into the counter-
current system allows the ascending limb of Henle to transport Na

out of it in excess of water. Hence, a lower tubular flow — due to a lower GFR — diminishes the amount of Na available for transport.

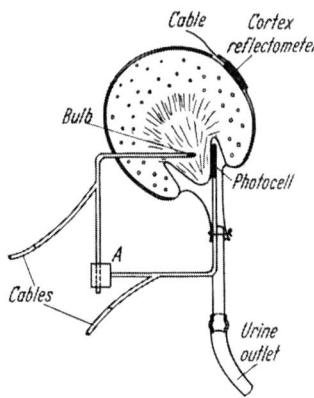

A disproportion between Na transport and medullary blood flow must therefore lead to a change in the concentration gradient in the medulla.

In shock there is definitely no volume flow through Henle's loops but still 25% of the normal medullary blood flow. This has been shown by actual recordings of medullary circulation times (4). The method used consisted of a photo-electric device inserted via the ureter in close proximity to the inner zone of the medulla. A small bulb providing the light source is pierced through the cortex to the medullary tissue. The passage time of Evans blue injected into the renal artery can in this way be directly measured

Fig. 10a. Determination of medullary and cortical circulation times from which corresponding blood flows are calculated. (From KRAMER, K., K. THURAU and P. DEETJEN)

(Fig. 10). Blood flow values are calculated from mean passage times and from the known volume of the vascular system. Cortical flow can be measured in a similar way by the use of reflectometers placed on the surface of the kidney. Normal values for dogs,

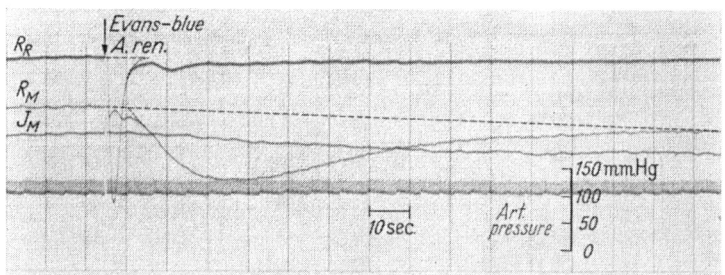

Fig. 10b. Original tracings from the devices shown in Fig. 10a. Note the widely different passage times of Evans blue injected into the renal artery in cortical and medullary tissue. (From KRAMER, K., K. THURAU and P. DEETJEN)

together with our findings in shock, are presented in Table 1. Here we see that the inner medullary blood flow, normally 0.5—1% of the cortical blood flow, is reduced in haemorrhagic shock to 20—27% of this value. The cortical blood flow shows a similar

Table 1. *Cortical and inner medullary blood flow during haemorrhagic shock and after reinfusion of blood in 3 dog experiments*

B. P. mm. Hg	Blood flow cortex ml./min.	Blood flow inner zone of medulla ml./min.	Cortex Δ BF %	Medulla Δ BF %
Control 110	455	3.85		
Haemorrhage . . . 60	185	0.92	— 59	— 76
Reinfusion 115	357	2.15	— 12	— 44
1 h. later. 115	333	1.39	— 27	— 64
Control 110	400	2.30		
Haemorrhage . . . 80	270	1.44	— 33	— 37
Haemorrhage . . . 40	44	0.63	— 89	— 73
Reinfusion 110	313	1.71	— 22	— 26
1 h. later. 115	208	1.20	— 48	— 48
Control 115	417	2.86		
Haemorrhage . . . 80	208	2.38	— 50	— 17
Haemorrhage . . . 45	73	0.57	— 82	— 80
Reinfusion 95	263	2.70	— 37	— 6
1 h. later. 95	244	2.13	— 41	— 26

reduction. In the post-infusion period, the blood flow in both cortex and inner medulla has only recovered to about 75% of normal (6).

The persistence of this small medullary flow in the absence of filtration supplying sodium led us to suspect that the solutes might be washed out of the medullary tissue depleting the osmotic gradient.

BOYLAN and ASSHAUER (1) studied the osmotic gradient in dogs under a variety of conditions. In the course of their study they determined the osmotic pressure of shock kidney slices in cortical and outer and inner medullary tissues taken after 3 hours' hacmorrhagic shock. They found a complete washout of the medullary solutes to isotonicity, indicating that in shock there is no functioning countercurrent system (Fig. 11).

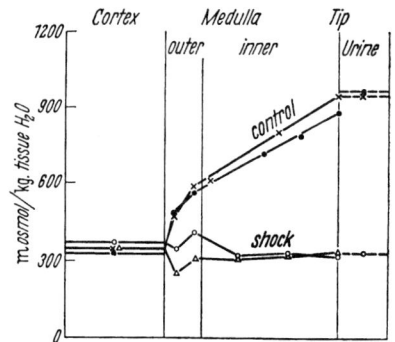

Fig. 11. Osmolapity in kidney slices taken from dogs following 48 hours' water deprivation in control and shock states. (From BOYLAN, J. W., and E. ASSHAUER)

Summary

1. Renal failure following circulatory shock develops because of persistent vasoconstriction which is just sufficient to prevent glomerular filtration.

Hypoxia of renal tissue has not been demonstrated in surviving cases.

2. During the low-pressure phase in circulatory shock the remaining blood flow through the medullary regions washes out the osmotic gradient built up by the countercurrent system of Henle's loops, so that a concentrated urine cannot be formed.

3. During recovery from circulatory failure the osmotic gradient of the medullary region can only be built up if sufficient fluid from the glomerular filtrate reaches the countercurrent system. The greater the GF, the faster the gradient is built up.

References

1. BOYLAN, J. W., and E. ASSHAUER: Unpublished data. — 2. DEETJEN, P., and K. KRAMER: Pflügers Arch. Physiol. (G.) (in press). — 3. KRAMER, K., and K. ULLRICH: Pflügers Arch. Physiol. (G.) 267, 251 (1958). — 4. KRAMER, K., K. THURAU and P. DEETJEN: Pflügers Arch. Physiol. (G.) 270, 251 (1960). — 5. KRAMER, K., and P. DEETJEN: Pflügers Arch. Physiol. (G.) 271, 782 (1960). — 6. KRAMER, K., and P. DEETJEN: Unpublished data. — 7. KUHN, W., and A. RAMEL: Helv. chim. acta 42, 628 (1959). — 8. LASSEN, N. A., O. MUNCK and J. H. THAYSEN: Acta physiol. Scand. 51, 371 (1961). — 9. MUNCK, O.: Renal Circulation in Acute Renal Failure. Oxford 1958. — 10. MUNCK, O., N. LASSEN, P. DEETJEN and K. KRAMER: Lancet (G. B.) (in press). — 11. OLIVER, J., M. MacDOWELL and A. FRACY: J. Clin. Invest. (U. S. A.) 30, 1305 (1951). — 12. PAPPENHEIMER, J. P., and W. B. KINTER: Amer. J. Physiol. 185, 371 (1956). — 13. SELKURT, E. E.: Klin. Wschr. (G.) 33, 359 (1955). — 14. TRUETA, J., A. E. BARCLEY, P. M. DANIEL, K. J. FRANKLIN and M. M. L. PRICHARD: Studies of the Renal Circulation. Oxford 1947. — 15. ULLRICH, K., and G. PEHLING: Pflügers Arch. Physiol. (G.) 267, 207 (1958). — 16. ULLRICH, K., K. KRAMER and J. W. BOYLAN: Progr. Cardiovasc. Dis. (U. S. A.) 3, 395 (1961). — 17. WIGGERS, C.: Physiology of Shock. New York 1950.

Renal blood flow and renal clearances during hemorrhage and hemorrhagic shock

By

E. E. SELKURT

We have been interested for some time in the changes in renal blood flow and renal clearance which occur during a standardized hemorrhagic shock procedure in the anesthetized dog (1). Fig. 1 shows the average trends in a group of five animals which showed comparable effects. The procedure was to bleed to 60 mm. Hg and to hold pressure here for 90 minutes. Then followed further bleeding to about 40 mm. Hg for an additional 45 minutes, whereupon blood was retransfused. The average of the blood pressure changes is shown at the top.

The second panel shows simultaneous clearances of PAH, creatinine, and direct blood flow measurements done by a venous outflow technique. Blood flow based on the clearance of PAH is shown here in two ways. The one labelled BF_{PAH} is simply the clearance of PAH plus the hematocrit volume. Above this is shown the blood flow computed by the Fick principle, namely:

$$\frac{BF_{PAH}}{\frac{A - V}{A}}$$

The clearance of creatinine is also shown at the lower left of the middle panel.

During control, BF_{PAH} averaged about 90 per cent of the simultaneous direct blood flow. Blood flow by the Fick method averaged about 20 per cent higher than the simultaneous direct blood flow. Since no correction was made for diffusion of PAH out of the red cells into the venous plasma, the true extraction ratio might be expected to be somewhat higher than those found in this series. Such a correction would bring the value down toward the direct blood flow measurement.

Upon hemorrhage, direct flow decreased to about one-third of the control value early in the hypotensive period. Urine volume dropped markedly, and the animals became extremely oliguric followed by anuria. The clearances based upon the low urine volumes, although markedly decreased, are not reliable and have not been portrayed in these experiments.

Although direct flow progressively decreased during oligemic shock, some flow persisted at all times, even though it reached the low value of about 7 per cent of control during the phase of lowest blood pressure. With transfusion, there was partial recovery

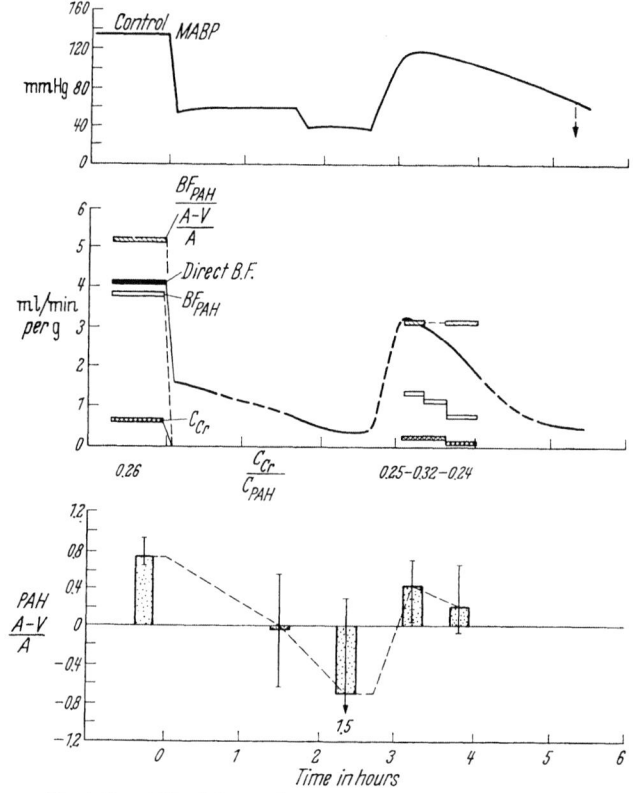

Fig. 1. Renal blood flow and clearance during hemorrhagic shock.

$$BF_{\text{PAH}} = C_{\text{PAH}} \times \frac{1}{1\text{-hemat.}} \; ; \; C_{Cr} = \text{clearance of creatinine}$$

of blood flow measured by the direct method. However, it was not maintained and, as normovolemic shock ensued, renal blood flow decreased more rapidly than the blood pressure as renal vascular resistance progressively increased. Blood flow based upon the clearance of PAH, namely BF_{PAH}, only partially recovered during this time, as did the clearance of creatinine. However, the blood flow computed by the Fick method showed recovery comparable to the direct blood flow, but again tended to remain higher as direct flow started to decrease. The creatinine clearance recovered to the degree of C_{PAH}, *but not to direct BF*.

The lower panel of the figure shows the changes in the extraction ratio of PAH. The columns represent the averages of the values obtained, with range of variation indicated by the vertical lines. Of interest is the decline in extraction of PAH to approximately O in the mid-point of the oligemic shock phase, and the finding of negative extraction ratios during the lowest phase of hypotension at the time of the most marked reduction in direct blood flow. Upon transfusion, the extraction of PAH was partially, and in a few instances, fairly completely restored, but this was not maintained, and the extraction ratio began to fall again as normovolemic shock progressed. We have been most interested in the negative extraction ratios which have been noted for PAH during the course of hemorrhagic shock. These observations may assume particular importance in the consideration of a dual circulation in the kidney, namely, a cortical one and a medullary circuit.

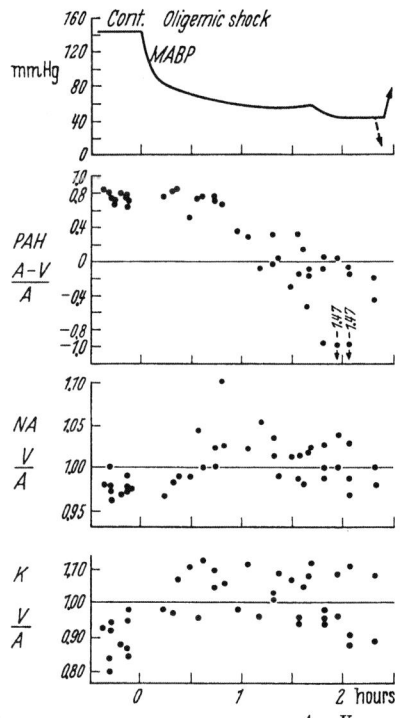

Fig. 2. Changes in extraction of PAH $\dfrac{A - V}{A}$, and electrolyte content (Na and K) in renal venous blood compared to arterial during oligemic shock

To analyze the situation further, let us look at Fig. 2. This contains a more recent series of five animals, grouped together for convenience, using approximately the same hemorrhagic shock procedure. In these, clearances were done but no direct blood flow measurements were made. 5% NaCl was infused for about 30 minutes prior to control and during the control periods. The procedures were similar enough to group 1 that we can assume that direct blood flow changes probably manifested the same trends. Since all of the animals in this group did not survive beyond the hypotensive period, only the changes are portrayed during oligemic shock. In the upper part of the figure is shown the trend of the mean arterial blood pressure as a result of hemorrhage. The second part of the figure shows the extraction ratios for PAH during the control and during oligemic shock. Note again, as in the first series, that negative extraction ratios of PAH are seen approximately one hour after completion of hemorrhage comparing with the results found in the first series.

We wonder if the phenomenon cannot be explained by a persistence of flow, although at a reduced rate, through zones of the kidney which might be particularly susceptible to the effects of a poor oxygen supply, namely, the loop of Henle and the parallel blood vascular system of the vasa recta. Because of countercurrent diffusion of oxygen, this may be a zone of relatively poor oxygen supply. Supporting this is the evidence of the low hematocrit existing in the vasa recta system, presumably supplying the loop of Henle portion of the nephron.

Although we are not in support of the notion that medullary circulation opens up in terms of a shunt mechanism (TRUETA) during hemorrhage, I feel that the evidence is at least adequate that there may be changes in regional circulation. Dr. KRAMER has shown in one experiment that a proportional reduction in cortical and medullary blood flow occurred. There exists further evidence which indicates that the cortical circulation may actually close off during hemorrhagic shock, while that through the medullary circuits, although reduced, may persist. The original work of TRUETA suggested this, and more recent work has supported this notion. Confirmatory evidence comes from stimulation of the nerve supply to the kidney, which would be expected to be a fundamental physiological influence evoked during hemorrhagic hypotension. As an example, the work of INSULL et al. (2) has shown that, during hemorrhage and stimulation of the sciatic nerve and the perirenal plexus, the juxtamedullary glomeruli were uniformly stained with injected Prussian blue, but that the peripheral glomeruli were not. They interpreted this to mean that there was regional cortical ischemia but continued flow through the medulla. This work done in the rabbit has been confirmed by BLOCK, WAKIM and MANN (3) and by KAHN et al. (4). Injection of epinephrine in the rabbit, as MONTAGUE and WILSON (5) have found, also produces a cortical ischemia but shows persistent medullary circulation by injection techniques (India ink). The excellent serial angiograms made by DANIEL et al. (6) in cats and dogs have given further evidence of the dual circulation in these kidneys, rapid in the cortex, but slow in the medulla.

We suggest that during shock there is in fact a closure of the cortical circulation but some persistence of the medullary circulation. The second group of animals supply some evidence for this conclusion. In the third part of the figure are shown the comparisons of sodium in the renal venous blood compared to the arterial inflow during the control and during oligemic shock. Note that, as the negative extraction ratios of PAH develop, there is an increase of the venous over arterial ratio of sodium, signifying a greater sodium content in the venous blood than in the entering arterial blood of the kidney. We interpret this to mean that the blood flowing from the kidney at this time is passing through a zone of hyperosmolarity. At the present time the only known region of the nephron where sodium would be expected in higher concentration than that existing in the arterial plasma is in the loop of Henle and the corresponding parts of the vasa recta system. With cessation of glomerular filtration following hemorrhage, the counter-current exchange system across the loop of Henle system comes to a halt. The continued perfusion of blood through this circuit then, in effect, washes away the hyperosmotic concentration, including that of sodium. It is noted in the bottom part of the figure that potassium shows the same trend, but since the clearance of potassium is somewhat more complex that that of sodium, we suggest that the removal of sodium presents the best evidence.

The negative extraction of PAH adds another facet to the problem. The negative extraction of PAH may mean that PAH concentrated in the nephron is leaking back into the circulation of the kidney, so that more leaves the vein than enters the kidney via the artery. In a more limited series, negative extraction of creatinine was observed. Because PAH is secreted and concentrated in the lumen of the nephron, it is theoretically possible that any site of the nephron might leak PAH and return it to the capillary and venous blood. It may be, however, that the loop of Henle system is the most likely for operation of this mechanism. One reason is the afore-mentioned evidence of the susceptibility of this region to anoxic damage. Secondly, since PAH secreted by the proximal tubules during the control periods may also be concentrated by counter-current exchange in the loop of Henle system, it has probably a higher concentration here than anywhere else in the nephron system. Hence the diffusion gradient (lumen → interstitial space → vasa recta) would be greatest.

Histological studies seem to favor this conclusion. Although we have not yet had an opportunity to examine the kidney in our series histologically, based upon the work of LUCKÉ (7) and others, it has been found that although cloudy swelling occurs in the proximal tubules the most marked changes in the anuric kidney of shock occur in the ascending limb of Henle and the distal convoluted tubule, giving basis for the once popular designation "lower nephron nephrosis". Although not necessarily typical of the present acute experiments, in the chronic changes that occur in the anuric shock kidney it has been observed that tubulovenous and tubulo-interstitial rupture may actually occur. When these are seen, they are most frequent in the boundary zone of the medulla, where the thick ascending limb of Henle is in intimate relationship to the vasa recta. Since changes have not been seen in the thin segment of the loop of Henle, it may well be that the most susceptible part of the nephron system is the thick portion of the ascending limb.

The concept that back-diffusion of PAH and creatinine occurs might require that back-diffusion of H_2O must needs occur from the loop of Henle system. Actually, this does not appear to be a primary necessity, although it might facilitate the diffusion process.

Alternatively, it is possible that the negative extractions may simply reflect a wash-out of PAH, creatinine, Na, etc., concentrated in the vasa recta loops during the control periods by the mechanism explained by Dr. KRAMER.

In conclusion, the present work supports the hypothesis of the operation of a counter-current system in the canine kidney. Finally, like that of Dr. KRAMER, our work suggests the need for a re-evaluation of the pathogenesis and treatment of the shock kidney.

Summary
During oligemic shock in the dog, renal blood flow is markedly reduced but never ceases entirely, even though urine formation stops and renal clearances are zero. Negative extraction ratios of PAH and creatinine, and higher concentrations of sodium and potassium in renal venous blood compared to that in the arterial inflow, provide evidence of "washout" of the zone of hyperosmolarity in the medulla of the kidney during oligemic shock. Back diffusion from the lumen of the nephron is considered as another possible explanation for negative extraction ratios of PAH and creatinine.

References
1. SELKURT, E. E.: Amer. J. Physiol. 145, 699 (1946). — 2. INSULL. W. Jr., I. G. TILLOTSON and J. HAYMAN Jr.: Amer. J. Physiol. 163, 676 (1950). — 3. BLOCK, M. A., K. G. WAKIN and F. C. MANN: A. M. A. Arch. Path. (U. S. A.) 53, 437 (1952). — 4. KAHN, J. R., L. T. SKEGGS and N. P. SHUMWAY: Circulation (U. S. A.) 1, 445 (1950). — 5. MONTAGUE, F. E., and F. L. WILSON Jr.: Amer. J. Physiol. 159, 581 (1949). — 6. DANIEL, P. M., C. N. PEABODY and M. M. L. PRITCHARD: Quart. J. Exper. Physiol. (G. B.) 36, 199 (1951). — 7. LUCKÉ, B.: Mil. Surgeon (U. S. A.) 99, 371 (1946).

The participation of the adrenal glands in endotoxin shock

By

B. HÖKFELT, S. BYGDEMAN, and J. SEKKENES

The object of this paper is to present in summary fashion some data on hormone production by the adrenal medulla and the adrenal cortex under conditions of endotoxin shock. Consequently, we shall be dealing with catecholamines, on the one hand, and corticosteroids, including cortisol and aldosterone, on the other. During the past decade, physico-chemical methods have been worked out, allowing qualitative and quantitative analysis of both these categories of hormones in adrenal venous blood.

Material and methods

Acute experiments were performed in 22 normal, adult cats of both sexes, anaesthetised with Nembutal (35 mg./kg. i.p.). After heparinisation, a cannula was inserted in the left lumbo-adrenal vein, and 3 to 15 ml. of blood from the adrenal were collected intermittently for the determination of catecholamines, cortisol, and aldosterone. Between collection periods, the adrenal venous effluent was returned to the animal via the left femoral vein as described by SCHAPIRO and STJÄRNE (39). Peripheral blood was drawn from a cannula in the left femoral artery. Blood loss was continuously measured, and replaced by transfusion of either blood or 6 per cent dextran in saline. The blood samples were centrifuged immediately after collection, and the plasma divided into proper portions for the respective analytical procedures. To prevent destruction of catecholamines, the plasma for this determination was acidified with an equal volume of 1.5 per cent trichloroacetic acid; precipitated proteins were removed after centrifugation.

Blood pressure was recorded continuously from the right carotid artery, using a Statham pressure transducer and a Grass polygraph. The right jugular vein was used for injections.

Serial haematocrit determinations were made, and the secretion rates were calculated from the hormone concentrations and the plasma flow per minute.

For the estimation of catecholamines in the plasma (0.5—2 ml.) and adrenal tissue, the fluorimetric procedure of EULER and LISHAJKO (15) was applied.

Plasma cortisol (0.2 ml. of plasma for adrenal blood, 2 ml. for peripheral blood) was determined by the method of Silber and Porter (*40*), as modified by Peterson et al. (*36*). Aldosterone concentrations (4—6 ml. of plasma) were measured by a double isotope dilution derivative technique similar to that of Kliman and Peterson (*29*).

In order to investigate the capacity of the adrenals to produce steroid hormones following death in endotoxin shock, the cannulated adrenal from representative animals was sliced and incubated with 7-^{3}H-progesterone in Krebs-Ringer-bicarbonate solution with added glucose (200 mg. %) (*38*) for 2 hours under air at 37° C. The steroids were extracted, purified, and isolated by paper chromatography according to Neher (*33*). The position of the compounds was determined by UV absorption, as well as by radioactivity as indicated on a Baird-Atomic strip scanner. The specific activity of cortisol was determined by colorimetry after reduction with blue tetrazolium, and counting in a Packard Tri-Carb Scintillation spectrometer. The amounts of aldosterone were too small to allow colorimetric evaluation, but could be calculated on the basis of counts of the eluted aldosterone fraction, using the specific activity of cortisol as an index.

Endotoxin, derived from Proteus, was made up to contain 1 mg./ml. of saline; 0.1—1 mg./kg. was injected intravenously during approximately 15 seconds. A single injection of 0.5—0.6 mg./kg. usually resulted in death within 3 to 6 hours.

Results and discussion

Adrenal medulla. Fig. 1 shows the typical changes produced by a lethal dose of endotoxin on mean arterial blood pressure and adrenal plasma catecholamines in the cat. The general blood-pressure response was similar to that observed by others in the anaesthetised dog (*44*). Thus, there was an initial fall, followed by a return towards pre-injection levels, and then a gradual fall until death ensued. The hypotensive phases were associated with a definite reduction in adrenal blood flow but, despite this, the minute output of catecholamines increased markedly, both in the first and in the final hypotensive phase. During the normotensive period, catecholamine secretion fell, but always remained above pre-injection levels. As to the relative proportions of adrenaline and noradrenaline, the latter hormone was predominant in most samples in 3 out of 4 cats; towards the end of the experiments the relative proportion of adrenaline increased almost invariably.

The catecholamine concentration in the peripheral blood was repeatedly found to be too low to contribute significantly to the amounts demonstrated in the blood from the adrenal vein.

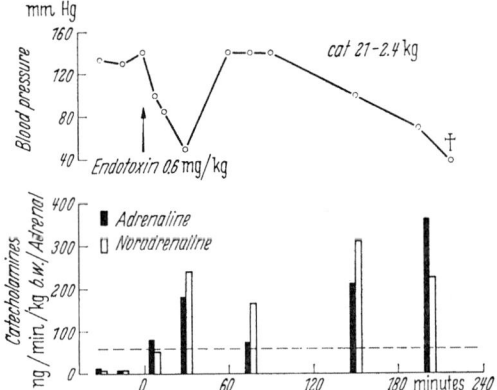

Fig. 1. Mean arterial blood pressure and adrenal plasma catecholamines following a lethal dose of endotoxin in the cat

An identical pattern of response for both blood pressure and catecholamines was also seen after smaller doses of endotoxin, doses which did not lead to death within an observation period of more than six hours (Fig. 2).

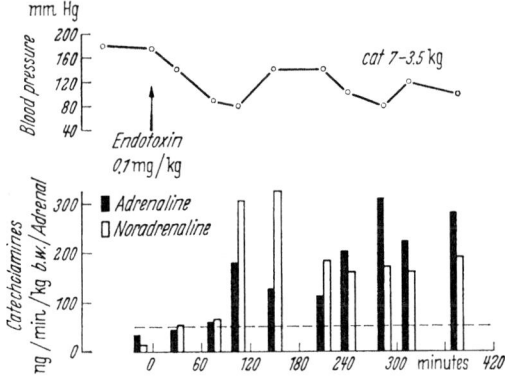

Fig. 2. Mean arterial blood pressure and adrenal plasma catecholamines following a non-lethal dose of endotoxin

Marked stimulation of the adrenal medulla following injection of endotoxin in the dog was reported by EGDAHL (13) and by NYKIEL and GLAVIANO (35). The increased catecholamine release was prevented by sectioning the splanchnic nerves (35), a finding which we have been able to confirm in the cat. Thus, adrenal stimulation in endotoxaemia involves a neurogenic mechanism. Direct stimulation of the gland by endotoxin per se, or products such as histamine (41) and potassium (37) released in the shocked animal, seems to be excluded.

In Egdahl's experiments, catecholamine production was not correlated to hypotension. Nykiel and Glaviano, on the other hand, found a rise in catecholamine secretion only in the presence of a significant decrease in arterial blood pressure. In view of the findings of Nykiel and Glaviano and ourselves, it seems reasonable to conclude that a baroceptor mechanism plays an important role in the catecholamine release occurring in endotoxin shock. This does not, however, exclude the possibility that other factors might also be active. Thus, for instance, it seems likely that with increasing anoxia, reflexes are initiated from carotid and aortic chemoreceptors, as well as from higher centres of the central nervous system (14).

After the injection of lethal doses of endotoxin in the rabbit, Heiffer et al. (25) recorded a blood-pressure response similar to that described above for the dog and the cat. During the initial blood-pressure fall, however, no increase in circulating catecholamines could be demonstrated, whereas elevated values were found during the following near-normotensive and the final hypotensive stage. In view of their findings, the authors discuss the possibility of a depression of the sympathetic nervous system, including the adrenal medulla, during the initial phases of endotoxin shock. To test this hypothesis, we compared in the same cat

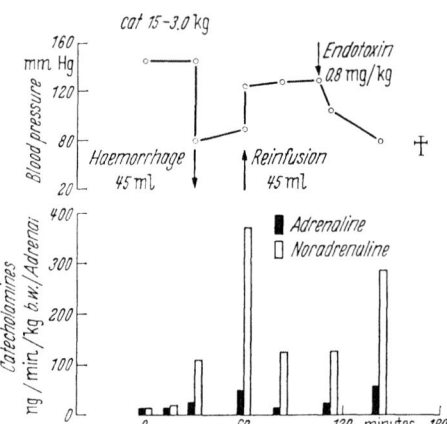

Fig. 3. Comparison of the changes in mean arterial blood pressure and adrenal plasma catecholamines produced by an acute haemorrhage and a lethal dose of endotoxin

the changes in catecholamine secretion following reduction of the blood pressure for 30 minutes by bleeding, with those induced during the first 30 minutes after endotoxin. As can be seen in

Fig. 3, the increase in catecholamine production is of the same order of magnitude under the two conditions. Similarly, hypotension as a result of acute haemorrhage approximately two hours after the injection of a lethal dose of endotoxin, evoked prompt stimulation of the adrenal medulla (Fig. 4), pointing to a highly efficient baroreflex mechanism.

As illustrated in Fig. 1, adrenal catecholamine secretion reaches maximal values in the terminal stage of endotoxin shock. This implies that the adrenal medulla and the neurogenic regulatory mechanisms involved continue to function

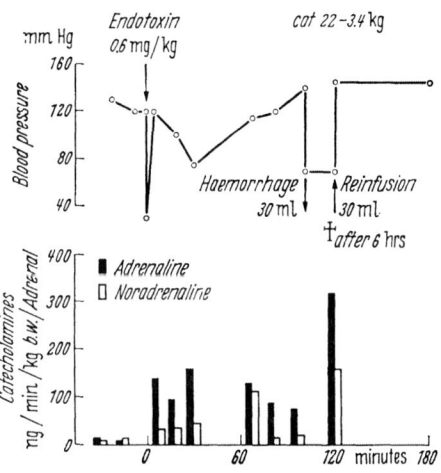

Fig. 4. Effect of acute bleeding on mean arterial blood pressure and adrenal catecholamine production in a cat pre-treated with a lethal dose of endotoxin

till death ensues. Identical findings have been reported in the terminal stage of haemorrhagic shock by WALKER et al. (42) and

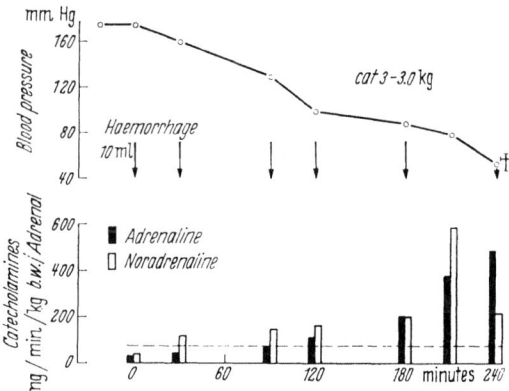

Fig. 5. Changes in mean arterial blood pressure and adrenal plasma catecholamines induced by repeated haemorrhages

GLAVIANO et al. (22), and are also demonstrated in Fig. 5. This figure may also serve to illustrate — although not very convincingly — that adrenal medullary stimulation might occur after a gradual decrease in blood volume before the arterial blood pressure reaches hypotensive levels. Several investigators (19, 43) have presented evidence showing that a dimunition in blood volume as such might induce stimulation of the adrenal medulla.

Following death in endotoxin shock, the adrenal tissue of the cat still contained adrenaline and noradrenaline in amounts not differing significantly from those in the controls (Table 1). This confirms earlier observations of the rapid resynthesis of adrenal medullary hormones in connection with increased release (28, 6, 7).

Table 1. *Adrenaline (A) and noradrenaline (N) in adrenal tissue μg./adrenal/kg. B. W.*

Operated controls		After lethal dose of endotoxin		
A	N	HRS	A	N
78	50	1	47	23
80	22	3	51	6
68	20	4	51	14
51	24	5	43	10
49	41	6	42	14
38	22	6	88	27

In the rabbit, depletion of adrenal catecholamines has been reported after lethal doses of endotoxin (25). It should, however, be emphasised that the adrenal medulla, even after depletion of its stored catecholamines, is still capable of producing considerable quantities of medullary hormones (7).

Adrenal cortex. Melby, Egdahl, and Spink have published a series of papers dealing with the effect of endotoxin on cortisol production and metabolism (30, 12, 13, 32). Measurement of cortisol in the effluent of the cannulated lumbo-adrenal vein in the unanaesthetised dog revealed that intravenous injection of endotoxin, in pyrogenic as well as lethal doses, produces a rapid increase in cortisol secretion. Adrenocortical secretory failure was never seen, but the response to exogenous ACTH was diminished after the administration of lethal doses. In this latter respect, endotoxin shock differs from haemorrhagic shock, in which the response of the adrenal cortex to exogenous ACTH has been found to be enhanced (27).

In some of our experiments (Table 2) the injection of endotoxin, even in lethal doses, evoked no increase in cortisol output. This lack of effect can almost certainly be explained on the basis of maximal cortisol secretion following the "stress" of adrenal-vein cannulation in the anaesthetised animal (26). In the last four animals, cortisol secretion rates tended to decline immediately prior to death. In view of this and of the afore-mentioned diminished response of the adrenal cortex to exogenous ACTH after endotoxin, it seemed of some interest to investigate the capacity of such adrenal tissue to produce cortisol *in vitro*. It can be seen that no difference existed in this respect between adrenals from control animals and those from endotoxin-treated cats. The

Table 2

Dose of endo-toxin mg./kg.	Adrenal cortisol secretion µg./min./kg. B.W.								Cortisol[1] after incu-bation
	Hrs after endotoxin								
	0	½	1	2	3	4	5	6	
0	0.7			0.8	0.8	1.0		1.3	3
0	1.6	1.7	1.0	1.5	1.3	1.0			5
0.2	0.8	1.1	1.0	1.0	1.1	1.1	1.1	1.0	6
0.5	1.4	1.2		1.3	1.5	[2]			10
0.6	1.3	1.6	1.3	1.7	0.9	[2]			2
0.7	1.0	1.5	0.9			0.9	0.3	[2]	9
0.8	1.6	1.0	1.0	[2]					7
1.0	1.7	1.0	[2]						4

[1] µg./100 mg. adrenal tissue/2 hrs
[2] Indicates death

possibility nevertheless remains that the adrenals *in vivo* might have had a decreased capacity to produce steroids, as a result of the severe anoxia occurring after administration of endotoxin. This would not have been revealed by the present incubation studies carried out under air supplying the necessary oxygen (*24*).

As to the mechanism whereby endotoxin leads to increased cortisol production, MELBY et al. (*32*) have shown that this effect is abolished by hypophysectomy. EGDAHL et al. (*12, 13*) have reported that endotoxin can cause stimulation of adrenocortical secretion in doses which exert no effect on body temperature, blood pressure, or catecholamine secretion. They suggest that endotoxin acts directly on the central nervous system to elicit ACTH release.

Mention should also be made of the fact that the high levels of cortisol demonstrated in the peripheral plasma after pyrogenic doses of endotoxin are entirely due to increased secretion from the adrenal gland (*32*). In the case of lethal doses of endotoxin, the high plasma levels of cortisol are to be ascribed partly to increased adrenal secretion and partly to retarded removal of cortisol from the plasma (*32*). Similar results were earlier obtained by MELBY and SPINK (*31*) in patients surviving shock due to infection as compared to those with fatal shock.

The secretion of aldosterone by the adrenal cortex seems to vary to a great extent in relation to haemodynamic changes in the body (*4, 5, 17*). Thus, increased aldosterone production has been shown to occur in the following 3 cases: after blood loss (*3, 16, 23*), after supradiaphragmatic constriction of the inferior vena cava, resulting in hepatic venous congestion (*2, 8, 34*), and in bilateral constriction of the common carotid (*20*).

In view of the fact that severe haemodynamic changes occur in endotoxin shock (*21*), it became of interest to determine how this condition would influence aldosterone secretion. Some of the results are presented in Table 3. In the non-injected control, no appreciable changes in aldosterone were observed. In one cat injected with a non-lethal dose of endotoxin and in two out of three cats given lethal doses, a marked increase in aldosterone was noted as hypotension developed. In the third cat, the pre-injection level of aldosterone was exceedingly high and was still high — as compared to the values in the other cats — 30 minutes after injection of endotoxin. The initial high level of aldosterone in this single cart might have been a transient response to cannulation of the adrenal vein *per se* (*10*).

Table 3

Dose mg./kg.	Adrenal aldosterone secretion (A) in ng./min.[1] and blood pressure (BP) after endotoxin							Aldosterone after incubation[2]
HRS	0	1/2	1	2	3	4	5	
0 A	25		24			28	31	150
BP	140		140			120	110	
0.2 A	19				20	43	45	—
BP	160				140	95	80	
0.5 A	21		47	66	51	3		330
BP	120		80	70	75			
0.8 A	22	71	20	3				410
BP	95	60	80					
1.0 A	118	66	3					230
BP	120	100						
	Haemorrhage Reinfusion					Haemorrhage		
0 A	17	77↑				19	70	
BP	150↓	70				145↓	75	

[1] ng. = 0.001 microgramme
[2] ng./100 mg. adrenal tissue/2 hrs
[3] Indicates death

The changes in aldosterone production as described occurred without corresponding changes in cortisol output, which might indicate that they were not initiated by ACTH. The same applies to the increase in aldosterone seen after haemorrhage (Table 3), which might be indicative of a common mechanism involved in the regulation of aldosterone secretion in haemorrhagic and endotoxin shock. There is a great deal of evidence that the raised aldosterone secretion following blood loss is regulated by a humoral mechanism. The studies of FARREL (*18*) indicate that such a factor originates in the head. One could speculate that the release of the presumed hormone might then be evoked either via the atrial stretch receptors, as described by ANDERSSON et al. (*1*), or via the receptors located at the thyro-carotid junction, and sensitive to changes in pulse pressure, as demonstrated by GANN et al. (*20*). However, recent experiments by DAVIS et al. (*9, 11*) indicate that haemorrhage is followed by a rise in aldosterone secretion in the decapitated dog as well. The authors have presented data which suggest a renal origin of an aldosterone-stimulating hormone.

On incubation, adrenals from cats expiring in endotoxin shock seemed to be able to synthesise aldosterone at least as efficiently as control adrenals. Thus, there is no evidence of an absolute aldosterone insufficiency under endotoxin shock, either on the basis of the aldosterone output in the adrenal vein or as judged by *in vitro* results.

Summary

The effect of endotoxin on the adrenal secretion of catecholamines, cortisol, and aldosterone has been studied in the cat, using physico-chemical procedures for hormone assays.

Lethal doses of endotoxin invariably induce increased secretion of adrenaline and noradrenaline. The catecholamine release is dependent on a neurogenic mechanism and seems, at least in part, to result from a fall in arterial blood pressure, implying involvement of baroceptors. This does not, however, exclude the participation of other mechanisms, such as chemo- and blood-volume receptors. The adrenal medulla continues to secrete large amounts of catecholamines in the terminal stage of endotoxin shock, and no evidence was obtained of a decreased reactivity of the sympathetic nervous system, including the adrenal medulla, during any phase of endotoxaemia.

In the anaesthetised cat, adrenal cortisol output is high — sometimes maximal — following cannulation of the adrenal vein and is either further elevated or not significantly altered during the first phase after the injection of a lethal dose of endotoxin; in the final stage, cortisol production tends to decrease. Aldosterone secretion, on the other hand, is usually not maximal initially and seems to increase significantly following injection of a lethal dose of endotoxin, possibly in relation to the development of hypotension. There was no evidence of absolute adrenocortical failure, either as regards cortisol or as regards aldosterone.

Acknowledgements

This work was supported by grants from the Swedish Medical Research Council and the Swedish National Association for the Control of Heart and Chest Diseases. We are grateful to Miss V. BRING, Mrs. M. GORDON, Mr. T. BORGE, and Mr. N. Å. PERSSON for their skilful technical assistance. The endotoxin used was kindly supplied by Dr. H. J. BEIN of CIBA Ltd., Basle.

References

1. ANDERSSON, C. H., M. McCALLY, and G. L. FARREL: Endocrinology (U. S. A.) **64**, 202 (1959). — 2. BALL, W. C., and J. O. DAVIS: Amer. J. Physiol. **191**, 339 (1957). — 3. BARTTER, F. C.: Scand. J. Clin. Laborat. Invest. **10**, 50 (1957). — 4. BARTTER, F. C., E. G. BIGLIERI, P. PRONOVE, and C. DELEA: In: Aldosterone: Report on Symposium, Geneva, June 1957. J. & A. Churchill (1958). — 5. BARTTER, F. C., I. H. MILLS, E. G. BIGLIERI, and C. DELEA: Recent Progr. Hormone Res. (U. S. A.) **15**, 311 (1959). — 6. BYGDEMAN, S., and U. S. v. EULER: Acta physiol. Scand. **44**, 375 (1958). — 7. BYGDEMAN, S., U. S. v. EULER, and B. HÖKFELT: Acta physiol. Scand. **49**, 21 (1960). — 8. DAVIS, J. O., M. M. PECHET, W. C. BALL, and M. J. GOODKIN: J. Clin. Invest. (U. S. A.) **36**, 689 (1957). — 9. DAVIS, J. O., C. CARPENTER, C. AYERS, and R. C. BAHN: Program, 42nd Endocrine Society Meeting, June 1960, p. 14. — 10. DAVIS, J. O., N. A. YANKOPOULOS, F. LIEBERMAN, J. E. HOLMAN, and R. C. BAHN: J. Clin. Invest. (U. S. A.) **39**, 765 (1960). — 11. DAVIS, J. O., C. C. J. CARPENTER, C. R. AYRES, J. E. HOLMAN, and R. C. BAHN: J. Clin. Invest. (U. S. A.) **40**, 684 (1961). — 12. EGDAHL, R. H., J. C. MELBY, and W. W. SPINK: Proc. Soc. Exper. Biol. Med. (U. S. A.) **101**, 369 (1959). — 13. EGDAHL, R. H.: J. Clin. Invest. (U. S. A.) **38**, 1120 (1959). — 14. EULER, U. S. v., and B. FOLKOW: Naunyn-Schmiedebergs Arch. exper. Path. (G.) **219**, 242 (1953). — 15. EULER, U. S. v., and F. LISHAJKO: Acta physiol. Scand. **51**, 348 (1961). — 16. FARREL, G. L., R. S. ROSNAGLE, and W. E. RAUSCHKOLB: Circulation Res. **4**, 606 (1956). — 17. FARREL, G. L.: Physiol. Rev. (U. S. A.) **38**, 709 (1958). — 18. FARREL, G. L.: Endocrinology (U. S. A.) **65**, 239 (1959). — 19. FOWLER, N. O., R. SHABETAI, and J. C. HOLMES: Circulation Res. (U. S. A.) **9**, 427 (1961). — 20. GANN, D. S., I. H. MILLS, and F. C. BARTTER: Fed. Proc. (U. S. A.) **19**, 605 (1960). — 21. GILBERT, R. P.: Physiol. Rev. (U. S. A.) **40**, 245 (1960). — 22. GLAVIANO, V. V., N. BASS, and F. NYKIEL: Circulation Res. (U. S. A.) **8**, 564 (1960). — 23. GOODKIND, M. J., W. C. BALL, and J. O. DAVIS: Amer. J. Physiol. **189**, 181 (1957). — 24. HAYANO, M., N. SABA, R. I. DORFFMAN, and O. HECHTOR: Recent Progr. Hormone Res. (U. S. A.) **12**, 79 (1956). — 25. HEIFFER, H. H., R. L. MUNDY, and B. MEHLMAN: Amer. J. Physiol. **198**, 1307 (1960). — 26. HILTON, J. G., D. C. WEAVER, G. MUELHEIMS, V. V. GLAVIANO, and R. WEGRIA: Amer. J. Physiol. **192**, 525 (1958). — 27. HUME, D. M., and D. H. NELSON: Surg. Forum (U. S. A.) **5**, 568 (1955). — 28. HÖKFELT, B., and J. McCLEAN: Acta physiol. Scand. **21**, 258 (1950). — 29. KLIMAN, B., and R. E. PETERSON: J. Biol. Chem. (U. S. A.) **235**, 1639 (1960). — 30. MELBY, J. C., R. H. EGDAHL, and W. W. SPINK: Fed. Proc. (U. S. A.) **16**, 425 (1957). — 31. MELBY, J. C., and W. W. SPINK: J. Clin. Invest. (U. S. A.) **37**, 1791 (1958). — 32. MELBY, J. C., R. H. EGDAHL, and W. W. SPINK: J. Laborat. Clin. Med. (U. S. A.) **56**, 50 (1960). — 33. NEHER, R.: An International Symposium on Aldosterone. p. 11. London: J. & A. Churchill Ltd. 1958. — 34. NEHER, R., and A.

WETTSTEIN: J. Clin. Invest. (U. S. A.) 35, 800 (1956). — 35. NYKIEL, F., and
V. V. GLAVIANO: J. Appl. Physiol. (U. S. A.) 16, 348 (1961). — 36. PETERSON,
R. E., A. KARRER and S. L. GUERRA: Analyt. Chem. (U. S. A.) 29,
144 (1957). — 37. RAPELA, C. E.: Rev. Soc. argent. biol. 24, 1 (1948). —
38. SAFFRAN, M., and A. V. SCHALLY: Endocrinology (U. S. A.) 56, 523
(1955). — 39. SCHAPIRO, S., and L. STJÄRNE: Proc. Soc. Exper. Biol.
Med. (U. S. A.) 99, 414 (1958). — 40. SILBER, R. H., and C. C. PORTER:
J. Biol. Chem. (U. S. A.) 210, 923 (1954). — 41. SPINK, W. W., and J. A.
VICK: Proc. Soc. Exper. Biol. Med. (U. S. A.) 106, 242 (1961). — 42. WALKER,
W. F., M. S. ZILELI, F. W. REUTER, W. C. SHOEMAKER, D. FRIEND, and
F. D. MOORE: Amer. J. Physiol. 197, 773 (1959). — 43. WALKER, W. F.,
W. C. SHOEMAKER, A. J. KAALSTAD, and F. D. MOORE: Amer. J. Physiol.
197, 781 (1959). — 44. WEIL, M. H., L. D. MACLEAN, M. B. VISSCHER, and
W. W. SPINK: J. Clin. Invest. (U. S. A.) 35, 1191 (1956).

Aldosterone and alterations in circulatory reactivity following endotoxins

By

H. J. BEIN

The pituitary-adrenocortical system and the sympathetic nervous system with the adrenal medulla are involved in the adaptation of the organism to any form of injury, including responses to endotoxins. Changes in the concentrations of corticosteroids and catecholamines in response to an endotoxin have been noted (for references see *4, 5, 6, 8, 9, 10, 12*). However, it is not yet known to what extent the fluctuations observed in the concentrations of the adrenal hormones are directly responsible for the consequences and course of endotoxin intoxication.

Though the mechanism of action of endotoxins is probably far more complex than is generally assumed, it is nevertheless possible to use the effects of endotoxin on definite physiological systems as a tool in testing possible antagonisms. On this basis, a number of investigators have shown that certain corticosteroids are capable of affording protection against death due to endotoxin [see e. g. ABERNATHY and SPINK (1957), TAUBER and GARSON (1958), MELBY et al. (1959)]. But whereas it had usually been assumed that only hydrocortisone and derivatives with similar pharmacological properties were effective in this respect, it now appears that the other genuine corticosteroid, namely aldosterone, is also able to afford protection (BEIN and JAQUES, 1960). In various species (regardless as to whether or not the animals are anaesthetised) and against various toxins, the doses required in the case of aldosterone are much smaller than for hydrocortisone or prednisolone (*2*). As noted in the case of other corticosteroids as well, the doses of aldosterone affording protection against death are much higher than the amounts secreted by the adrenal veins under the influence of endotoxins (HÖKFELT, 1961). Experiments in which endotoxin is administered in one single lethal dose therefore require doses of corticosteroids exceeding physiological amounts. Of course, such experimental conditions are not representative of endotoxin liberation as normally encountered, nor can they

imitate the hormone production which occurs in response to endotoxin poisoning. Nevertheless, it is interesting to note that, with
single doses of aldosterone, animals can be protected against
massive endotoxin inundation which would otherwise have proved
fatal and that such protection can even be achieved when the
aldosterone is given not prior to the endotoxin, but afterwards, i. e.
up to 1 hour later (2).

In experiments on anaesthetised cats, aldosterone not only
affords protection against death due to endotoxin but — in contrast
to other corticosteroids — it also restores reactivity towards
endogenous pressor amines after this reactivity has been altered
under the influence of endotoxins (2).

The experiments to be described here were carried out on
anaesthetised cats (Dial CIBA 30 mg./kg. i. p. and 30 mg./kg. s. c.)
and dogs (morphine 0.25 mg./kg. s. c., urethan 0.75 g./kg. p. o.).

As frequently reported in the relevant literature, the arterial
pressure drops after intravenous administration of endotoxin. In
the majority of experiments with cats, the arterial pressure — following an intravenous dose of endotoxin — shows a sharp drop
which is generally of only short duration; it then rises again and
finally declines slowly once more. Sometimes, between the injection
of endotoxin and the primary fall in blood pressure, there is a latent
period which may exceed one minute. In a few animals the pronounced primary drop in pressure does not occur, and circulation
may suddenly collapse after a latent period of 1 to $1^{1}/_{2}$ hours.
Primary respiratory failure as a cause is very unlikely, since death
cannot be prevented by artificial respiration.

As borne out by reports in the literature, dogs are usually much
less susceptible to endotoxins than cats; furthermore, most of them
show pronounced and early tachyphylaxis. This was also the case
with the endotoxins used by us, which were of the polysaccharide
type obtained from Proteus[1]. Whereas all cats died after approximately 1 to 2 hours, the anaesthetised dogs survived the observation time of 6 to 8 hours, even when we injected more than 10 times
the lethal dose for cats. In spite of this species difference, both cats
and dogs showed changed circulatory reactions towards adrenaline
and noradrenaline under the influence of endotoxin, which seems
to indicate a common denominator.

In the cat, the rise in blood pressure due to noradrenaline is
diminished and may even be abolished.

---

[1] I should like to express my thanks to Dr. F. W. KAHNT for his kindness
in supplying the endotoxins used in our experiments.

In some cases this occurs as rapidly as 5—10 minutes after
administration of the endotoxin (see Fig. 1), whereas in certain
other cases a latent period of more than $^1/_2$ to 1 hour is observed.
The loss of reactivity towards noradrenaline is not due to general
unresponsiveness of the blood vessels, as it may occur at a moment
when reactivity towards hypertensin shows hardly any decrease
(Fig. 1). When the dose of noradrenaline is increased, hyporeactivity
can be overcome at this stage of intoxication, and the blood pressure
will rise again.

mm Hg

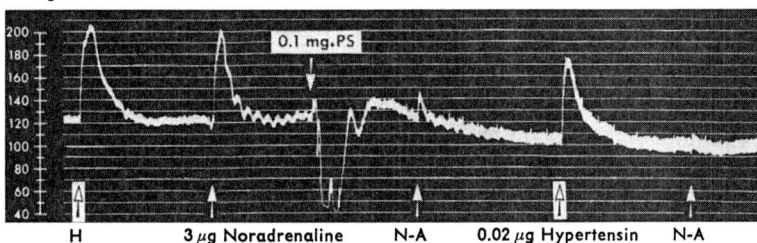

Fig. 1. Cat. Blood pressure, measured by means of a mercury manometer in the right carotid
artery. Inhibition of the pressor response to i. v. adrenaline (N—A, 3 μg./kg. i. v.) after 0.1 mg./
kg. i. v. Proteus endotoxin (PS). The blood pressure effect of 0.02 μg./kg. i. v. hypertensin (H)
is diminished to a far lesser extent. The doses of noradrenaline and hypertensin chosen were
such as to have approximately the same effect on the blood pressure before injection of the
endotoxin. Time indicated in units of 1 min

The effect of adrenaline is also modified by endotoxins in a most
typical manner in that an actual reversal of blood pressure takes
place (Fig. 2). In some experiments this phenomenon could be
observed almost immediately after the endotoxin injection; in
other experiments it developed only after a considerable latent
period (more than $^1/_2$ to 1 hour). The development of this phenomenon is independent of the height of the arterial blood pressure;
it also occurs despite artificial respiration.

As with noradrenaline, the quantitative angle also plays a
significant role. As a rule the dose used was 2 or 3 μg./kg. i.v.
adrenaline, a dose which in most experiments leads to an increase
in pressure which is always reversed by the endotoxin. When
higher doses of adrenaline are employed — e. g. 10 μg./kg. i. v. — reversal may occur after a longer latent period than with smaller
doses, or may even be absent altogether.

The mechanisms underlying the reversal of the action of adrenaline on the blood pressure and the diminution in the action of
noradrenaline observed in response to endotoxins are anything
but clear from a pharmacological point of view. Although these

effects bear some resemblance to those of a sympathicolytic, there is no proof that the action of the endotoxin can be regarded as identical with that of a real sympathicolytic. Obviously, special experimental conditions are required.

In the cat the toxic effect of the endotoxin and its influence on the activity of adrenaline are weaker when chloralose instead of

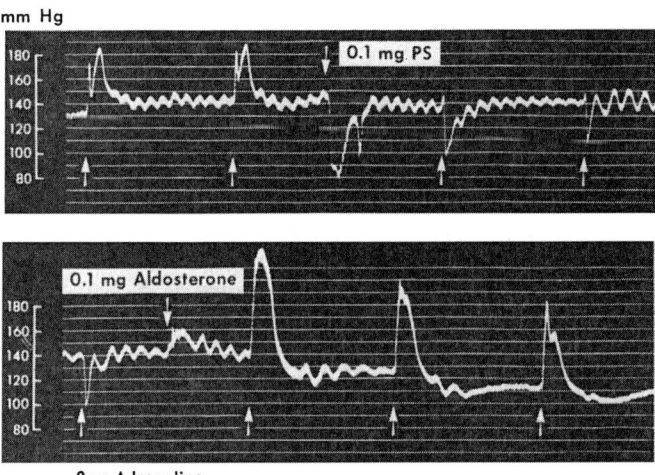

Fig. 2. Cat. Blood pressure (same technique as in Fig. 1). Reversal of the pressor response to adrenaline, 2 μg./kg. i. v., after i. v. administered Proteus endotoxin (0.1 mg./kg. PS).Following aldosterone, the pressor response to adrenaline is in this experiment immediately restored. Time indication see Fig. 1

Dial is used for the anaesthesia or when the experiments are carried out on spinal cats. A diminution in the pyrogenic effect of endotoxins in chloralose anaesthesia has incidentally already been described earlier (7). It may be that the endotoxin acts indirectly by involving other systems in the body or that Dial reinforces the effect of the endotoxin.

After pre-treatment with reserpine (1 mg./kg. s. c. daily for three days, and 3 mg./kg. s. c. on the day of the experiment) no inhibition of the rise in blood pressure due to adrenaline and noradrenaline occurs following administration of the endotoxin — but, instead, an additional sensitisation. The action of the endotoxin may possibly depend on the presence of catecholamines, since the storages should be depleted by the reserpine pre-treatment; on the other hand, it may also be that some blocking action of reserpine on the nervous system plays the more important role.

Aldosterone not only affords protection against death due to endotoxin, but one may say that it also normalises the action of noradrenaline and adrenaline on the blood pressure which has been altered by the endotoxin. Its full effect may either develop only after a latent period or — in other experiments — very rapidly (Fig. 2). In this connection, it is not necessary that the pressure reduced by the endotoxin should also be "normalised" by aldosterone. In our experiments, the influence of aldosterone on the blood pressure proved completely inconsistent; sometimes the pressure rose, sometimes it showed no significant change, and occasionally it actually declined in response to aldosterone.

We do not yet know which of the many factors determining the arterial blood pressure is the one basically affected by the endotoxin and by aldosterone. As the blood flow through a peripheral vessel is altered by the endotoxin and restored by aldosterone, we can assume that both compounds may affect the function of the peripheral vessels directly. However, it might be that an action is also exerted on the heart.

The increase in the blood flow through the femoral vein, which is typical following such small doses of adrenaline in the cat as

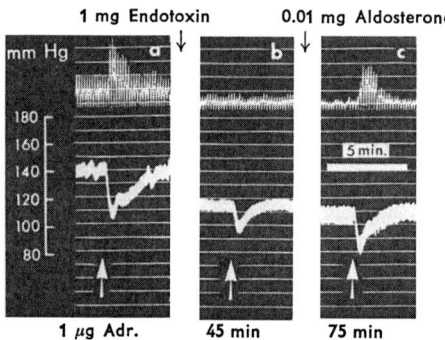

Fig. 3. Dog. Blood pressure in the right carotid artery (Hg manometer, lower tracing) and blood flow through the left femoral vein, recorded with the aid of a photo-electric drop counter[1] (upper tracing). The increase in flow following low doses of adrenaline (1 μg./kg. i. v.) is suppressed after endotoxin (1 mg./kg. i. v.), but reappears after aldosterone (10 μg./kg. i. v.). a) Before, b) 45 min. and c) 75 min. after endotoxin

well as in the dog, disappears after the administration of endotoxin but reappears after aldosterone (Fig. 3). In order to exclude as far as possible any reactions due simply to changes in pressure,

[1] I should like to take this opportunity to thank Dr. H. H. WAGENER for constructing the blood flow meter.

we used — in contrast to the experiments reported before — doses of adrenaline which had a small and invariably lowering effect on arterial pressure. The effect of aldosterone on the peripheral blood flow itself is quite as inconsistent as its effect on the arterial blood pressure, i.e. the blood flow after being diminished by the endo-toxin does not necessarily increase again in response to aldosterone. This clearly proves that the vascular reactivity of the dog is also changed by the endotoxin and restored by aldosterone, though the blood pressure raising effect of adrenaline is diminished to a far lesser extent than in the cat.

We could not observe a similar restoration of circulatory re-actions with prednisolone as is the case with aldosterone. In spite of prophylactic treatment with prednisolone in doses that afford protection against death due to endotoxin, reversal of the action of adrenaline nevertheless occurs. Thus, aldosterone and predni-solone differ from each other also with regard to their anti-endo-toxic activity. The fact that prednisolone, like aldosterone, pro-longs the survival time after administration of the endotoxin without changing the blood pressure reaction chosen as test object, indicates that the altered reactivity towards adrenaline and nor-adrenaline cannot, or at least cannot primarily, be the cause of death due to endotoxin, but that the altered reactivity is only one facet of the action of endotoxins. It is therefore clear that the importance of the alteration in the reactivity of the circulatory system towards catecholamines during endotoxin poisoning — whether it take the form of a diminution or an enhancement — must be generally re-examined.

Finally, efforts should be made to determine to what extent the known pharmacological properties of corticosteroids participate in their anti-toxic activity. Since aldosterone has no anti-inflamma-tory action, nor does it delay the healing of wounds (3), these particular properties can hardly be decisive.

In the course of systematic screening, other steroids with an activity similar to that of aldosterone have been found. This applies for instance to 19-oxo-progesterone, which has the following chemical formula:

According to findings made by P. A. DESAULLES[1], this steroid has neither anti-inflammatory nor salt-retaining effects, so that these two actions do not seem to be a primary requisite for prolongation of the survival time after endotoxin administration in cats or for normalisation of the reactivity of the circulatory system towards catecholamines. The anti-toxic action of steroids may thus be regarded as a pharmacological action *per se*.

Summary

1. In the anaesthetised cat, lethal doses of bacterial endotoxins cause an alteration in reactivity towards adrenaline and noradrenaline which is restored by aldosterone but not by hydrocortisone or prednisolone.
2. Similarly, in the anaesthetised dog aldosterone normalises vascular effects of adrenaline which have been altered by the endotoxin.
3. Reference is made to certain of the experimental prerequisites upon which the changed circulatory reactivity of adrenaline and noradrenaline following lethal doses of endotoxin was found to depend.
4. The anti-toxic action of corticosteroids can probably be regarded as a pharmacological property *per se*, since steroids exerting no anti-inflammatory or salt-retaining activity have been found which in the anaesthetised cat behave similarly to aldosterone.

Acknowledgements

My warmest thanks are due to Mr. C. SCHMID for his most accurate technical aid.

References

1. ABERNATHY, R. S., and W. W. SPINK: Proc. Soc. Exper. Biol. Med. (U. S. A.) 95, 580 (1957). — 2. BEIN, H. J., and R. JAQUES: Experientia (Switz.) 16, 24 (1960). — 3. DESAULLES, P. A., W. SCHULER, and R. MEIER: Experientia (Switz.) 11, 68 (1955). — 4. HEIFFER, M. H., R. L. MUNDY, and B. MEHLMAN: Amer. J. Physiol. 198, 1307 (1960). — 5. HÖKFELT, B.: See the present volume, p. 151. — 6. MANGER, W. M., J. L. BOLLMAN, F. T. MAHER, and J. BERKSON: Amer. J. Physiol. 190, 310 (1957). — 7. MEIER, R., H. J. BEIN, and R. JAQUES: Internat. Arch. Allergy (Switz.) 11, 101 (1957). — 8. MELBY, J. C., I. C. BOSSENMAIER, R. H. EGDAHL, and W. W. SPINK: Lancet (G. B.) 1959/I, 441. — 9. NYKIEL, F., and V. V. GLAVIANO: J. Appl. Physiol. (U. S. A.) 16, 348 (1961). — 10. PEKKARINEN, A.: The Biochemical Response to Injury. p. 217. Oxford: Blackwell 1960. — 11. TAUBER, H., and W. GARSON: Proc. Soc. Exper. Biol. Med. (U. S. A.) 97, 886 (1958). — 12. WALTON, R. P., J. A. RICHARDSON, R. P. WALTON JR., and W. L. THOMPSON: Amer. J. Physiol. 197, 223 (1959).

---

[1] I should like to express my sincere thanks to Dr. P. A. DESAULLES for giving me permission to mention his results.

Discussion

ADAMS-RAY: I would like to create some more confusion and perhaps introduce some new rays in the rainbow of catecholamines. Several years ago, our chairman indicated that there must be catechol cells outside the adrenal medulla, and he actually found them in the prostate.

Much aided by his interest and encouragement, NORDENSTAM and I[1] found cells in the human skin giving a chromaffin reaction. This (slide) is one of them with the protrusions filled with *colourless* granules, giving fluorescence in U.V. light an a positive ferri-ferricyanide reaction[2]. We have some indications that these cells contain vasoconstrictor substances. They do not stain in inflammatory vasodilated red skin, especially after X-ray treatment. In electron-microscopic studies[3], they were found to be lying in close contact with the smooth muscle cell and with unmyelinated nerve fibres. The ultrastructure of the granules closely resembles that of the granules of the adrenal medulla.

Preliminary results of incubation with dopa indicate that, as the cells of adrenal medulla, they are then easier to demonstrate.

The skin being difficult to study because of its content of other granulated cells and nerves, we — BLOOM, VON EULER, LISHAJKO, RITZÉN, ÖSTLUND, and myself[4]—have looked into the heart of *Myxine glutinosa* which contains a very large amount of catecholamines but no nerves or mast cells. It has been possible to show that there is a great quantity of these cells in the heart, that the granules contain catecholamines which can be liberated by reserpine, and that the granules have the same ultrastructure as those of the adrenal medulla.

HOWARD: I should like briefly to confirm some of the observations made by Dr. BEIN relative to the potential value of aldosterone in the treatment of septic shock. In our laboratory, septic shock has been produced in the cat under Dial-urethane anaesthesia (BONDOC, BESKID, WOLFERTH). A standard experiment was developed utilising in respective experiments 10 mg./kg. of heat-killed Proteus or 2.5 mg./kg. of *E. coli* endotoxin (Difco) intravenously. These doses were selected as producing death in 100% of cats in 6—16 hours. A dose of aldosterone (0.1 mg./kg.) was selected as being the largest amount that in itself produced no fatality in the cat. The aldosterone was given as a single intravenous injection 30 minutes after the bacterial insult.

Aldosterone was found to lengthen survival time (16 hours to 9 days) after infusion of Proteus. The ultimate mortality rate remained 100%. Following infusion of *E. coli* endotoxin, aldosterone resulted in an ultimate survival rate of 46%. Those cats which did not survive died after a lapse of 18 hours to 4 days.

[1] ADAMS-RAY, J., and H. NORDENSTAM: Lyon chir. 52, 125 (1956).

[2] ADAMS-RAY, J., G. BLOOM, and M. RITZÉN: Acta morph. Neerl. Scand. 2, 131 (1960).

[3] RHODIN, J., J. ADAMS-RAY, and H. NORDENSTAM: Zschr. Zellforsch. (G.) 49, 275 (1959).

[4] BLOOM, G., E. ÖSTLUND, U. VON EULER, F. LISHAJKO, and M. RITZÉN: Acta physiol. Scand. (in press.)

NICKERSON: Dr. BEIN is opening a Pandora's box with the pressor and depressor responses to adrenaline and noradrenaline, because the responses in the intact cardiovascular system are so complex. Comparing the dose-response curves for both adrenaline and noradrenaline in rabbits before and after endotoxin, we found only potentiation of the pressor responses. The difference might be in the species or the dosage. We employed sublethal doses of endotoxin. The picture is complicated also by the fact that the blood-pressure records he has shown indicate an inhibitory effect of endotoxin on alpha-receptors, whereas the blood-flow measurements indicate an inhibitory effect on beta-receptors, which would give just the opposite effect on blood pressure. The only experiments which we have on a relatively simplified system, isolated aorta strips, show only sensitisation to catecholamines by endotoxin. This does not occur if the exposure to endotoxin is in a simple salt solution; but in the presence of whole blood or blood cells, endotoxin clearly potentiates responses to adrenaline.

SPINK: I would like to put a question to Dr. HÖKFELT. How soon after injection of endotoxin can you detect a rise in the blood concentration of catecholamines? This relates to our findings on the mechanism of endotoxin shock that I shall discuss in more detail shortly. Within a very few minutes after the injection of endotoxin we have found a rise in the blood histamine in the dog and in the monkey. The information on your slides suggested that the rise in catecholamines was not detected until 30 minutes after the injection of endotoxin. As a matter of fact, it is not unlikely that several humoral factors make their appearance after the injection of endotoxin, including serotin, histamine, and the catecholamines. All of these probably play some role in the vascular activity that takes place after the administration of endotoxin.

HÖKFELT: Figure 4 illustrates a fact which I did not mention in my paper. In the cat, the rapid injection of a lethal dose of endotoxin is followed — within a minute or so — by a very marked but transient drop in blood pressure. As can be seen, adrenal venous blood collected in immediate connection with this event shows a pronounced increase in catecholamine output. If I am not mistaken, this occurs at the time when histamine is supposed to be released, and the increased catecholamine secretion at this time could therefore be due to the liberation of histamine.

In order to find out a little more about the mechanism involved in this transient "pre-initial" blood-pressure fall, we performed the following experiment. A rapid fall in blood pressure was induced by haemorrhage, and then the level was restored within a minute or two by reinfusion of the blood. When the adrenal catecholamine output was then measured, no change could be observed as compared to the pre-haemorrhage values. Thus, it seems possible that histamine or a similar substance is involved in the catecholamine release immediately following the injection of endotoxin. At all events, the adrenal medulla shows a rapid, marked response after endotoxin.

BEIN: I think that the differences observed as between Dr. NICKERSON and myself may depend entirely on the dose of endotoxin; whereas doses which do not provoke the death of animals may enhance the action of adrenaline, we have always used doses of endotoxin which killed the animals. We have also observed a diminution in the blood-pressure response towards adrenaline in rabbits after lethal doses of endotoxin.

In the course of this meeting it has frequently been stated that endotoxin is in one way or another connected with adrenaline and histamine; however, endotoxin liberates a variety of other substances as well, such as slow-reacting substances, etc. All these reaction products may change the substrates, so that the reactivity of the latter may be altered in consequence.

JAQUES and I have not found any significant change in the action of histamine on the blood pressure or on the blood flow through the femoral vessels. We found the same to be true for the action of serotonin, except when serotonin caused a rise in blood pressure which was then subsequently abolished, i. e. similar to the blood-pressure rise after adrenaline.

HALPERN: Assuming that endotoxin behaves as a histamine releaser, it is a very peculiar one if it really releases histamine in such a short time. An important histamine releaser like 48/80, when injected intravenously into an animal, requires about 60—120 seconds before one can see the first effect on the blood pressure and before histamine appears in the circulation. Therefore the mechanism of the release of histamine by endotoxin, if such a release does in fact occur, must presumably be quite different as compared with that of the typical and classical histamine releasers.

UVNÄS: I should have said something similar to what you did, Dr. HALPERN. I wonder if we really know what we are talking about when we discuss endotoxin. I think we are dealing with agents from different bacteria which therefore may have different actions. Moreover, I suppose that the animal species also vary in their reponses to endotoxin. Some years ago, I investigated an endotoxin preparation as regards its histamine-liberating properties in rat mast cells. This endotoxin preparation had no effect at all on these cells.

HÖKFELT: As to the remark by Dr. UVNÄS concerning the delay in catecholamine release after histamine, may I again point out that the rapid, transient blood-pressure fall after endotoxin does not appear immediately after the injection, but only after a minute or two.

Reflex mechanisms and the central nervous system

By

E. NEIL

The cardiovascular system in the resting body normally operates under tonic restraint, reflexly engendered from sensory endings situated in the systemic arterial walls, in the walls of the cardiac chambers and the great veins. The nature of this reflex restraint has been most fully documented by experiments which make use of the accessibility of the carotid sinus, the anatomy of which permits its vascular isolation and perfusion. The characteristics of the reflex cardiovascular responses obtained by altering local conditions in the innervated carotid sinus are qualitatively similar to those which may be obtained (with more difficulty) by selective alteration of the local circumstances in the other systemic arterial mechanoreceptor areas, viz: the aortic arch, the root of the right subclavian artery, and in parts of the common carotid artery itself. Correspondingly the effects of altering conditions in the carotid bifurcation detailed below can be taken as approximately representative of the systemic arterial mechanoreceptor reflexes as a whole.

Vascular isolation of the innervated carotid sinus permits us to alter the mean perfusion pressure, the pulse pressure and the rate of pulsation at will. A rise of perfusion pressure causes: (1) a fall of systemic pressure, (2) some cardiac slowing, (3) some fall of cardiac output, (4) some decrease of arteriolar resistance, and (5) some increase of venous capacity. A fall of sinus perfusion pressure produces the opposite effects on the circulation. Such cardio-vascular changes are chiefly the result of synaptic connections between the central ends of the sinus nerve fibres and the neurones of the medullary centres. Thus, sinus nerve stimulation causes an inhibition of the medullary vasomotor centre, which is reflected in a decreased discharge of thoracolumbar sympathetic fibres. As these sympathetic fibres supply both the heart (on which they exert both chronotropic and inotropic effects) and the systemic arterioles and veins (on which they exert a tonic vasoconstrictor effect) it is simple to understand that the arterial blood pressure is reflexly depressed by sinus nerve stimulation. In the past, measurements of cardiac output in these circumstances have been relatively few and have been of doubtful accuracy. In the last decade, however, convincing evidence has accrued that sinus nerve stimulation causes a fall of cardiac output. As the arterial blood pressure is mainly governed by the cardiac output and the arteriolar resistance, a change of blood pressure may be brought about by either or both of these factors. Previously the sinus reflex response was identified as wholly due to a change in the arteriolar resistance. Nowadays it is acknowledged that changes in venous capacity and cardiac output make a notable contribution to the cardiovascular response to sinus reflexes.

The cardio-inhibitory centre in the medulla is probably identical with the dorsal motor nucleus of the vagus. It is stimulated reflexly by the sinus nerve afferents; most of the cardiac slowing evoked in sinus reflexes occurs via this mechanism.

Mechanoreceptors are found in the adventitia of the sinus wall. They are responsive to deformation; the deformation which they ordinarily experience is provoked as a pulsatile expansion of the vessel wall by the systolic ejection of the heart. Indeed, if this normal expansion be prevented by enclosing the sinus in a rigid cast, changes of intraluminal pressure themselves cause no activity of the sinus nerve endings. Abnormal forms of deformation of the sinus wall, such as can be produced by external mechanical stimulation, by tugging of the carotid artery or by the topical application of vasoconstrictor drugs, will of course also prove effective in provoking extra activity from these mechanoreceptors. Impulse activity can be recorded by placing the sinus nerve on electrodes; a salvo of impulses occurs with each pulse beat. The frequency pattern and duration of these bursts depends not only on the mean blood pressure level but also, as might be expected from knowledge of the behaviour of other mechanoreceptors, on the rate and amplitude of the pulse pressure. If the degree of pulsation be reduced in the sinus segment by incorporating an air reservoir in the perfusion circuit, two notable changes occur even though the mean perfusion pressure has remained unaltered: (1) the number of fibres discharging decreases; (2) the peak frequency with which each unit discharges is lessened. These results are of importance in interpreting the circulatory responses to mild but continued bleeding. It is well known that an experimental animal or a patient submitted to operation may maintain the same level of mean arterial blood pressure despite the inevitable blood loss which such procedures entail. It is also well documented that cardiac acceleration and vasoconstriction of the gut and skin aid the maintenance of the mean systemic blood pressure despite the progressive decline of the cardiac output which occurs in these circumstances. As the mean arterial blood pressure has not altered, one cannot account for reflex tachycardia and vasoconstriction by considering the *mean* blood pressure as the sole stimulus of the mechanoreceptors. However, the reduction in pulse pressure which inevitably results from even mild bleeding leads to a more sparse discharge from the mechanoreceptors; this in turn causes reflex tachycardia which further reduces the pulse pressure. Owing to these changes the mean blood pressure may be maintained, although deepening pallor and an ever-accelerating heart rate should warn the experienced anaesthetist that the circulatory reserves are being encroached upon. Naturally *all* the cardiovascular mechanoreceptors participate in this reflex adjustment of the cardiovascular system, for all of them are sensitive to deformation occasioned by the phasic action of the heart.

When haemorrhage is more profound, resulting in an obvious fall of mean blood pressure, these reflex adjustments are intensified. Although the mean pressure does fall, it shows less change than does that of a similar animal, whose buffer nerves have been sectioned, which is subjected to the same procedure in terms of blood loss. Correspondingly the heart and brain of the "intact" animal submitted to bleeding enjoy a better pressure head of blood supply which enables them to function more efficiently in the circumstances. The reflex mechanism presumably serves an emergency purpose; less vital parts of the circulation are temporarily shut down — thus the blood supply of skin and gut is reduced. Herein may lie one of the problems of irreversible haemorrhagic shock, for one organ which serves a vital function in metabolism and in detoxication is the liver. Profound vasoconstriction of the splanchnic bed must have a particularly deleterious effect on the liver, which receives the majority of its blood and oxygen supply from the portal vein. The portal circulation possesses two sets of resistance vessels which are constricted in these conditions; the reduction in portal flow may well account for the failure of the liver to dissimilate lactate and other unwanted metabolites.

It must be clearly understood that the maintenance of vasoconstriction in sustained hypotension is dependent upon the continued viability of the vasomotor centre. There is little evidence, however, that vasomotor failure is responsible for the state of shock. The electrical stimulation of afferent pressor nerves (such as the chemoreceptor afferents) evokes definite rises of the systemic blood pressure until the end. Indeed, it is arguable that the state of arteriolar vasoconstriction, so beneficial in an emergency in helping to sustain the blood pressure, becomes an arrant nuisance in long-standing states of hypovolaemic hypotension by throttling the nutrient supply to tissues such as the liver and the kidneys. The role of the baroreceptors in inhibiting mesencephalic reticular structures is perhaps worthy of mention. KOCH was the first to note that hypertension in the vascularly isolated carotid sinus of an unanaesthetised dog provoked a behavioural reaction similar to sleep. Later experiments by DELL showed that the baroreceptor afferents depressed the activity of the ascending reticular formation at midbrain level, thereby depressing conscious alertness. Systemic hypotension not only reduces this baroreceptor inhibition of the reticular system but simultaneously increases chemoreceptor afferent activity, which directly stimulates the mesencephalic reticulum. Such alteration in the afferent pattern of activity which the brain stem receives presumably contributes to the causation of restlessness, a feature so often documented as a symptom of early shock. One must in this context allow that many of the neurogenic features of shock may have a central origin. There are, after all, few things more emotionally disturbing than to see one's blood distributed over a wide area, particularly when this experience is accompanied by the sight of widespread tissue injury and the conscious and unconscious acknowledgement by the central nervous system of the receipt of nociceptive stimuli. Cortico-hypothalamicofugal barrages presumably reinforce sympathetic activity and indeed in the early stages of injury probably outweigh the reflex effects described above. It is also worth noting that widespread constriction of the skin vessels produced by emotional or by reflex mechanisms in hypotension will set in motion an increased impulse traffic from "cold" receptors which, by hypothalamic relays, will further increase the shut-down of the skin circulation. Such considerations help us to explain the common subjective complaint of subjects in the early stages of shock that they feel cold.

Cardiac receptors exist in the atrial and ventricular walls. Thanks to converging evidence from electroneurography, perfusion studies and drug responses, it is clear that some if not all of these receptors function as mechanoreceptors in much the same way as LUDWIG envisaged ninety-five years ago. They exert a tonic restraint on the cardiovascular system, qualitatively similar to that exercised by the arterial receptors. In hypovolaemia their lessened activity contributes to the prevailing state of reflex vasoconstriction. In addition, the left atrial receptors have been identified as the fingers of the afferent arm of a reflex mechanism affecting the secretion of the antidiuretic hormone. Ordinarily they are believed to exercise a mild degree of tonic restraint upon ADH secretion; in oligaemia it has been suggested that the increased secretion of ADH owes some of its origin to the reduction in afferent impulse traffic from the atrial receptors. It is doubtful whether this is of much importance in shock, where G. F. R. and R. P. F. are in any case so profoundly reduced.

Some suggestions that the right atrial receptors may be concerned with the reflex regulation of aldosterone secretion are not very relevant here. Whereas some support can be found for the proposition that high pressures in the right atrium inhibit aldosterone secretion, it has recently been shown that a fall in right atrial pressure such as might occur in hypovolaemia does not *per se* lead to an increase in aldosterone output. In oligaemia it seems likely that the reflex increase in aldosterone secretion which occurs results from a diminution in the afferent impulse activity of vagal mechanoreceptors situated in the thyrocarotid area.

Before leaving the cardiac receptors it must be noted that many of the cardio-sensory nerve endings remain to be investigated. Thus, those that signal myocardial ischaemia have received little attention. It is possible that the forcible approximation of the ventricular walls which occurs in a heart which possesses a negligible end-systolic reserve may stimulate sensory nerve endings of high threshold which may contribute to the syndrome of cardiovascular shock. Subendocardial haemorrhages have been noted in such circumstances.

Chemoreceptors

The chemoreceptors of the carotid and aortic bodies are profoundly stimulated in haemorrhagic hypotension. The oxygen usage of the epithelioid cells is very high — three times that of brain cells, weight for weight. Ordinarily their blood flow is 2,000 ml./100 g. /min. and their oxygen tension must be close to that of arterial blood. In hypotension there results stagnant anoxia; a thunderous discharge of afferent impulses is thereby aroused. These impulses cause reflex vasoconstriction and hyperpnoea. The glomus response to hypotension is sensitised by acidaemia. One of the dramatic features of hypotension is that section of the sinus nerves causes a further fall of blood pressure — due to interruption of the chemoreceptor afferents.

Summary

This review of the reflex regulation of cardiovascular mechanisms in hypotension provides ample evidence that reflex vasoconstriction is likely to be the first circulatory response to a fall in blood pressure. Such vasoconstriction, whilst useful in maintaining systemic blood pressure and therefore cerebral blood flow at as high a pressure as can be produced, nevertheless brings in its train the results accruing from splanchnic asphyxia.

The effects of emotional stress on the circulation through voluntary muscles

By

A. D. M. GREENFIELD

In this communication I would like to deal briefly with the effects in man of emotional stress on the muscular circulation. It has, of course, been known for a long time that emotional stress causes an increase in forearm blood flow (WILKINS and EICHNA, 1941), and some years ago I was able to observe a fall in forearm vascular resistance during an emotional faint (GREEN-FIELD, 1951). Although it seemed probable that vasodilator nerves to muscle, evidence for which had been obtained in post-haemor-rhagic fainting by BARCROFT and EDHOLM (1945), were also involv-ed in the emotional faint, no direct evidence was available. A humoral agent or vasoconstrictor release might also have contrib-uted. It is not easy to provoke an emotional faint under obser-vational conditions that allow the mechanism to be fully analysed.

Since this time, Dr. FOLKOW and Dr. UVNÄS and their co-workers have clearly demonstrated in the dog and cat a powerful system of cholinergic vasodilator fibres, distributed with the sympathetic nerves to the vessels of skeletal muscle, and capable of being stimulated by electrodes suitably implanted in the brain and brain stem, but not influenced by the afferent stimuli which affect the vasomotor centre and adrenergic sympathetic outflow. The ob-servations of ABRAHAMS and HILTON (1957) that stimulation of areas of the brain which cause muscular vasodilatation in anaesthet-ised cats causes "flight or fight" reactions in conscious cats sug-gested that emotional stress might stimulate the cholinergic vasodilator system.

Many observations have accumulated to show that the blood flow is increased in the forearm in emotional stress (BROD, FENCL, HEJL and JIRKA, 1959) and it has been shown by several independ-ent methods that, while there is regularly an increased flow through the muscles, the flow through the skin is often little changed (BLAIR, GLOVER, GREENFIELD and RODDIE, 1959; FENCL, HEJL, JIRKA, MADLAFÓUSEK and BROD, 1959).

The evidence that cholinergic vasodilator nerves contribute to this emotional vasodilatation will now be reviewed.

1. In some experiments, the size and duration of the dilatation in the forearm and the associated changes in arterial pressure and in blood flow in the hand are of a type which is quite unlike the changes following intravenous infusions of adrenaline.

2. The vasodilatation is usually less pronounced, or entirely absent, in the sympathectomised arm. BLAIR et al. (1959), in 11 experiments on 5 unilaterally sympathectomised subjects, found a smaller peak flow, and lower plateau of flow, on the sympathectomised side. BARCROFT, BROD, HIRSJÄRVI and KITCHIN (1960), however, found little difference between the average of 15 observations on 8 patients with cervical sympathectomy and the average of 20 similar tests on 11 normal persons.

3. In the arm with the deep nerves blocked, the resting level of flow is, of course, raised. During stress, the peak flow and the plateau level of flow are on average rather higher on the blocked side, but the increase in flow is much less on the blocked than on the normal side (BLAIR et al. 1959). Analysing their results in a different way, BARCROFT et al. (1960) also found that the increase in flow was relatively smaller in the arm with stellate block than in the normal arm.

4. Both groups found a reduction in the response after atropine. BLAIR et al. (1959) found in 16 experiments that the absolute size of the response was invariably smaller in the arm into which atropine had been administered intra-arterially than it was in the simultaneously observed control arm. BARCROFT et al. (1960), measuring the effects of mental arithmetic before and after atropine, found that the ratio of stress flow to resting flow was always less after atropine than it had been before. They also, in very carefully controlled experiments in which the efficiency of the intra-arterial atropine was tested before and after with acetylcholine, found a reduced response in all but 2 of 20 tests on 12 subjects.

5. The action of adrenergic sympathetic vasomotor nerves can be effectively blocked by the infusion of bretylium tosylate into the brachial artery. Under circumstances where this substance has been proved to be effective, there is no reduction in the response to emotional stress in the injected, as compared to the opposite non-injected arm (BLAIR, GLOVER, KIDD and RODDIE, 1960).

6. Dr. W. E. GLOVER, Dr. R. G. SHANKS and I have found that the vasodilator action of intravenously administered adrenaline, and the transient vasodilator action of intra-arterially administered adrenaline, can be blocked in an arm which has received a suitable

intra-arterial dose of dichloroisoproterenol. In such an arm (Fig. 1), the increase in blood flow with emotional stress is usually less than in the control arm, but the increase is usually considerable, and has not yet been observed to be abolished. These observations confirm the conclusion of BARCROFT et al. (1960) that a humoral mechanism is partly responsible for the peripheral circulatory changes, and are compatible with the conclusion of BLAIR et al. (1959) that cholinergic vasodilator nerves are also partly responsible.

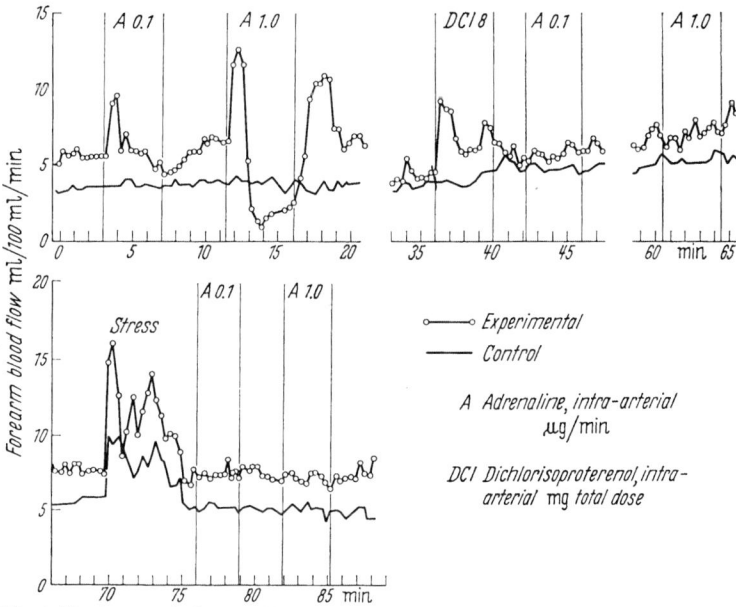

Fig. 1. The increase in forearm blood flow with emotional stress was in this experiment as great in the forearm in which the vasodilator action of adrenaline was blocked by DCI as it was in the contralateral control forearm

References

ABRAHAMS,V. C., and S. M. HILTON: J. Physiol. (G.B.) 140, 16P—17P (1957).
BARCROFT, H., J. BROD, Z. HEJL, E. A. HIRSJÄRVI, and A. H. KITCHIN: Clin. Sc. (U. S. A.) 19, 577 (1960). — BARCROFT, H., and O. G. EDHOLM: J. Physiol. (G. B.) 104, 161 (1945). — BLAIR, D. A., W. E. GLOVER, A. D. M. GREENFIELD, and I. C. RODDIE: J. Physiol. (G. B.) 148, 633 (1959). — BLAIR, D. A., W. E. GLOVER, B. S. L. KIDD, and I. C. RODDIE: Brit. J. Pharmacol. 15, 466 (1960). — BROD, J., V. FENCL, Z. HEJL, and J. JIRKA: Clin. Sc. (U. S. A.) 18, 269 (1959).
FENCL, V., Z. HEJL, J. JIRKA, J. MADLAFÓUSEK, and J. BROD: Clin. Sc. (U. S. A.) 18, 491 (1959).
GREENFIELD, A. D. M.: Lancet (G. B.) 1951/I, 1302.
WILKINS, R. W., and L. W. EICHNA: Johns Hopkins Hosp. Bull. (U. S. A.) 68, 425 (1941).

Discussion

UVNÄS: Dr. NEIL, you mentioned the Bezold-Jarisch reflex. Of course, there are many drugs that activate this reflex, and many speculations have been made as to the nature of the chemoreceptors involved. Now many of the drugs which activate the Bezold-Jarisch reflex are vasoactive drugs. Is it possible that the reflex can be due to activation of stretch receptors secondary to the vascular actions of the drugs?

It was very interesting to hear about Dr. GREENFIELD's speculations as to the possible role of the sympathetic vasodilator fibres in man, since we have been interested in the significance of these fibres for several years. Dr. GREENFIELD's colleague, Dr. GLOVER, visited us a year ago just when we were trying to activate the vasodilator fibres in conscious cats by emotional stimuli. We tried to irritate the cat in various ways, e. g. by exposing it to dogs, rats, and other — as we supposed — annoying things. No vasodilatation could be observed until Dr. GLOVER entered the room and barked like a dog! Immediately the cat's muscle blood flow increased. Unfortunately, we were not able to repeat the vasodilator response and therefore could not determine by atropinisation whether the blood-flow increase was really due to vasodilator nerve activation.

But there is another question I would like to ask Dr. GREENFIELD. We have found in our cats that, when we increase blood-flow in the skeletal muscles, a change occurs in the oxygen uptake of the muscles. If we increase blood-flow by activating vasodilator fibres, at the same time a decrease in the oxygen consumption is observed. Now if we produce the same increase of blood-flow in the muscle by inhibiting vasoconstrictor tone, an increase of oxygen uptake occurs. If you plot increase of blood-flow against change in oxygen consumption, you will find that when sympathetic constrictor tone is inhibited, there is a rather good correlation between increase of blood-flow and increase of oxygen consumption. On the other hand, if you increase blood-flow by activating the dilator fibres, oxygen consumption goes down to 50 or 60% of the initial level, independently of the magnitude of the blood-flow increase. How is one to explain these differences?

NEIL: In reply to Dr. UVNÄS's question as to where the veratrine is active; well, there are many places where a muscular action (in the heart for instance) might contribute to the stimulation of the receptor. I think, however, that the veratrine does hit the receptor itself rather than that it first exerts effects secondarily to changes of flow or local distortion produced by a muscular action. We have Dr. BACQ here, after all, who is one of the world's authorities on veratrine, and I think he would agree that the drug has a direct action on the receptor membrane. I myself have for the last few years been studying the carotid body recording from the chemoreceptors. Veratrine exerts a stimulant effect on these receptors which long outlasts the drug's influence on carotid body vessels or on carotid body flow. There are similar experiments by DAWES and his co-workers on the coronary mechano-receptors in which the reactivity of these fibre endings to veratrine was directly recorded. So I would say, and perhaps Dr. BACQ would add something, that this drug exerts a direct effect on receptor nerve endings. Of course, this is the importance of the Bezold-Jarisch reflex: veratrine is being used as a tool to show up the cardiovascular reflex effects of these cardiac receptors. None of these cardiac nerve endings, when stimulated, produces tachycardia and vasoconstriction — a reflex response which has been ascribed to these receptors by BAINBRIDGE. That idea still persists in the literature, but the Bainbridge reflex does not come from the heart; it comes, I think, from the lung parenchyma, and I could substantiate that if it comes up later.

GREENFIELD: I am very interested to hear about Dr. UVNÄS's experiments. I haven't any explanation to offer, but these experiments perhaps provide another piece of evidence to add to those he has already obtained that the vasoconstrictor and vasodilator fibres of muscles may not act on the same vessels and may therefore not act in quite the same way on muscle metabolism.

FOLKOW: There is one type of depressor reflex which, I believe, the surgeons often see and which is elicited by the manipulations during, for example, operations in the abdominal cavity. Mostly, I think, these reflex depressor reactions are very brief and don't cause much trouble, but sometimes, as I have heard from Dr. GELIN, they can be prolonged and difficult to handle, and the patient may occasionally go into something which can be called a shock condition; this applies especially to patients whose myocardium is in a poor state from the start. Dr. GELIN, Dr. LINDELL, Dr. STENBERG, and I have tried to analyse these depressor responses, and the general pattern seems to be the same as that observed in response to baroreceptor stimulation. Weak stimulation generally causes only a reflex bradycardia; but with more intense afferent stimulation generalised inhibition of sympathetic tone also occurs, causing — among other things — relaxation of the venous side with pooling of the blood. This often leads to a marked decrease in cardiac output as judged by the fact that the pulse pressure may be reduced to about 20—30% of the original value. Usually, this depressor response is eliminated as soon as the manipulation stops, but sometimes it is prolonged. The afferent fibres appear to join the sympathetic abdominal nerves and not the vagal nerves. It has been suggested that these depressor fibres might come from the Pacinian corpuscles of the mesenteries and abdominal organs. BRONK studied the fibres of these corpuscles some years ago, and recently SARNOFF et al. discussed whether they might be identical with the abdominal "depressor" fibres. However, the fibres from the Pacinian corpuscles are thick, myelinated A fibres, with a stimulation threshold similar to that of the somatomotor fibres. On the other hand, the afferent fibres causing the depressor responses in the patients had a stimulation threshold about 50 times higher than that of the motor fibres. This suggests that they are very *thin* fibres. We believe that they may be identical with the fibres mediating pain sensations on distension of the abdominal viscera, rather than that they are specific cardiovascular mechanoreceptors. It is known that pain fibres make reflex connections with the nervous cardiovascular control, and both pressor and depressor reflexes have been reported here.

GREGERSEN: My question for Dr. NEIL was whether or not he has had an opportunity to determine the threshold, or oxygen level, at which this discharge is triggered ?

NEIL: On the chemoreceptors ?

GREGERSEN: Yes.

NEIL: Oh yes! The problem is complicated by the effects of anaesthesia. One inevitably has to use an anaesthetised preparation, and the local circulation of the glomus is affected by sympathetic reflexes which themselves are

182   Discussion

susceptible to the depth of anaesthesia. I think, from my work, that the important factor responsible for initiating chemoreceptor impulse discharge is a cutting down of their blood flow, which produces local changes in the glomus oxygen tissue tension. There is no simple answer to your question, but I would say this — that from the moment you can depict any change in the systemic blood pressure to a lower mean value, then the chemoreceptors are already beginning to increase their activity, and at this time there is no alteration which you can demonstrate in arterial tension or content of oxygen. But the receptors are extremely susceptible to stagnant anoxia, and I think this is more important than their response in anaemic anoxia, such as is produced by haemodilution or mild degrees of anoxic anoxia as seen at moderate altitudes.

BEIN: I would like to ask Dr. FOLKOW how he elicited these reflexes he spoke about.

FOLKOW: Firstly, we stimulated the afferent fibres to an adequate degree simply by pulling on the mesenteries or the intestine, but then we isolated fine afferent nerve trunks and stimulated them directly with an electrode by way of a square-wave stimulator enabling us to vary the voltage, frequency, and pulse duration. The voltage needed, at a given pulse duration, to excite the actual "depressor" fibres in the abdominal visceral organs was about 50 times higher than the voltage needed to activate the A fibres of the skeletal muscles; so the fibres appear to be very thin indeed.

BEIN: Some years ago, we made similar experiments and recorded the action potential from the afferent fibres coming from the intestine. Pulling the intestine evokes discharge of action potentials, but only in the thin afferent fibres; I would agree that the fibres coming from the Pacinian corpuscles are not involved. Interestingly enough, you can block the action potentials already in the periphery by ganglionic blocking drugs. After a ganglionic blocker, you can pull the intestine without eliciting discharges in the afferent nerves[1]. We also found that anaesthesia plays an important role in eliciting action potentials in these thin afferent intestinal nerves in contrast to the thick afferent nerves.

BACQ: The intensity and even the presence of the Bezold-Jarisch reflex depends on the ionic pattern in the blood, as I demonstrated in the case of striped muscle in 1939; and JARISCH has done all the work on the vascular reflex elicited by veratrine. If you inject a subliminal dose of veratrine, you can produce the reflex by injecting small amounts of potassium ions, and you can block the action of veratrine by a previous injection of calcium ions. This, I believe, may be very important, because in many states of shock there is an increase in the potassium ion concentration in the blood, mainly when anuria is also present. I feel that too little attention has hitherto been paid to the ion concentration (potassium and calcium) in the blood.

Now I have a remark to make on Dr. GREENFIELD's experiments. One can easily block the effect of acetylcholine with atropine or the effect of adrenaline with dichloroisoproterenol when the mediators are injected into the blood, but it takes a much higher concentration of atropine or of the other inhibitor to block the effect if the mediator is liberated at the periphery. Hence, I am not completely convinced by this experiment that, for instance, with dichloroisoproterenol he had blocked the beta receptors in the vessels of the forearm and the possible adrenergic vasodilator component.

[1] H. J. BEIN: Helvet. physiol. acta 9, C15—C16, 1951; H. J. BEIN and R. MEIER: Anaesthesist (G.) 3, 25—31, 1954.

GREENFIELD: I entirely agree with Dr. BACQ about this. The blocking of substances administered intravascularly is not evidence that the same substances are blocked when released at nerve endings. The points I would make are these: firstly, in our experiments with atropine, we find a reduction in the response to emotion, and this difference we interpret to mean that we have at any rate partially blocked the cholinergic pathway. We don't know what would happen if we completely blocked it. The effect would presumably be greater. Secondly, in the experiments with DCI, we are trying to block circulating adrenaline, and we are testing DCI against adrenaline arriving in the circulation, so that in this particular instance I don't think the problem arises. We test with circulating adrenaline for the blocking action of DCI against circulating adrenaline.

NICKERSON: I would like to raise one point relating Dr. GREENFIELD's remarks to the general shock problem which we are discussing. The condition he has described may or may not be referred to as shock, depending on one's personal preference. However, we should make a clear distinction between this and the type of shock referred to in most of the remainder of the discussion. Some workers make the distinction of primary versus secondary shock. We tend to refer to the picture presented by Dr. GREENFIELD as vasodilator as opposed to vasoconstrictor shock, and it is clinically useful to distinguish between these as warm and cold shock. From a clinical standpoint, the condition he has discussed can usually be readily treated by positioning the patient so that gravity facilitates the venous return, whereas the other type of shock associated with vasoconstriction is much less affected by such manoeuvres.

STRÖM: I would agree with Dr. GREENFIELD that a cholinergic vasodilator reaction in skeletal muscle during emotional stress may be of importance in the development of shock. It might be of pathogenetic significance and have therapeutic implications, as it appears that the increased blood flow caused by cholinergic vasodilator activation is metabolically inactive and therefore ought to be counteracted pharmacologically. Although I agree with Dr. GREENFIELD on this first point, I don't feel certain that his evidence is good enough to warrant a conclusion that cholinergic vasodilator activation may really be *quantitatively* important in shock. Vasodilatation in skeletal muscle might be caused by constrictor inhibition, dilator activation, systemic overflow of adrenaline from the adrenals, or — and this is the most important factor — by local muscular activity. In order to analyse this problem, you use ganglionic blockade or surgical sympathectomy, intra-arterial injections of atropine, sympathetic blockade, and deep forearm-nerve blockade. And in each experimental situation you find a small difference, but the quantitative importance of cholinergic vasodilatation is still difficult to state in a quantitative manner. During emotional stress, there is intense arousal and increased skeletal muscular activity. In order to rule out an effect of increased muscular tone on forearm blood flow it may be necessary not only to use deep forearm blockade, which is seldom complete, but also to use local curarisation and to observe the effect by, for example, electromyography or local oxygen extraction.

KRAMER: I would like to raise another question. Yesterday, Dr. RUSHMER showed a somewhat puzzling effect on the heart rate during haemorrhage, namely bradycardia. I would like to put a question to Dr. NEIL. You certainly remember the work of Dr. LANDGREN. LANDGREN found in graded pressure studies in dogs that at a pressure of about 60 mm. Hg the discharge from the carotid sinus reaches a minimum and then increases again. In our laboratory, Dr. SCHOLDERER and Dr. MÜHL repeated these experiments on the depressor nerve and found in about 50% of cases that a decrease in pressure — from 70 down to 30 — caused a definite and sometimes striking increase in output from these aortic receptors. So my question is now: could it be possible that these increases in discharges at low pressure might account for Dr. RUSHMER's findings on the conscious dog? We never see this bradycardia in the anaesthetised dog, and in the normal dog it seems possible that these cardioinhibitor systems may have caused bradycardia.

FINE: There are data showing that, except terminally, vasodilatation is not present in haemorrhagic shock or in endotoxin shock. This evidence derives from haemodynamic data, measured effluent from organs, and haemogobin content of the tissues examined, including the muscles. As clinicians we seek ways to counter the excessive damage caused by vasoconstrictor activity. This seems to be the significant physiological abnormality. Since Dibenamine is a notably effective protective agent, one would like to explain the eventual outcome of irreversible shock in terms of excessive vasoconstrictor activity. But it is difficult to do so, because reserpine has failed to afford protection and because other compounds that are not anti-adrenergic also appear to work. Whether a reduction in vasoconstrictor activity should be a major therapeutic objective remains unanswered. The French school and PENNER and BERNHEIM have posed the problem of excessive vasoconstrictor activity in a dramatic way by showing a vast and universal sympathetic discharge in response to the injection of a minute quantity of endotoxin into the cerebral ventricles. We have reproduced the phenomenon of massive haemorrhage and necrosis of the gut, which they describe, and have been able to block it by coeliac ganglionectomy. We have also blocked the Shwartzman reaction in the kidney produced by endotoxin by denervating the renal pedicle.

NEIL: There are several points that have struck me. One is that at the beginning I would agree with Dr. GREENFIELD. I think it is possible that there may be in trauma an emotional concomitant which may well cause a corticohypothalamic initiated vasodilatation. This, together with the blood loss, produces a big fall in blood pressure which in turn sets in motion vasoconstrictor reflexes of cardiovascular origin. This vasoconstriction is likely to be a progressive phenomenon; for, once mechanoreceptor reflexes have caused vasoconstriction of the skin, then the "cold" receptors in the skin start discharging, and this evokes a hypothalamic response of further vasoconstriction. Presumably this is one reason why, in a clinical case of shock, the patient complains of feeling cold; his peripheral thermoreceptors are telling him he is cold.

These afferent reflexes from the abdomen I have not had time to discuss. There are of course many thin fibre afferents in both vagal and splanchnic sympathetic trunks which come from the viscera. A particularly vivid cardiovascular reflex can sometimes be evoked from the gall bladder during surgical operations; traction on the gall bladder causes the heart to slow or even to stop. We know well, too, that some spinal men, though they have no conscious sensation of bladder pressure, may nevertheless learn to realise that the bladder is full when they get flushing of the face, which may be accompanied by vasoconstriction of the feet.

Now I would like to turn to Dr. KRAMER's interesting question about Dr. RUSHMER's bradycardia or at least Dr. RUSHMER's dog's bradycardia. I do of course know of LANDGREN's work; some of it was performed while we were in the same laboratory. I think, to be fair, that Dr. KRAMER has obviously read the paper more recently than I. I did not know that LANDGREN got the reversal at such high pressures as 60 mm. Hg. However, these sinus receptors are after all deformation receptors and, after a certain fall of pressure in the isolated sinus subjected to static perfusion, one might get abnormal stresses in the sinus segment which may lead to baroreceptor firing. I have not seen much evidence of this with the sinus — only two or three times in many experiments — but I am interested in Dr. KRAMER's findings with the aortic arch and its nerve supply. There is, however, a reflex provoked by the stagnant anoxia of haemorrhage which is perhaps even more likely to cause an occasional bout of bradycardia, and that is the chemoreceptor primary effect on the heart. Now you might be thinking that this does not fit in. It is a complicated story and goes as follows:

First perfuse the isolated innervated chemoreceptor carotid area with anoxic blood; the animal hyperventilates and the heart rate response is variable. Secondly, if you control the breathing response by artificial ventilation, chemoreceptor stimulation now causes bradycardia. Now if you do a third experiment by stimulating the chemoreceptors in a dog whose pulmonary vagi have been cut, then the breathing increases markedly as a reflex response to chemoreceptor stimulation, but the heart rate shows slowing as in the second experiment. These experiments have been done by Professor DALY of London. They show you that you are setting in motion a chain of reflexes. If there is not much respiratory response to chemoreceptor stimulation, then the cardiac response is slowing. If, however, the hyperpnoea is vivid, the primary chemoreceptor cardiac chronotropic reflex is masked by tachycardia evoked by pulmonary afferent vagal effects arising from the distended lungs which are moving more vigorously.

I think the bradycardia of Dr. RUSHMER's dog may well be due to chemoreceptor stimulation by haemorrhage. I cannot remember whether Dr. RUSHMER recorded respiratory events at the same time.

RUSHMER: In some of the animals, yes.

NEIL: Was the respiratory response to haemorrhage very marked?

RUSHMER: No, it was not in most animals.

NEIL: Well, you will get the bradycardia. I think from my experience, which is not the same as Dr. KRAMER's, that this is the more likely explanation.

GREENFIELD: I would like to thank Dr. STRÖM for his remarks, with many of which I entirely agree. With respect to the effect of atropine during emotional stress, I think different workers have found different things. In our experiments, we found a reduction of forearm vasodilatation in all of 16 experiments, and BARCROFT, BROD et al. found a reduction in 18 out of 20 experiments. My guess is that the relative contributions to this response of 1) humoral agents, 2) vasoconstrictor release, and 3) vasodilator activation vary in size with the particular conditions and the particular sort of emotional stress which is being applied. With respect to Dr. STRÖM's very important point about whether the vasodilatation is partly secondary to contraction of the voluntary muscles, I'm afraid I do not have as good an answer as I would like to have. However, after emotional stress, when we tell the subject that everything is perfectly all right, that he need not worry and can relax, the blood flow in the forearm falls precipitously. After any sort of exercise which produces a similar elevation of blood flow the return of flow to normal is very much slower. Further, the increase in blood flow is much smaller in a sympathectomised arm than it is in the contralateral normal arm, although the somatic outflow to the muscles of both is intact. So I do not think that muscular contraction plays much part in the elevation of muscle blood flow during emotional stress.

Hemorrhagic and post-hemorrhagic shock

By

J. M. HOWARD

Clinical surgery has provided an almost unlimited experience in the treatment of hemorrhagic shock in man. In spite of this opportunity, the number of careful clinical studies in man is distressingly small. Studies in man have almost been limited to World War I, World War II, and the Korean War and to a very few very careful civilian studies such as that led by COURNAND and GREGERSON during World War II. Nevertheless, progress has been outstanding. Transfusion has solved the major problems in the treatment of hemorrhagic shock in the younger patient. Most of the problems at present, numerically speaking, exist in the older group of patients who obviously tolerate blood loss less efficiently than do their younger counterparts. Progress being made in the freeze-storage of blood and in understanding plasma reactions will further solidify progress in transfusion.

It is essential to recognize how few studies have been done in man. It is not at all certain that the studies in animals are pertinent in many respects to the problems of man. For instance, much of the work in animals has been done on dogs. Long-continued hemorrhage in the dog, particularly with retransfusion therapy, leads to engorgement of the splanchnic bed with subsequent hemorrhage into the gastro-intestinal tract. Too many patients have been lost after prolonged hemorrhage and after transfusion, but the syndrome of splanchnic engorgement and secondary intestinal hemorrhage has not been documented in man. Neither has the anaerobic bacterial overgrowth of the liver been observed in man. These facts alone raise serious criticism of the work which you and I have done on the dog and make it imperative that man himself be studied to an increasing extent. This is perhaps the most important observation which I have to make.

Gradual blood loss is obviously tolerated by man far better than rapid blood loss. It is not unusual to see a patient come into the hospital with a hemoglobin concentration of 5 grams per cent, the loss being secondary to gradual gastro-intestinal bleeding. Such a patient may tolerate this loss of approximately two-thirds of his red cell mass fairly well. Two factors are involved. One is the *gradual* diminution in blood volume. The other is the fact that as his red cell mass falls, his plasma volume, by replenishment, tends to stay fairly constant. The total blood volume deficit, therefore, is not as great as would occur from the same loss of red cell mass due to rapid hemorrhage. Similar observations have been made with acute blood loss where the blood volume itself was maintained using dextran. Under such circumstances, if a patient is bleeding from multiple wounds of the soft tissues, dextran has been infused in an effort to maintain the blood volume at an approximately normal level. Under these circumstances the hematocrit falls approximately 5 volumes per cent per 500 cc. of dextran administered. As the hematocrit falls acutely in the presence of a normal blood volume, the pulse rate tends to rise, although the blood pressure remains normal. This sequence is tolerated fairly well by the patient so long as the hematocrit stays above twenty-five volumes per cent. However, if the hematocrit falls rapidly below 25 volumes per cent, the pulse rate rises sharply and although the blood pressure is maintained, the patient develops respiratory distress and may, indeed, go into a Cheyne-Stokes type of respiration.

Although the patient can tolerate the rapid loss of the red cell mass fairly well, provided his total blood volume remains normal, he does not tolerate the loss of volume of whole blood nearly as well. Many studies indicate that, in the absence of anesthesia and alcohol, peripheral vasoconstriction and an increased cardiac rate can maintain a blood pressure at a normal level until approximately 20% of the blood volume has been lost. Although this varies with the size of the individual, twenty per cent of an adult's blood volume would be in the range of 1,000 cc. When between 20 and 30 per cent of the blood volume has been lost, the blood pressure starts to fall, and by the time that 45 per cent of the blood volume has been lost the blood pressure is unobtainable.

One of the most useful concepts that has evolved is the concept of the state of "compensated shock". Such a patient has lost perhaps 20 per cent of his blood volume but has maintained a normal blood pressure. Under these circumstances his tissue perfusion is by no means normal. Furthermore, his compensatory mechanism is functioning perhaps maximally. Under these circumstances the loss of any additional blood may precipitate a profound hypotension. Furthermore, the administration of anesthesia prior to the correction of the blood volume deficit may precipitate a profound state of "decompensated shock". By some means, not clearly understood, anesthesia blocks the compensatory mechanism, a blockade that may prove fatal.

The young man, as studied in the Korean battle casualty, tolerates hemorrhage well for a short time. In our observation of five thousand battle casualties in Korea, we were dealing with an average evacuation time to the forward hospital of three and a half hours after injury. Type 0 blood was used without cross-match. Under these circumstances, where one was working with a previously healthy young man with a short period of time lapse between injury and resuscitation, irreversible hemorrhagic or wound shock was not apparent. Continued hypotension, in the absence of injury to the heart or central nervous system, represented continued hemorrhage or inadequate transfusion. Under these circumstances the only organ which was recognized to decompensate was the kidney, leading to acute post-traumatic renal insufficiency. It is impossible to state with certainty that anoxia is the cause of post-traumatic renal insufficiency, but it is fair to say that, with the exception of transfusion reaction, the syndrome followed only after profound injury and profound hypotension. Furthermore, the observation seemed valid that in the young man who had been previously healthy, only the kidney could be delineated as an organ whose loss of function appeared irreparable.

As we have studied in man the function of each organ after injury, abnormalities of function have been detectable. Hemorrhagic shock accentuates these functional deviations, both as to magnitude and as to duration. Decompensation of an organ in a young man (soldier) has not been found after hemorrhagic shock – except for the kidney. Only the kidney's function, not the blood pressure, was sometimes irreversible.

In Korea the mortality rate, as described by the U. S. Army's Surgical Research Team, in a selected group of casualties is demonstrated in Tables 1, 2 and 3. The overall mortality rate of those casualties reaching medical aid fell to 2.4%.

The high fatality rates following abdominal injury, in contradistinction to the considerably lower rates after injury to the extremity, reflect first and foremost the fact that anesthesia had to be given to patients with massive abdominal injuries before the blood volume deficit was corrected. In other words, anesthesia and operation were necessary parts of hemostasis. With injury limited to the extremity, it was usually possible by means of a tourniquet to obtain hemostasis, after which the blood volume could be corrected prior to anesthesia and operative injury. The relative role of infection was also different. Pertinent to this comparison is

Table 1. *Korean battle casualties (admitted to forward hospital) with an unobtainable blood pressure*

Site of injury	Total		Receiving 15 or more pints of blood			Receiving less than 15 pints of blood		
	Number	Case fatality rate %	Number	Deaths	Case fatality rate %	Number	Deaths	Case fatality rate
Abdomen . .	14	65	10	9	90	4	0	0
Abdomen and extremity .	8	38	7	3	43	1	0	0
Extremity only . . .	16	13	9	2	22	7	0	0
Total or average	38	37	26	14	54	12	0	0

Table 2. *Case fatality rate of Korean battle casualties who required 15 or more pints of blood and plasma expander*

Site of injury	Total		Case fatality rate %	Number dying of continued hemorrhage	Case fatality rate including continued hemorrhage %
	No.	Deaths			
Abdomen	24	19	79	11	62
Abdomen and extremities . . .	29	12	41	3	35
Extremities . . .	29	12	17	1	14
Chest	7	3	43	1	33
Total or average .	89	39	44	16	32

Table 3. *Incidence of renal failure in Korean battle casualties who required 15 or more pints of blood[1]*

Site of injury	Number living 3 days or longer	Anuria %	Oliguria %	Non-oliguric azotemia %
Abdomen . . .	9	22	11	11
Abdomen and extremity . .	14	28	0	7
Extremity. . .	19	0	11	22
Chest	1	0	0	0
Total	43			
Average. . .		14	7	14

[1] Based on 60 consecutive casualties requiring over 15 pints of blood. Thus, of the 43 casualties who lived, 35% (anuria 14%, oliguria 7%, and azotemia 14%) developed clinically significant post-traumatic renal insufficiency.

the observation that insufficient attention has been given in the laboratory to methods of obtaining hemostasis without general anesthesia. I refer to such possibilities as inserting a balloon catheter up the femoral artery and into the aorta above the celiac axis as a means of partially or temporarily occluding the aorta. This might stop bleeding in the abdominal viscera while transfusion is carried out and while the patient is prepared for anesthetic and operative control of the hemorrhage. Another area of potential value is hypothermia, for this offers definite protection against anoxia.

One of the great deficiencies in studying hemorrhagic shock in man or in animals rests in the deficient methods of measuring blood volume. The author and his colleagues have studied many patients in an effort to measure their blood volume by means of dilution of dye, tagged albumin, or radiochromium-tagged red cells. It is my honest belief that these methods are inadequate in the injured man and that other investigators might interpret our data differently than we have interpreted it. This appears at present to be the greatest defect in methodology currently apparent in shock studies. Working in the Korean experience, PRENTICE and associates spent months trying to identify the fate of massive volumes of blood administered. After clinical "overtransfusion" of several thousand cubic centimeters of blood, the measured blood volume sometimes reflected a deficiency of one or two thousand cubic centimeters! This has not been explained. The "additional" blood could not be found.

MOORE has correctly emphasized the limitations and the value of the hematocrit in estimating blood loss. Initially, there is no change in the hematocrit with acute blood loss. Thereafter, a gradual hemodilution occurs. After a rapid loss of 20—30% of the blood volume (approximately 1,000—1,500 cc.), the hematocrit falls for 24—36 hours, stabilizing then with a total blood volume depleted by approximately 15%. If the initial loss is less (10—15%), the hematocrit stabilizes within 8—24 hours (MOORE).

In older, arteriosclerotic patients, particularly in those patients undergoing operation or those who have recently undergone operation (24—48 hours previously), blood volume deficiency is not the only problem and many of these patients may die in spite of transfusion. Neither vasoconstrictors nor hydrocortisone, as adjuncts to transfusion, have answered the therapeutic needs. Current studies have been directed more and more toward evaluating myocardial failure as a fundamental aspect of the refractory shock (post-transfusion) syndrome in the geriatric patient.

The classical studies by COURNAND, RICHARDS, GREGERSON and their associates in 1943 and thereafter demonstrated some of the changes in the patients with acute hemorrhage. Their patients were studied by cardiac catheterization. It was found that venous oxygen saturation was elevated in some of their patients. There was also an elevated blood lactate level. These findings have been interpreted as reflecting tissue anoxia associated with arterio-venous shunts. After a period of three or four hours, mild acidosis developed with pH falling to about a level of 7.28. In the presence of low blood volume, normal venous pressures were found, but the cardiac output was low. They also found an increased arterio-venous carbon dioxide difference, suggesting again a slow or poor tissue perfusion. In their most severely shocked patients, the blood volume deficit was approximately 40%. They did not always find an increased perfusion resistance. They did find a decreased renal blood flow. Pertinent to the immediate discussion, they found a decreased cardiac output in patients after acute hemorrhage. The fundamental defect in acute hemorrhage is the decreased blood volume with a decrease in venous return to the right heart.

This type of cardiac failure is well recognized, but the type that exists in older patients does not appear to be due to the same deficiency. I refer specifically to the geriatric patients who continue to run a hypotension following transfusion. Many of these patients have by all criteria a normal blood volume yet maintain a refractory hypotension. In our experience the central venous pressure in four patients was normal or elevated. They were acidotic and this acidosis appears to be metabolic in origin. The lactic acid concentration rises in the blood, the pyruvate concentration rising to a lesser extent. These patients may or may not have electrolyte changes which would produce cardiac failure.

Dr. TZIROS, in our department, has been studying the serum electrolyte changes in patients undergoing various degrees of hemorrhage and operative trauma. His studies have been performed hourly during operation and for several hours thereafter. He has paid particular attention to those patients who are refractory to treatment of the shock. The electrolyte changes have been correlated with changes in the electrocardiogram. In a study of almost 100 patients now he finds a predictable rise in the concentration of phosphate in the blood. Not infrequently there is a fall in sodium concentration and a rise in potassium concentration. In an occasional patient, we have found a sharp drop in the concentration of calcium. We have not documented the relationship of the fall in calcium to the electrocardiographic changes but have demonstrated its relationship to a marked tachycardia. The trend has been toward the occasional finding of a fall in serum calcium and a fall in serum sodium concentrations with a concomitant rise in the concentration of serum potassium. At least two patients have responded rather dramatically to the infusion intravenously of calcium gluconate after the blood pressure had failed to respond adequately to transfusion. We have incompletely documented the finding of cardiac failure in the patient with refractory shock after hemorrhage and operation, but this is the direction in which our work will continue.

Along similar lines in animals, GUYTON studied mild, moderate, and severe hemorrhagic shock. In each type, irreversibility could be produced after various periods of time. He measured the total basal oxygen consumption by the animal and later measured the oxygen consumption during shock. He was then able to calculate the total oxygen deficit, which progressed during the shock phase. In experiments with animals in the various planes of shock, he was able to reach an irreversible stage when the total oxygen deficit reached 120–150 mls per kilogram. He also reported that in hemorrhagic shock so long as the cardiac output remained above a certain critical value, which appeared to be about $1/3$ to $1/2$ normal, circulatory deterioration would not occur and the various compensatory factors of the circulation could bring about recovery. SIMEONE and colleague also found in the dog that the oxygen tension of the heart fell in hemorrhagic shock and was slow to respond to transfusion. Our studies in the dog indicate that with the blood pressure down to 30 mm. of mercury systolic (secondary to hemorrhage) the coronary blood flow falls to approximately 50%. Norepinephrine administration results in a sharp rise in the coronary blood flow, the flow rising above the normal level when the blood pressure is titrated back to its normal level. SIMEONE concurred in this finding but found that pyruvate extraction by the myocardium, low in hemorrhagic shock in the dog, was not increased by norepinephrine. The myocardial contractile force decreased late in the shock phase. STRAWITZ and associates subjected dogs to hemorrhage to a pressure of 40 mm. of mercury and maintained this level for three and five hours. Oxidative phosphorylation by the dog's cardiac mitochondria was reduced to only a modest extent. They did not believe that this finding could explain the myocardial failure which accompanies the long hemorrhagic hypertension.

Several investigators have been working with an organic buffer T. H. A. M., tris (hydroxymethyl) amino-methane. DARBY

and associates produced acidosis in dogs by giving lactic acid intravenously or by increasing the CO_2 concentration in the ventilating
gas. T. H. A. M. intravenously was effective in raising the arterial
blood pH, increasing the plasma CO_2 combining power, increasing
the ventricular contractile force, and increasing the response to
norepinephrine. NAHAS and associates studied the buffering effect
of T. H. A. M. on A-C-D blood and its effect on the survival of
dogs transfused after massive hemorrhage. When severe hemorrhagic shock was produced in the dogs, rapid retransfusion of
citrated blood resulted in deaths in acidosis. The addition of
T. H. A. M. with the retransfusion significantly increased survival
and lessened the state of acidosis.

Renal failure, as a sequel to severe injury and profound hemorrhagic shock, cannot be overlooked. The studies by the U. S. Army's
Surgical Research Team in Korea documented the various degrees
of renal failure which occur in man. Some casualties developed a
fatal oliguria. Others developed a modest oliguria but a striking
azotemia. Others maintained a normal urinary volume but were
found to maintain a reduced glomerular filtration rate and reduced
renal blood flow for days thereafter.

These are but some of the areas of ongoing studies in the field of
hemorrhagic shock. This report has emphasized work in the human
and has indicated that secondary cardiac failure may well play
a major role in the refractory shock phase in the geriatric patient.
Attention has also been called to the fact that additional efforts
might be well extended toward methods of controlling intra-abdominal hemorrhage short of anesthesia and operative intervention
so as to permit the replacement of blood volume before adding the
secondary insults. In the young man, renal damage, but not
irreversible shock, is the sequel to massive hemorrhage and injury.

Summary

Too few studies have been done in man. It is well proved that hemorrhagic shock in the young man responds to transfusion and refractory shock is
seldom a problem. In the older man, transfusion after a period of hemorrhagic
shock may not *always* restore the blood pressure. Perhaps cardiac failure is
sometimes superimposed.

Acute renal failure is the obvious syndrome of great concern after
profound hemorrhagic shock. Its pathogenesis and prevention are urgent
problems.

Finally, new techniques for measurement of blood volume in the injured
man are urgently needed.

References

1. ARTZ, C. P., J. M. HOWARD, Y. SAKO, A. W. BRONWELL and T. PREN-
TICE: Ann. Surg. (U.S.A.) **141**, 285 (1955). — 2. SAKO, Y., C. P. ARTZ, J. M.
HOWARD, A. W. BRONWELL and F. K. INUI: Surgery (U.S.A.) **37**, 602 (1955).
— 3. ARTZ, C. P., J. M. HOWARD and J. P. FRAWLEY: Surgery (U.S.A.)
37, 612 (1955). — 4. HUGHES, C. W.: Surgery (U.S.A.) **36**, 65 (1954). —
5. PRENTICE, T. C., J. M. OLNEY Jr., C. P. ARTZ and J. M. HOWARD:
Surg. Gyn. Obstetr. (U.S.A.) **99**, 542 (1954). — 6. STRAWITZ, J. G., and
H. HIFT: Surg. Forum, Vol. VII. American College of Surgeons, 1957. —
7. DARBY, T. D., et al.: Fed. Proc. (U.S.A.) **19**, 103 (1960). — 8. NAHAS, G. G.:
Clin. Res. (U.S.A.) **8**, 231 (1960). (Abstract). — 9. NAHAS, G. G., et al.: Fed.
Proc. (U.S.A.) **19**, 54 (1960). (Abstract). — 10. MOORE, F. D.: Metabolic
Care of the Surgical Patient. Philadelphia and London: W. B. Saunders
Co. 1959. — 11. COURNAND, A., R. L. RILEY, S. E. BRADLEY, E. S.
BREED, R. P. NOBLE, H. D. LAUSON, M. I. GREGERSON and D. W. RICHARDS:
Surgery (U.S.A.) **13**, 964 (1943). — 12. TZIROS, D.: Unpublished
data. — 13. GUYTON, A. C.: Cardiac Function in Shock. Presented at the
Shock Symposium, December 1960, Walter Reed Medical Center, Washing-
ton, D. C. — 14. SIMEONE, F. A.: Keynote Address. Presented at the Shock
Symposium, December 1960, Walter Reed Medical Center, Washington, D.C.
— 15. VOWLES, K. D. J., F. E. BARSE, W. J. BOVARD, C. M. COUVES
and J. M. HOWARD: Ann. Surg. (U.S.A.) **153**, 202 (1961).

The effect of hypovolaemic (stagnant) and arterial hypoxia on the distribution of cardiac output in dogs and rats

By

L. TAKÁCS

In previous experiments performed at our department, the circulation of the heart [TAKÁCS (1)], kidney [GÖMÖRI, KOVÁCH, TAKÁCS, FÖLDI, SZABÓ, NAGY, and WILTNER (2), TAKÁCS and KÁLLAY (3, 4)], and hind extremities [TAKÁCS (5)] of *dogs* was compared under various conditions of hypovolaemic (stagnant) and arterial hypoxia. Though in ischaemic or traumatic shock and in dehydration a low cardiac output may be observed, and in arterial hypoxia (art. saturation about 60 per cent) an elevated cardiac output, a similar redistribution of the cardiac output was established in both instances, i.e. the coronary fraction of the cardiac output increased while the renal and limb fractions

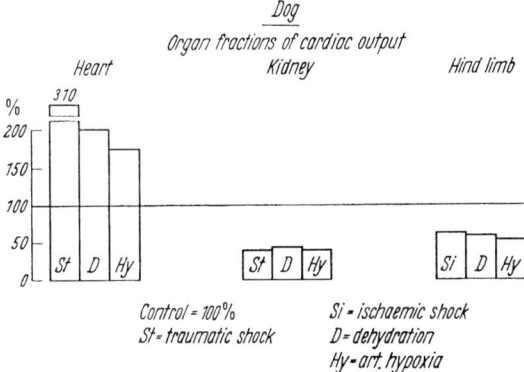

Fig. 1. Effect of traumatic shock, ischaemic shock, dehydration, and arterial hypoxia on the heart, kidney, and hind-limb fractions of the cardiac output in dogs

decreased (Fig. 1). We assumed that tissue hypoxia would probably produce similar alterations in the distribution of the cardiac output in dogs.

In the present experiments the circulation of *rats* after haemorrhage, in ischaemic shock [TAKÁCS, KÁLLAY, and SKOLNIK (6)], and in arterial hypoxia was compared.

13*

The experiments were carried out on rats anaesthetised with sodium pentobarbital (40 mg./kg. i.p.), each group consisting of 10—30 animals. In the first group determinations were made 5—20 minutes after a 23 ml./kg. level of haemorrhage had been reached, and in the second group 1—2.5 hours after both hind extremities had been ligated for three hours. The third group was made to inhale a gas mixture of low oxygen tension for 8—10 minutes. Though arterial saturation fluctuated between 35 and 75 per cent (mean value: 56 per cent), similar alterations were observed.

The blood pressure was measured directly in the carotid artery, and the cardiac output was ascertained by Hamilton's dye-dilution method: 0.3 ml. of 1.5 per cent Evans blue was injected into the femoral vein; blood samples were taken from the carotid artery every 0.66 seconds. The dye concentration was determined with a Beckman DU spectrophotometer, by diluting 20 μl. blood to 3.0 ml.

Organ fractions of the cardiac output were studied by the indicator fractionation method of SAPIRSTEIN (7), using Rb[86]. "This technic depends on the fact that all organs — other than the brain — have virtually the same extraction ratio for Rb[86] as the whole body during the first minute after a single intravenous injection of the label." [SAPIRSTEIN (7)]. The advantage of SAPIR-STEIN's method consists in the fact that the flow fractions of the cardiac output of small animals can be measured simultaneously.

By thus measuring the blood pressure, cardiac output, and organ fractions of the cardiac output, it was possible to calculate the blood flow and the vascular resistance in different organs.

Results

A definite decrease in blood pressure was observed in all three groups (Fig. 2). In the case of hypoxia, this finding is somewhat surprising, as it is well known from results obtained in larger mammals that the blood pressure tends to increase. The decrease only ensues in the final stage (circulatory collapse). In rats, however, a fall in blood pressure was generally observed during the early phase of hypoxia. After cessation of respiration the blood pressure began to increase again, and finally circulatory collapse occurred.

The cardiac output decreased in haemorrhage and in ischaemic shock, while total peripheral resistance actually increased slightly. In arterial hypoxia the cardiac output remained unchanged, and a corresponding decrease in total peripheral resistance was observed.

The alterations in the circulation of the heart and kidney are shown in Figs 3 and 4. The myocardial blood flow diminished in the group with haemorrhage and also in the group with ischaemic shock, whereas in arterial hypoxia it showed no change. Only in hypoxia was an alteration – i.e. a decrease – in resistance observed. The

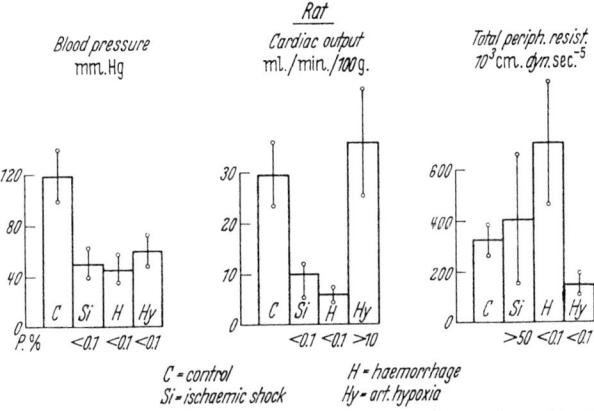

Fig. 2. Effect of ischaemic shock, haemorrhage, and arterial hypoxia on blood pressure, cardiac output, and total peripheral resistance in rats

heart fraction of the cardiac output increased in shock and after haemorrhage, but in arterial hypoxia no alteration could be detected (Fig. 3).

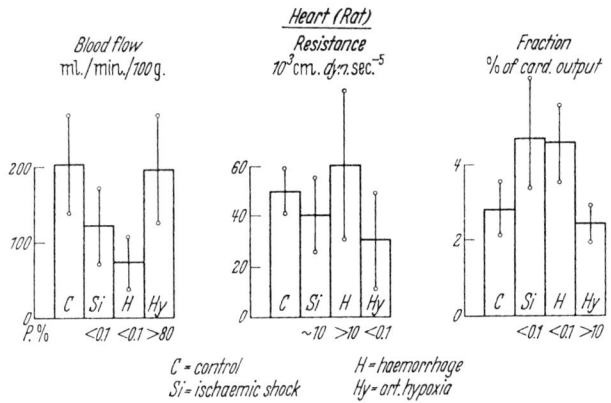

Fig. 3. Effect of ischaemic shock, haemorrhage, and arterial hypoxia on the coronary circulation of rats

The renal blood flow and the renal fraction of the cardiac output were found to be lowered after haemorrhage and in shock. In arterial hypoxia the blood flow and the renal fraction of the

cardiac output were unaltered and a decrease in vascular resistance
was found (Fig. 4).

The circulation in the other organs after haemorrhage and in
shock is characterised by a definite decrease in blood flow and an
increase in vascular resistance. In arterial hypoxia, however,
the blood flow was unchanged, while a diminution in circulatory

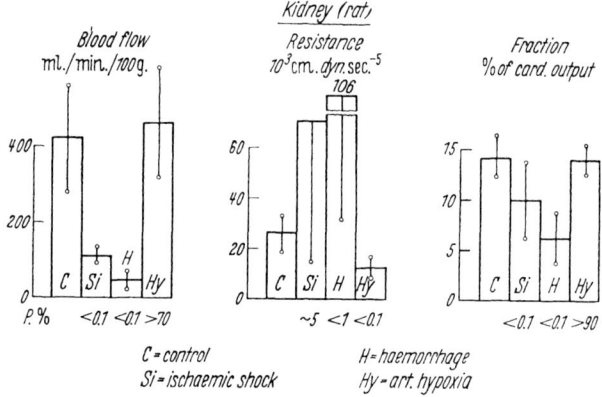

Fig. 4. Effect of ischaemic shock, haemorrhage, and arterial hypoxia on the renal
circulation of rats

resistances was recorded; the organ fractions of the cardiac output were essentially unchanged — except for a slight decrease in
the liver fraction. In animals with shock and haemorrhage, several
organs showed changes.

Our data obtained after haemorrhage corresponded essentially
to the results of SAPIRSTEIN, SAPIRSTEIN, and BREDEMEYER (8).

Our experiments indicated that after haemorrhage and in
ischaemic shock, i.e. in stagnant, hypovolaemic hypoxia in rats,
the distribution of the cardiac output was essentially similar to
the alterations observed in dogs. In the case of arterial hypoxia in
rats, however, a peculiar phenomenon was observed: while a
significant decrease occurred in the blood pressure, the cardiac
output and organ fractions of the cardiac output remained unchanged. Owing to arterial hypoxia a general vasodilatation
seemed to occur in which the various organs participated to an
approximately similar degree. This vasodilatation, unlike that
observed in dog and man, was not offset by an increase in cardiac
output, with the result that hypotension developed.

It may be assumed that the redistribution of the cardiac output
can be regarded as a process of readjustment by which the blood

flow in certain organs is enhanced. It is possible that, in the absence of "shifts" in the circulation, anaesthetised rats are unable to adapt themselves to arterial hypoxia to the same degree as other species in which such "shifting" is detectable.

Conclusions

It may be concluded that: 1) in dogs the pattern of redistribution of the cardiac output is similar both in shock and dehydration (hypovolaemic, stagnant hypoxia) as well as in arterial hypoxia; 2) on the other hand, in rats the circulatory alterations after haemorrhage and in ischaemic shock (stagnant hypoxia) are different from those occurring in arterial hypoxia.

Thus it seems that in dogs tissue hypoxia of different origin may cause essentially identical circulatory regulation, whereas in rats the mechanisms differ.

References

1. TAKÁCS, L.: Acta physiol. Acad. sc. Hungaricae 11, 55 (1957). — 2. GÖMÖRI, P., A. G. B. KOVÁCH, L. TAKÁCS, M. FÖLDI., G. SZABÓ, Z. NAGY, and W. WILTNER: Acta med. Acad. sc. Hungaricae 16, 37 (1960). — 3. TAKÁCS, L., and K. KÁLLAY: Acta physiol. Acad. sc. Hungaricae 12, 375 (1957). — 4. TAKÁCS, L., and K. KÁLLAY: Acta med. Acad. sc. Hungaricae 10, 309 (1957). — 5. TAKÁCS, L.: Acta physiol. Acad. sc. Hungaricae 11, 189 (1957). — 6. TAKÁCS, L., K. KÁLLAY, and J. SKOLNIK: Acta med. Acad. sc. Hungaricae 14, 457 (1959). — 7. SAPIRSTEIN, L. A.: Amer. J. Physiol. 193, 161 (1958). — 8. SAPIRSTEIN, L. A., E. H. SAPIRSTEIN, and A. BREDEMEYER: Circulation Res. (U.S.A.) 8, 135 (1960).

Observations on haemo-respiratory effects of acute haemorrhage

By

H. Bjurstedt and J. C. G. Coleridge*

The following experiments were undertaken in order to study the effects of acute haemorrhage on pulmonary function, blood gases, and the acid-base balance.

Methods

All experiments were performed on dogs lightly anaesthetised with chloralose and heparinised. 250—450 ml. of blood was allowed to escape from one cannulated femoral artery, the following parameters being continuously and simultaneously recorded before, during, and after the period of haemorrhage: (1) arterial blood pressure; (2) pulmonary ventilation; and (3) the arterial pH and O_2 saturation. The last-mentioned parameters were recorded by continuously passing arterial blood in a loop from the femoral artery through a glass-reference-electrode assembly and a photo-electric oximeter cuvette and back to the systemic circulation via the femoral vein (cf. Barr, Bjurstedt and Coleridge, 1959). In a number of experiments the animals were artificially ventilated with a Starling pump, and tubocurarine was given intravenously and repeatedly as needed to suppress spontaneous respiration. In the artificially ventilated animals, the end-tidal P_{CO_2} was also recorded by means of an automatic sampling device in connection with an infra-red CO_2 analyser.

Results and discussion

Fig. 1 shows some typical effects of acute, moderate haemorrhage (250 ml. between vertical lines 1 and 2) on pulmonary ventilation and on arterial O_2 saturation and pH during air breathing. Hyperventilation occurs during the period of bleeding and is associated with an increase in the arterial O_2 saturation and a marked alkaline shift in the pH tracing. The latter changes are in part explained as secondary to the hyperventilation. The hyperventilation, in turn, may be assumed to be partly of chemoreflex origin, since it has been shown by Landgren and Neil (1951) that the afferent impulse activity in the carotid chemoceptor fibres increases in response to a lowering of the arterial pressure. However, some

---

* Present address: Department of Physiology, University of Leeds, England.

hyperventilation also occurred when the animals were bled during O_2 breathing, indicating that also other mechanisms might have been involved, e. g. a reflex influence from peripheral baroceptors.

The post-haemorrhagic decrease in pulmonary ventilation seen in Fig. 1 is typically associated with a slow return of the arterial pH and O_2 saturation towards pre-haemorrhagic levels. The further

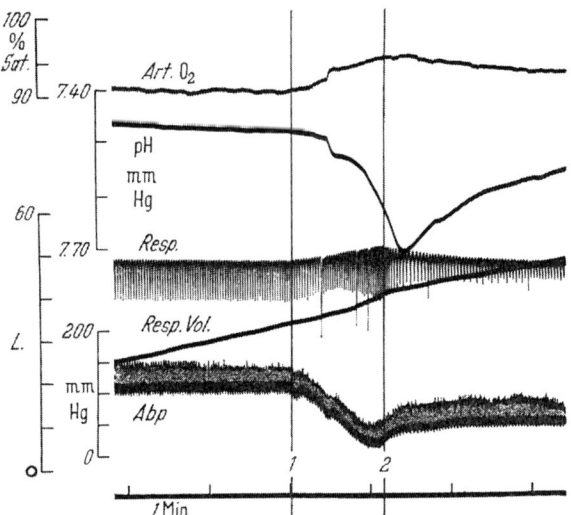

Fig. 1. Dog, chloralose, 14 kg. Effects of acute haemorrhage (250 ml. between vertical lines 1 and 2), during air breathing. From below upwards: arterial blood pressure (Abp); gas meter tracing (Resp. Vol.), the slope of which increases with the respiratory volume (calibration at the extreme left, in litres; each step in the tracing represents an expiration); thoracic respiratory movements (Resp.), inspiration downwards; arterial pH; arterial O_2 saturation

course of the arterial pH was usually a progressive shift in the acid direction, whereas the O_2 saturation showed less consistent changes. Eventually, the pulmonary ventilation showed a secondary, though not complete, recovery, whereas the arterial acid-base balance was characterised by a continuously increasing degree of acidosis.

In order to make it possible to distinguish between primary and secondary changes in pulmonary ventilation and acid-base balance, especially in the post-haemorrhagic period, another series of experiments was undertaken in which the animals were bled under artificially controlled ventilation and the end-tidal P_{CO_2} was recorded together with the arterial pH and other parameters.

In these experiments it was observed that, during the period of haemorrhage, there was a gradual decrease both in the end-tidal

P_{CO_2} and in the hydrogen ion concentration, although pulmonary ventilation was kept constant. The decrease in end-tidal P_{CO_2} was sometimes quite marked (Fig. 2). These changes must clearly be ascribed to a relative overventilation, because of a reduced total blood flow through the lungs. It may be inferred, then, that the marked alkalosis observed in the spontaneously breathing animals (cf. above) is the result of at least two factors, viz. pulmonary hyperventilation and reduced pulmonary blood flow.

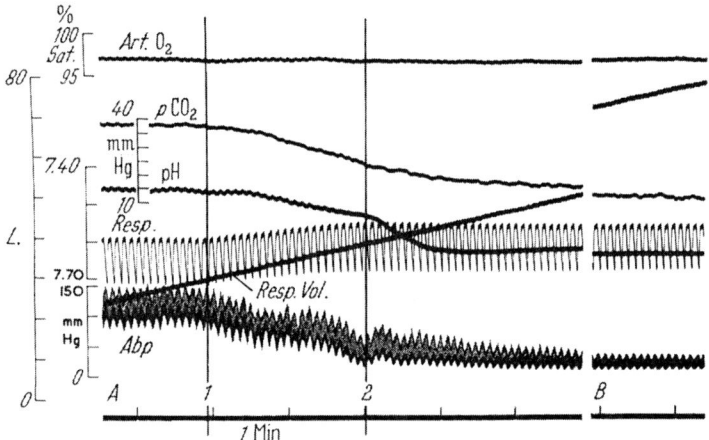

Fig. 2. Dog, chloralose, 15 kg. Effects of acute haemorrhage (450 ml. between vertical lines 1 and 2), during O_2 breathing, constant artificial ventilation. Recordings as in Fig. 1 with the addition of end-tidal P_{CO_2}. Interval of 6 min. between records A and B

By comparing the degree of arterial alkalosis (computing the arterial P_{CO_2}) with the concomitant decrease in end-tidal P_{CO_2} at the end of the period of haemorrhage during constant, artificial ventilation it should be possible to calculate the extent to which under-perfusion of ventilated alveoli may lead to the development of an alveolar dead space. In this context we shall, however, leave aside such effects of haemorrhage as may cause impairment in the efficiency of pulmonary function via uneven ventilation/perfusion ratios among the alveoli (cf. GERST, RATTENBORG and HOLADAY, 1959).

Turning instead to the post-haemorrhagic changes in arterial acid-base balance and in end-tidal P_{CO_2}, it was observed that there was still a tendency towards acidosis, although pulmonary ventilation was kept at the pre-haemorrhagic level (Fig. 3C). The end result was invariably a marked arterial acidosis, even if a given shift in pH required a considerably longer time to develop than in the case of the spontaneously breathing animals. The end-tidal P_{CO_2}, however, remained at a level lower than normal throughout the post-haemorrhagic period, exhibiting only a partial recovery. These changes are interpreted in terms of a progressive development of acidosis from reduction of the buffering capacity of the blood, i.e. an acidosis of metabolic origin.

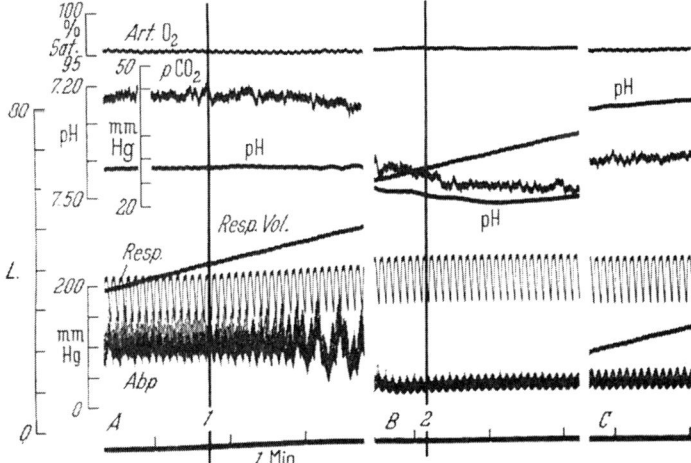

Fig. 3. Dog, chloralose, 15 kg. Late effects of acute haemorrhage (450 ml. between vertical lines 1 and 2), during O_2 breathing, constant artificial ventilation. Recordings as in Fig. 2. Intervals of 2 min. 40 sec. between records A and B, and 15 min. between records B and C

It can be inferred, then, that at least part of the acidosis occurring in the spontaneously breathing animals is also caused by accumulation of acid metabolites in tissues and blood. However, since a post-haemorrhagic depression of respiration was usually observed in these animals, it must be assumed that the acidosis seen here is of a combined nature, i.e. both respiratory and metabolic.

It is well known that central structures involved in various regulative processes are sensitive to changes in the hydrogen ion concentration, and that, for example, excessive acidosis may irreversibly depress the function of such structures. There are also indications that the responses of peripheral vessels to various vasoactive agents are modified by local changes in the hydrogen ion concentration. Extended studies of haemo-respiratory functions in different types of shock would therefore seem to be needed in order to investigate the functional connections between cardiovascular changes and alterations in the acid-base balance.

Summary

Effects of acute haemorrhage were studied in lightly anaesthetised dogs by means of continuous and simultaneous recordings of arterial pH and O_2 saturation, end-tidal P_{CO_2} and pulmonary ventilation. In spontaneously breathing animals, haemorrhage caused an initial hyperventilation followed by hypoventilation and a persistent trend towards acidosis. In experiments with constant, artificial ventilation, haemorrhage produced a marked and persistent lowering of the end-tidal P_{CO_2}, whereas the arterial pH eventually changed in the acid direction. Different mechanisms capable of producing acidosis after haemorrhage are discussed.

References

1. BARR, P.-O., H. BJURSTEDT, and J. C. G. COLERIDGE: Acta physiol. Scand. 47, 16 (1959). — 2. GERST, P. H., C. RATTENBORG, and D. A. HOLADAY: J. Clin. Invest. (U.S.A.) 38, 524 (1959). — 3. LANDGREN, S., and E. NEIL: Acta physiol. Scand. 23, 158 (1951).

Discussion

NICKERSON: Dr. HOWARD mentioned more or less together two items discussed at a recent conference by Dr. GUYTON. One is the relationship of lethality in haemorrhagic shock to oxygen debt, and the other is the matter of possible myocardial involvement. Mortality rate was well correlated with total oxygen debt during the bleeding period, but no real distinction between myocardial and peripheral contributions was apparent. The evidence for myocardial inadequacy did not seem to be convincing for periods of the shock process other than the terminal decompensation. I would also like to ask Dr. TAKÁCS a question about methodology. We attempted to utilise the Sapirstein method in haemorrhagic shock in dogs, and we were quite discouraged to find that clearance of the Rb^{86} from the blood was much delayed. In normal animals, most of it was gone within about two minutes. However, in shocked animals, a very appreciable percentage remained in the blood stream 5 to 10 minutes after the injection. Unequal extraction and recirculation of this material could give a very incorrect picture of the distribution of blood flow. I would like to know the extent to which the Rb^{86} persisted in the blood of his rats and the time at which the animals were sacrificed.

HOWARD: STRAWITZ and HIFT studied the function of mitochondria of the myocardium of dogs before and after the development of irreversible haemorrhagic shock. They found a decreased ATP production and an increased inorganic phosphate accumulation under the conditions of irreversibility.

TAKÁCS: We performed control experiments on dogs and rats. In normal dogs, 90—96 % of the injected Rb^{86} disappears from the blood after 2 minutes. While in 1 minute after the injection of Rb^{86}, more than 90% of the isotope disappears from the blood of normal rats, after haemorrhage with blood pressure of 20—30 mm. Hg, 91% of the injected isotope disappeared only after 2 minutes. Consequently, these latter rats were killed after $2—2^{1}/_{2}$ minutes.

ALLGÖWER: As a "bloody clinician" one is always confronted with the necessity for evaluating clinical parameters of the patient in order to assess the severity of the impending or actual shock. Personally, I have attained some peace of mind by using five criteria, and I would just like to ask Dr. HOWARD whether he, in the light of his 5,000 cases, would agree with these five criteria. Four of them were mentioned by Dr. FINE yesterday, i. e. pulse rate, blood pressure, urine flow, and peripheral circulation. I have a fifth criterion, which is probably the most useful in the clinical situation and which up to now has not been sufficiently used, namely careful evaluation of the "time factor" of the other four factors. If you consider the changes in heart rate, blood pressure, and urine flow as well as the changes in the peripheral flow, you get a much more dynamic picture and a far clearer prognostic insight than from one or two unrelated observations. I don't know whether Dr. HOWARD or the group as a whole would agree with such an empirical view.

HOWARD: About the only other guide we have is the response of the blood pressure to a change in position. If a patient sits up, his blood pressure may drop, often indicating a residual blood-volume deficit. ARTZ used a tilt table in an effort to develop this concept. Another guide, but one that doesn't come along at the right time, is the response to anaesthesia. A dramatic drop in pressure with anaesthesia is an indication that the blood volume may not have been restored. The value of the haematocrit has been "run down" too much. It is true that there is little immediate change in the haematocrit after haemorrhage, but a gradually falling haematocrit over a period of hours implies a blood-volume deficit. Again, I am pessimistic about the value of actual blood-volume measurements (by present techniques) *in the injured man*. I am not sure that each of us would interpret each other's data in the same way.

NICKERSON: I might add one other sign which we have found very useful in clinical studies — the rate of capillary filling in the nailbed after the blood has been expelled by pressure. This is hard to quantitate exactly, but we have found quite a clear distinction between the individual who is hypotensive with vasodilatation and the patient who is in real danger from hypotension associated with vasoconstriction.

BREWIN: I think the other simple clinical sign to bear in mind is the observation of the veins in the neck. This is important, particularly when you are replacing the blood loss by transfusion. You must watch the neck veins and if they become distended the patient certainly has had enough.

HÖKFELT: Dr. HOWARD, with respect to the question of heart failure in shock, in your experience there was no beneficial effect from treatment with either cortisone or hydrocortisone. I just wonder if you have as yet been able to test the usefulness of aldosterone and perhaps have some data on it. I raise this question, because there is some evidence that aldosterone is a sort of circulatory hormone. Dr. BEIN gave some evidence to this effect yesterday, and I also want to recall the recent investigations in Dr. SAYERS's laboratories at Western Reserve in Cleveland. They found that the functional capacity of the isolated rat heart-lung preparation is markedly increased by the addition of aldosterone to the perfusion fluid[1].

GROSS: May I just add that to my knowledge this work of SAYERS et al. has not so far been confirmed by others. SAYERS's group worked with aldosterone isolated from the urine, but as far as I know their observations were not checked with synthetic aldosterone. The isolated heart-lung preparation used by this group seems to be highly sensitive, as concentrations of their aldosterone as low as 10^{-10} were claimed to be active. Such low concentrations of d-l-aldosterone showed no direct stimulatory effect on the isolated rabbit atria[2].

HOWARD: We have not used aldosterone in the treatment of haemorrhagic shock, nor have we used it clinically in any form of cardiac failure.

BACQ: I would like to ask Dr. HOWARD a question. During the first stages of myocardial infarction, there is a very considerable fall in blood pressure, and I would like to know if he believes that this may be a reflex of the Bezold-Jarisch type. One argument in favour of this is that, in two cases of acute cardiac infarction we saw, a very dangerous *increase* in blood pressure occurred following injection of calcium and naturally we discontinued this kind of therapeutic essay.

---

[1] Amer. J. Physiol. **199**, 221 (1960).

[2] J. V. LEVY and V. RICHARDS: Clin. Res. (U.S.A.) **9**, 143 (1961).

HOWARD: You mean that an increase in blood pressure, i.e. hypertension, resulted from the calcium injection?

BACQ: Yes, an increase in blood pressure — which was very low — occurred in response to the calcium injection.

HOWARD: Several of us in Korea (STRAWITZ, ARTZ) studied the effect of calcium infusion. I refer to the effect of one or two grammes of calcium gluconate given intravenously. The effect on the normal person seemed minimal. There was perhaps a transient increase in depth of respiration or a sense of warmth of the skin. Most of the injured and shocked patients showed no significant response. However, an occasional hypotensive patient, remaining hypotensive after transfusion, showed a striking and persistent return of blood pressure to normal after calcium had been given. We have not detected a hypertensive response, except for perhaps a moment or so.

BOCK: I should like to refer to the paper by Dr. BJURSTEDT and to the deviations of pH in both directions which he has described. You remember that yesterday, in the discussion following Dr. BEIN's paper, Dr. NICKERSON reported on experiments on the vascular responsiveness to pressor drugs in endotoxin shock and that his findings were in contrast to those of Dr. BEIN. It might be that these conflicting data are due to species differences or to differences in the experimental set-up. Our own experiments on haemorrhagic and endotoxin shock in the conscious dog have shown, however, that in the same animal species and under the same experimental conditions the pressor reaction to noradrenaline and angiotensin may be enhanced or diminished. Furthermore, also in the course of the same experiment, an originally increased pressor reaction may become more and more decreased in a later stage. It also happens that in a state of shock the response to angiotensin is increased and the response to noradrenaline decreased, and vice versa. It might well be that these changes could be related to the changes in pH described by Dr. BJURSTEDT. I remember a recent paper by MEESMANN[1] indicating that a change in pH towards the acid side decreases the reaction to pressor drugs, such as noradrenaline and angiotensin, by varying degrees. Correction of the pH re-established the original response.

BOHR: We have studied the effect of the pH on the responsiveness of the vascular bed. Rabbit ear and rat hind-leg preparations were perfused with Krebs solution at a constant flow rate. The response to the intra-arterial injection of epinephrine was recorded as a rise in perfusion pressure. In every case, when the pH of the perfusion fluid was changed from 7.4 to 6.9 , the response increased in magnitude. Conversely, an increase in pH from 7.4 to 7.9 was accompanied by depression of the epinephrine response. These results, which conflict with the concept that acidosis is responsible for a decrease in responsiveness in the intact animal, add to the complexity that must be reckoned with in considering the pathogenesis of irreversibility in shock.

HOWARD: I should like to ask Dr. GREGERSEN to recall his early studies on man. You explained that, as shock developed, the pH of the blood fell and the lactic acid concentration rose. At what stage in the shock picture did you first detect this?

GREGERSEN: The pH was of course measured in patients by the team at Bellevue and also in our experiments on dogs, but I do not now recall the timing details, etc. in relation to other events, which would answer the

---

[1] Verhandlungen der Deutschen Gesellschaft für Kreislaufforschung, 1961.

question raised. Perhaps I in turn may raise another query. Why is there so little evidence of a real depression in oxygen consumption in man, whereas in the dog it is pronounced? Is it perhaps that oxygen consumption is seldom measured in such advanced stages of shock, because transfusion and resuscitation take priority, or is it because the dog can tolerate a much greater reduction in the cardiac output? In relation to body size the dog's cardiac output is of course much higher to start with than in man. Another difference mentioned here is that in man the peripheral resistance seldom rises much, if at all. Is that in accord with your observations, Dr. LILLEHEI?

LILLEHEI: I have had no experience in measuring total resistance in man.

GREGERSEN: In the dog we found large increases in peripheral resistance. I wonder if it is sufficient to assume that this is a species difference. It might also be the experimental procedure used to produce shock — though, as you may remember, Dr. FINE, we used various types, including simple haemorrhage.

FINE: These patients are in a state of severe vasoconstriction.

GREGERSEN: Well, the thing that puzzled me was that the marked evidence of intense peripheral vasoconstriction in man was not reflected in the total peripheral resistance.

FINE: We have recently taken a close look at the amount of data published on clinical shock. It is extraordinarily small. We simply do not have enough information. Aside from your data and those of RICHARDS and COURNAND during World War II, there has since been hardly anything apart from the data obtained by JOHN HOWARD and his staff in Korea in 1950 to 1952.

GREGERSEN: Yes.

FINE: Putting it all together, we find that we simply cannot draw any general conclusions on man until we get a lot more clinical data.

GREGERSEN: Dr. FINE, you may have seen the report Dr. CONLEY, Dr. LEIGH, and I prepared in the winter of 1940—41 and submitted to the National Research Council in April 1941, in which we did exactly the same thing. There was then an extreme paucity of reliable physiological data on man in shock. Although the report is 20 years old, I have been inclined to have it reproduced, because several investigators have asked me for it. It might be interesting for comparison with your review of clinical data on shock. I, too, would like to support what Dr. HOWARD says, and I believe that intensive studies on shock in man with all the new techniques available would be most rewarding.

SPINK: I might point out that my associates have shown in the monkey that endotoxin does cause a gradual decline in total peripheral resistance, which approaches the changes that occur in man. This gradual decline in peripheral resistance in the monkey differs from the findings in the dog.

FINE: There is vasoconstriction just the same.

SPINK: We have been impressed by the vasoconstriction that occurs initially, and then the subsequent appearance of vasodilation.

FINE: There may be a terminal vasodilation. But for all practical purposes they are in vasoconstriction as long as they are in shock.

GILBERT: I should like to support the comments that Dr. SPINK has just made. I would first like to recall that one would expect, not only from the baroreceptors but also from the intrinsic elasticity of the vessels, an increase in vascular resistance in any type of hypotension. This does not seem to occur to a striking degree in haemorrhagic hypotension. There are some data, but we need more to be sure. Furthermore, in endotoxin shock in the monkey we have found a progressive drop in total peripheral resistance instead of the expected rise. In the eviscerated dog, the same situation has been found to obtain using constant perfusion. There are few data in man that I know of. A few years ago, using the dye dilution technique in patients with hypotension associated with serious infection — some gram-positive and some gram-negative — we found the cardiac outputs to be at the normal basal level in four or five cases despite a definite hypotension, and therefore the calculated total peripheral resistance was normal or reduced. Now, this does not mean to say that these people were adequately perfused for the situation in which they were, since they were all quite sick, and three of them died. I think we are oversimplifying events when we just consider constriction of resistance vessels as a universal phenomenon in shock. There is certainly constriction in some beds, and there may be disproportionate constriction in some types of vessels, as was hinted at yesterday by several people including Dr. FOLKOW. Therefore, I think there is a need to focus our attention on *perversions* of constriction — such as intense venous constriction, perhaps, or arteriolar dilation — occurring in different vascular beds at different times in the progression of shock.

LILLEHEI: Much has been learned about total vascular resistance, as well as resistances in individual organs, by clinical studies in man and experimental studies in the dog during total cardiac by-pass using a pump-oxygenator. In general, resistance to flow appears to increase in more or less direct proportion to the length of time of total by-pass, although there are of course individual variations in the different organ systems. Moreover, despite the fact that high flow or "normal" cardiac output is being pumped into the patient or animal, complications also increase proportionately with the length of time of the by-pass. These complications occurring post-by-pass, such as oliguria, anuria, gastro-intestinal bleeding, and neurological defects, closely resemble the findings seen in the animal following prolonged shock. Indeed, I believe that prolonged cardiac by-pass, more than one hour, is a form of controlled clinical shock. However, before going into the causes and possible preventatives of such "controlled" shock, I think we should await Dr. SENNING's paper to-morrow in which this problem will be covered. Further discussion of the problem will then be more appropriate at that time.

HOWARD: Dr. GREGERSEN made some remarks about oxygen consumption. In man, there are two opposing factors. If the circulation remains adequate after injury, oxygen consumption increases. If the circulation collapses, oxygen consumption probably decreases simply on the basis of lack of tissue perfusion. The resultant changes in total oxygen consumption may very depending upon the magnitude of injury and the degree of circulatory competence.

VON EULER: Perhaps we could now resume the discussion on renal problems which was postponed yesterday.

BULL: Dr. KRAMER described the production of renal failure in experimental haemorrhagic shock. How readily can this be obtained? I had understood that it was difficult. If so, has Dr. KRAMER some special technique differing from other methods?

In the clinical field, I have for several years been interested in the early recognition of renal damage after injury. The most sensitive practical test, to my mind, is the osmolarity of hourly or eight-hourly specimens of urine, freezing-point determination being practical on small specimens. Disturbances are common, more common in burns than in other injuries, and the earliest finding is diminished concentration with low or sometimes normal volume. In the mildest cases there is recovery even during the transfusion period a few hours after injury, but other patients do not improve for several days, and they have moderate rises in blood urea; at that stage they are diagnosed as suffering from renal damage, but actually the situation has been present throughout. The severe cases proceed to established low osmolarity and renal failure. However, what urine is produced is often well regulated in respect to sodium and potassium. Sodium can be strongly reabsorbed and sufficient potassium is often excreted to make hyperpotassaemia rare. How does this fit with the suggestion of the altered balance of counter-current and medullary flow? I should have thought that overaction of a few surviving nephrons would be an alternative explanation. The histological finding of many damaged nephrons would also fit with this.

KRAMER: The method we use is extremely simple. We induce a haemorrhage which extends over about one hour, and then we wait for $3^1/_2$ hours and infuse in about 20—30 minutes. Then we observe the glomerular filtration rate, the osmotic U/P, and sometimes the blood flow. As I have shown in dogs which had pressures of 40—45 mm. Hg during the haemorrhagic period, we do not find any real recovery. The filtration rate is low, but in dogs which have about 60 mm. Hg pressure during the haemorrhagic period we find a recovery. This is the answer to your first question. Now to the problem of sodium excretion and the counter-current system: we found that there is an isotonic urine immediately after the re-infusion in those dogs in which the filtration rate during shock was zero. The sodium concentration is now sometimes equal to, but usually below, that of the plasma. We believe that the effectiveness of the counter-current system depends on the volume of fluid entering it. In shock, this volume is severely reduced, and so therefore is sodium transport. This may explain our occasional finding of a urine sodium concentration approximating that of the plasma.

BULL: I would only say that the results are a little different in treated patients, in that the initial stage of failure is often not one of isotonic urine with respect to sodium, but of retention of sodium.

GROSS: Yesterday, Dr. KRAMER also mentioned renin and asked if it might be of importance in the kidney during shock. So far all that is known from a few data in the literature is that renin secretion might be increased in shock, but there is no exact information about the degree of this elevated secretion, and we don't know anything about the possible participation of renin either in the regulation of renal haemodynamics or in the maintenance of systemic blood pressure. All we can say is that renin is probably also secreted from the normal kidney into the systemic circulation and that its secretion rate is higher from the shocked kidney. Thus renin may liberate its reaction product angiotensin also outside the kidney. This brings me to the paper of Dr. HÖKFELT, who mentioned yesterday that the kidney might play a role in the regulation of aldosterone secretion. No doubt you all know that it was demonstrated recently that angiotensin definitely stimulates aldosterone secretion if it is infused intravenously. Now we have the complex situation that in shock an increased secretion of three different humoral substances is observed, i.e. adrenergic substances, aldosterone, and angiotensin. It might be that there is a connection between these three, at least between angiotensin and aldosterone, and the problem now confronting us is to demonstrate that the increase in aldosterone secretion really is dependent on the increase in angiotensin secretion.

MIGONE: Regarding the so-called "dualism" of the renal circulation, I should like to stress the importance of a distinction between the old concept of TRUETA and modern views on the medullary circulation of the kidney. According to TRUETA, during tourniquet shock or adrenaline stimulation, renal ischaemia was limited to the cortical tissue, while the blood was diverted directly from the afferent to the efferent arterioles, by-passing the glomerular capillary. In fact, in the acute condition of renal ischaemia, such vascular by-pass remains a hypothetical implication.

According to the concept of TRUETA, during the renal ischaemia of shock, the medullary blood flow has to be increased and accelerated and the a—v O_2 difference decreased to a zero value. I don't think that this applies to humans. The decrease in PAH excretion demonstrated by SELKURT could perhaps be explained by the prevalent medullary circulation of the blood along Henle's loops, which cannot excrete PAH. In fact, the renal ischaemia of shock, owing to the progressive increase in resistance in the peripheral vessels, is more intense in the cortex, but it is also present — albeit to a lesser degree — in the medullary region. Here the blood is circulating along the juxtamedullary nephrons, whose principal portion consists of the Henle's loops extending up to the tip of the papilla, whereas the convoluted portion is poorly developed. On the other hand, in the peripheral cortex, the convoluted tubules are more in evidence and the Henle's loops are shorter. I should like to ask Dr. KRAMER whether his observations *in vivo* have revealed a slowing-down or stagnation of medullary blood flow under conditions of shock.

KRAMER: The TRUETA mechanism is found in rabbits, and, as we have heard yesterday, rabbits are peculiar animals. HERMANN REIN used to say: "A rabbit isn't an animal, it's a flower." Possibly there is some truth in this. We usually have nothing to do with rabbits when we want to study any kind of circulation that involves stress. You only have to hold it up by the ears and it dies! As we all know, in dogs we don't see this kind of diversion of blood through the juxtamedullary vessels. As for your other question, I think I can answer it very simply. We have tried to measure the sensitivity of medullary vessels and cortical vessels separately by photo-electric methods, and we found that continuous infusion of adrenaline or noradrenaline into the renal artery caused vasoconstriction in the medullary vessels at lower concentrations of adrenaline than in the cortical vessels. So we feel that the medullary vessels may be somewhat more sensitive. The difference is not very great, but it was possible to demonstrate it quite distinctly. In our shock experiments, we saw that the blood flow is still present in the medullary region — otherwise we couldn't have the wash-out (shown in Fig. 11). We have seen that the blood flow is still present, but that it is reduced to about 20—25% of normal (see Table 1).

BING: In connection with studies on the kidney in shock, it has been mentioned by Dr. HOWARD that kidney lesions were seen in his young patients and that no other organ was damaged in a similar way. We also know from the lectures by Dr. KRAMER and Dr. SELKURT that the renal lesions might be due to some pressor substance. In this connection I would like to show the results of some experiments by Dr. KAZIMIERCZAK and myself on the place of formation of renin in the kidney.

The first slide[1] shows a section of a rabbit kidney on which a separation of different parts of the renal tissue has been performed by a form of micro-surgery. In this way it was possible to isolate parts of the outer cortex containing only the cortex corticis and parts of the Bowman capsules. Such segments were found not to contain renin. On the other hand, segments containing glomeruli, afferent arterioles, and the tubular tissue surrounding them do contain renin. This must mean that renin is located in one or more of these structures. The first of the possibilites can be discarded, as it was found that isolated glomerular capillary loops contain insignificant amounts — less than 0.5% of the total quantity of renin. Renin must thus be located either in the afferent arterioles or in the proximal or distal convoluted tubules, which are lying close to these vessels.

In order to get further information, we compared the amount of renin in preparations containing glomeruli, distal parts of the afferent arterioles, and the surrounding tubular tissue, including parts of both proximal and distal convoluted tubules (Fig. 1 A), with the amount found in similar segments from which the proximal tubules had been removed (Fig. 1 B). Since removal of the proximal tubules was found not to influence the renin content, renin must be located either in the distal convoluted tubule, including the macula densa, or in the afferent arteriole or in both. Further information was obtained by determining the renin content of preparations in which both the distal and the proximal convoluted tubules were removed from the arterioles (Fig. 1 C). Such isolated afferent arterioles contain from less than 10% to about 40% of the renin. This again means that the macula densa, containing part of the distal tubules, accounts for about 60% to well over 90% of the renin.

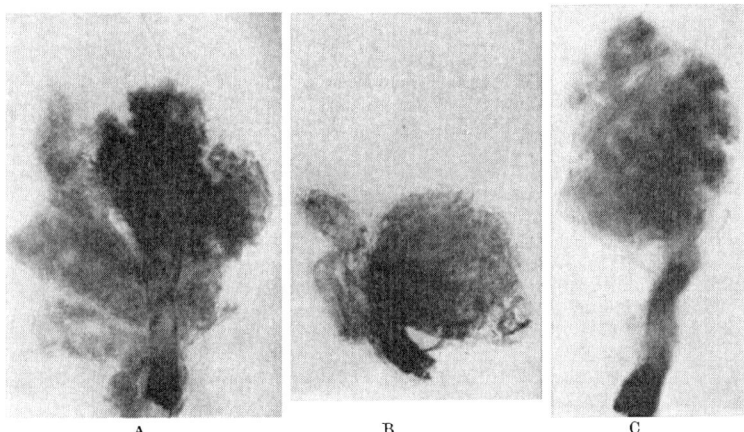

A   B   C

Fig. 1. In A the distal portion of the afferent arteriole and the capillary loop are surrounded by both proximal and distal convoluted tubules. In B the proximal tubules have been removed leaving the macula densa, including part of the distal tubule. In C both proximal and distal tubules have been removed

In conclusion, it can be said that most of the renin is located in the macula densa, while a smaller part is found in the afferent arteriole. From

[1] The first part of these experiments was published in Acta path. microbiol. Scand. **50**, 1 (1960) and the second part is in press *ibidem*.

Discussion 213

these places renin can easily obtain access to the lumen of the vessel. In shock, such passage need not be due to secretion, but may be the result of damage to the cells involving diffusion through abnormally permeable cells. It has thus been shown by KEMP[1] that lactic acid dehydrogenase is released from the cat kidney during haemorrhagic shock.

Release of renin with formation of angiotensin would account for vaso-constriction in the arterioles and glomerular capillary loops. But this is not the only effect of angiotensin, since it has been shown by LEYSSAC, ULRIK LASSEN, and HESS THAYSSEN[2], working at the institute of Prof. HANS USSING in Copenhagen, that angiotensin inhibits active sodium transport. These experiments were performed on 0.2 mm. thick ^{22}Na-loaded cortical slices from rabbit and rat kidneys, which were flushed in a well counter with non-radioactive Ringer's solution. At 0° only a slow decline in counting rate, presumably due to passive leakage of sodium, was found, but at a temperature of 37° the authors observed an acceleration in the ^{22}Na efflux rate representing active sodium transport.

When, instead of the usual Ringer's solution, a Ringer's solution containing angiotensin in a concentration as low as 10^{-12} M was used for flushing the slices, almost complete inhibition of active sodium transport was noted; and it was shown that the inhibition was rapidly reversible when flushing with the angiotensin-containing solution was followed by flushing with the angiotensin-free solution.

Whether these two effects of angiotensin — vasoconstriction and inhibition of active sodium transport — play any role in the pathogenesis of the shock kidney has still to be shown.

HÖKFELT: As Dr. GROSS just mentioned, and as touched on in my previous paper, it is becoming evident that the kidney can influence aldosterone secretion. That this is so was clearly demonstrated by a remarkable case recently studied in co-operation with Dr. E. ASK-UPMARK and Dr. S. BJÖRK and Dr. V. BJÖRK in Uppsala. The patient was a 17-year-old boy with coarctation of the aorta starting directly below the left renal artery — but not involving it — and extending downwards to include the right renal artery. At operation, a by-pass was introduced in the region of the abdominal aorta, and an attempt was also made to restore the blood supply to the right renal artery. Post-operatively, the patient did well for about a week, but then gradually went into shock, and it was realised that the cause was a haemorrhage into the abdomen. At re-operation, 3$^1/_2$ litres of blood were removed. Within a few days, severe hypertension developed (260/160 mm. Hg) and, in addition, polyuria, hypokalaemia, and alkalosis. In view of recent findings that hypertensin increases aldosterone production[3], it was thought that the right kidney might be involved by way of the renin mechanism. An aortogram was therefore performed and showed very poor right kidney circulation, and it was obvious that a Goldblatt mechanism might be operating. Urinary aldosterone was determined and found to be over 100 μg./24 hours (normal range 2—19 μg.). It was decided to remove the right kidney. As a result of this intervention, the blood pressure became normal, the urinary volume returned to normal, hypokalaemia and alkalosis disappeared, and the urinary aldosterone, measured a few days ago, was 5.6 μg./24 hours.

[1] Acta path. microbiol. Scand. (in press).
[2] Biochim. biophysica acta (U.S.A.) 48, 602 (1961).
[3] GENEST et al.: First International Congr. of Endocrinology, Copenhagen, July 1960, p. 173; LARAGH et al.: J. Amer. Med. Ass. 174, 234 (1960).

Shock, Symposium   14a

GELIN: In connection with Dr. KRAMER's presentation of his kidney studies, I would like to emphasise one factor operating in traumatic shock and in prolonged haemorrhagic shock — a factor due to changes in the flow properties of blood when increased viscosity of plasma and aggregation of cells with increased separation of plasma flow and cell flow enter into play. In other presentations here, it has been demonstrated that kidney blood flow is maintained fairly well despite lowering of blood pressure and blood volume.

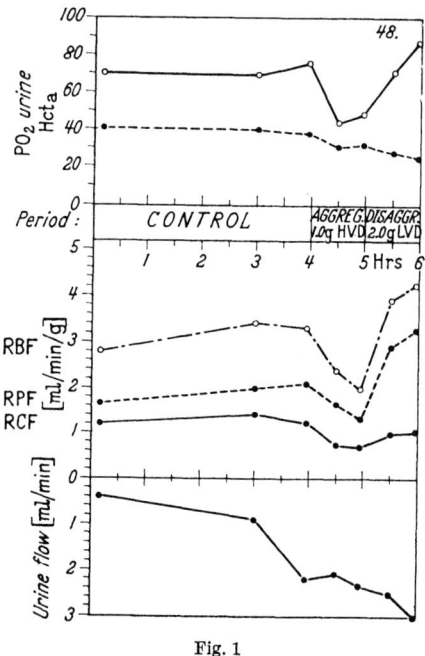

Fig. 1

In co-operation with Dr. PAPPENHEIMER and Dr. RENNIE, we have studied the flow disturbances induced by high-viscosity dextran and reversed with low-viscosity dextran (LVD) in dogs having 100% oxygen respiration. The dogs were catheterised in the ureter and in the renal vein and artery. Radioactive Diodrast and creatinine clearances were determined, as well as the arterial blood pressure, oxygen tension in the arterial blood, renal venous blood, and pelvic urine. The following slide shows 3 periods of study: a control period, a second period with induced flow disturbances, and a third period with reversed flow changes. After infusion of high-viscosity dextran (HVD) the total renal blood flow dropped. This drop was more pronounced for the red-cell flow than the plasma flow, despite an increase in the blood pressure from 140 to 160 mm. Hg. The oxygen tension dropped markedly when these flow changes were induced, but increased again when they were reversed by the infusion of low-viscosity dextran. This increase was relatively more pronounced for plasma flow than for cell flow. The red-cell flow increased, however, to pre-experimental values. The oxygen tension increased at the same time as the flow. These data indicate that these flow disturbances are due to shunting of cells and to stasis of cells.

SELKURT: I should like to say a few words in reply to Dr. MIGONE's question and comments. Regarding the action of the renal vascular shunt mechanism, I think we should abandon the idea that flow is increased through the medullary zones during shock and other experimental procedures (TRUETA shunt). It seems to me more accurate to say that flow may persist to the medulla and that it may, in fact, even be reduced. The evidence for this is particularly good in the rabbit kidney. As has already been stated, in this species cortical blood flow actually shuts down but probably persists in the medulla during renal nerve stimulation. In the dog Dr. KRAMER has presented evidence that both cortical flow and medullary flow appear to be reduced proportionately. I believe that this conclusion was based on only one experiment and, unfortunately, we should have more information. It should nevertheless be emphasised that there is a persistence of flow through the medulla, but at a reduced rate, and probably a shut-down in the cortex. At all events, there will be no increase in flow through the medulla.

My other comment has to do with the extraction of PAH. I heartily agree that the early decrease in PAH extraction following haemorrhage could very well mean that the blood is passing largely through the vasa recta system, away from the tubular secretory zones of the cortex. If hypotension is prolonged, this could, in fact, lead to an actual wash-out of the PAH stored in the medulla during the control period of elevated arterial pressure. This, as we have been told, might account for the negative PAH extraction found late in oligaemic shock.

KRAMER: I would like to make a few remarks to Dr. BING. I am afraid that the interpretation of the angiotensin experiments is somewhat presumptuous. These experiments are on slices, are they not? Now if you just follow the loss of sodium from these slices and find the loss reduced by angiotonin, it could well be that the permeability is changed and not the active transport. If possible, I would suggest doing similar experiments with kidney slices and angiotonin, measuring O_2 consumption by the Warburg technique. If the O_2 consumption decreases, your argument will be much stronger. Meanwhile, I think the interpretation should be regarded with caution.

Clinical aspects of traumatic shock

By

J. P. BULL

The nearer one gets to clinical injuries the less happy one is about the use of the word "shock". This embarrassment is not so much with regard to its precise definition but that its use implies the assumption that there is a single definite state or syndrome — like a diagnosable disease or injury — which is there to be recognised if only we know how to do it.

We have tried to side-step this difficulty in studies at the Birmingham Accident Hospital by starting from the practical problems of treating injuries as they are presented day by day. In this we have followed the well-worn track of distinguished predecessors such as COURNAND and RICHARDS and NOBLE and GREGERSEN nearly 20 years ago at Bellevue Hospital, New York, GRANT and REEVE with the British Army in World War II, and PRENTICE and his colleagues in Korea.

We attempted to investigate the illness of trauma and its treatment; the early stages of this illness might equally be called "shock". A surgical colleague, Mr. RUSCOE CLARKE, had been impressed by the good results following blood transfusion in war injuries, and we decided to look again at the role of blood loss in peace-time accidental injuries and at the effect of its replacement by blood transfusion. This approach had the great procedural advantage that blood loss is both measurable and treatable, and the most rational treatment — replacement of the loss by transfusion — is itself measurable. Dr. ELIZABETH TOPLEY worked with RUSCOE CLARKE to select aspects most likely to yield useful results within the technical possibilities of investigation and in the clinical situation where the primary concern must always be the welfare of the patient. She applied her previous experience of the conduct of controlled trials to the formidable problems of arranging adequate comparisons of injuries of various severities investigated and treated in different ways. The studies extended over several years; other members of the team were FLEAR, a biochemist; MARY FISHER, a clinical investigator; and DAVIES, an expert in the use of radioisotopes.

Logically the first requirement was to establish reliable techniques for measuring blood loss. In view of the delay and incompleteness of haemodilution after blood loss, measurements of haemoglobin or haematocrit are not sufficient. Two main approaches were used: the first was to measure the blood remaining in the circulation, comparing it with the expected normal before injury with suitable correction for amounts transfused; the second was to measure independently the amount lost from the circulation.

(1) For measurement of circulatory volume TOPLEY first used labelling of plasma with T.1824. This was soon superseded by labelling of red cells with P^{32} and later Cr^{51} tagging. Comparison of the methods in normals and especially in injured patients showed that the red cell methods were more reliable than plasma labelling. P^{32} and Cr^{51} were of comparable precision for volume measurements, but since we were also interested in survival of red cells Cr^{51} was usually preferred (DAVIES and TOPLEY, 1959). In our hands the accuracy of the method was about $\pm 10\%$ — or about $^1/_2$ litre in an adult. The blood loss inferred from these measurements depends also upon assuming a normal value before the accident; in many cases we checked this later by a follow-up convalescent value.

(2) External blood loss at the place of accident is not easily measured — though sometimes the information can be obtained directly or by the appearance of clothing or dressings.

In closed injuries the swelling of limbs can be measured. Where practical, fluid displacement and comparison with the normal limb gives a good estimate accurate for the leg to 50—75 ml. An alternative is circumferential measurement with a tape. There are various possible techniques; we preferred measuring at a series of standard intervals. Such calculations were accurate to approx. 250 ml. for the thigh or approx. 150 ml. for the leg. An approximate guide, which has been found very useful in teaching, is to show what various volumes of swelling look like on a normal person. Areas of felt can be cut to have a volume of $^1/_2$ litre, 1 litre, 2 litres, etc., and when wrapped around a normal body they show approximately what swelling such a volume of haemorrhage would cause. It may be doubted whether these swellings can be considered as volumes of blood lost, but when such areas are operated upon the major content is blood and not oedema; the haematocrit is seldom raised, and the extent of the later spread of staining confirms that the major content is blood.

The usual procedure has been to use as many of these clues as possible to estimate the blood loss of each patient and to see whether the estimate of circulatory volume — in practice, red cell volume — checks with this estimate. Blood is transfused to replace the loss, and later circulatory volume estimates provide a check on the calculation and information on possible further bleeding. In almost all cases these various pieces of evidence fit together consistently. There is thus no appreciable mysterious loss in the types of skeletal and limb trauma of all severities which we have investigated. There may of course be a later anaemia due, for instance, to infection, but we are speaking now only of the first few days after the injury. An important finding, however, is that the losses so measured are often very great. Sometimes losses are internal, as for instance after rupture of the spleen.

Having established adequate estimates of blood loss, we tried to see what correlation there was with the classical symptoms and signs of shock. GRANT and REEVE made a very useful summary of these signs, the most extreme group being that of cold hypotension, with other patterns of hypertension and rapid pulse occurring in some cases. Dr. FISHER (1958) made observations of these various signs in 50 injured patients at the actual time of blood volume measurement. Broad associations of blood pressure and pulse rate with blood volume were found, but no particular combination of signs was sufficient to diagnose the amount of bleeding.

Frequent syndromes were:

1. Hypotension — often with cold skin, often with tachycardia. Such patients had on average a blood volume 50—60% of normal.

2. Tachycardia — with normal blood pressure, the skin might be warm or cold. Such patients had on average a blood volume about 70% of normal.

3. Hypertension — with fast, normal or slow pulse. Such patients had a blood volume about 80% of normal. It is interesting to note that the average age of these patients with a hypertensive response was not different from that of the rest.

4. Normal pattern — > 70% blood volume.

These patterns were altered by anaesthesia and do not have the same significance in the post-operative period.

On the basis of blood volume and clinical studies on a total of 145 injured patients, the following aids to clinical assessment of blood loss were recognised (TOPLEY, 1958).

Injury   Type of fracture
                Likely vessel and soft-tissue damage
                External bleeding
                Swelling

Circulation   Pulse more than 90 per minute
               Systolic blood pressure less than 100 mm. Hg
               Pallor and/or coldness of skin
               Level of external jugular vein
Red cell volume estimates
Haemoglobin level: day 4—14.

With increasing experience of these in relation to direct estimates, blood volume determinations are found to be less often required. Injuries confined to the limbs seldom need help from blood volume estimation, but there remain a number of multiple injuries, injuries with losses greater than 3 litres, and intra-abdominal and intra-pelvic injuries, where they continue to be of great value.

The *effects* of replacement of blood loss were studied in three grades of injury. In the most minor grade some cases which were transfused were compared with others not transfused. In the more severe injuries different degrees of adequacy of transfusion were compared. The results confirmed that replacement of blood loss tended to correct the various "shock" syndromes and also improved the subsequent clinical course. We would not of course claim that all functions always return to normal. Many of the patients had symptoms relating to the particular areas or special severity of injury. It also may well be that there remain altered functions which we do not usually investigate. GRABER (1960) has described disturbances of homeostatic mechanisms even after adequate transfusion.

Our biochemical studies confirm the improvement with correction of blood volume (FLEAR and CLARKE, 1955). There is little evidence of water retention or of sodium retention. Nitrogen excretion does rise somewhat in fully transfused, as well as under-transfused patients, but positive nitrogen balances appear to be more easily achieved in transfused patients. This dissociation of electrolyte and nitrogen metabolism provides further support for the view that the syndrome of trauma should not be considered as either unitary or inevitable.

The studies described here have explored the orthodox view that blood loss is the most important causative factor in traumatic shock and that it is best treated by blood replacement. This may be thought so generally accepted as not to need saying again, but when one looks at the recent publications on the subject it appears that it may be forgotten. Recent studies describe tests on anti-histamines, anti-serotonin, corticoids, and noradrenaline for the treatment of shock. The test conditions used to provide a criterion of success are usually the withholding of blood replacement after haemorrhage for so long that the circulation can barely recover again. This is clearly an interesting field of research, but such situations need not be at all common in clinical traumatic patients. If we were studying, for instance, asphyxia, we might well design a machine which limited the oxygen supply to maintain 70% oxygen saturation, so that deprivation for, say, 1 hour produced a situation which could not then be relieved by oxygen. We might then perhaps call this irreversible anoxia, or even perhaps normoxaemic asphyxia. We might explore whether Coramine or digitalis prolonged survival or whether pre-treatment with anti-adrenaline was helpful, but we would be very foolish to conclude that these were any substitute for a clear airway and oxygen given as soon as possible to patients with asphyxia.

Most major injuries are multiple injuries involving fractures of several parts of the skeleton, and many functions are disturbed, including psychological, reflex, and endocrine changes. Various combinations of symptoms and signs result. If blood loss is corrected early, many of these symptoms return to near normal with minimal general disturbance. Surgery is usually then successful in patching up the skeletal damage, and this also applies if the damage is to solid organs such as spleen, liver or kidneys. The major injuries which still most frequently give clinical trouble are those complicated by injures to other essential organs, in particular damage to brain or lung. These are the cases which most often die, but not from traumatic shock. Some people do, however, still die without such complications, and some of their deaths are correctly attributed to "shock". Autopsy of such cases reveals unrecognised, untreated blood loss.

Summary

1. Studies on the illness of trauma following civilian injuries are reported.

2. Various techniques are described for measurement of blood loss; this is often greater than would be expected clinically. The losses so measured are consistent with careful repeated blood volume determinations, and there is little evidence of any mysterious loss of blood in the types of skeletal trauma investigated.

3. The classical symptoms and signs of shock were carefully observed in 50 patients at the time of blood volume measurements. Broad associations of blood pressure and pulse rate with blood volume were found, but no particular combination of signs was sufficient to diagnose the amount of bleeding.

4. Assessment of the effects of replacement for blood loss have included serial photographic records which show the characteristic appearance — difficult to make quantitative — of patients who have not been adequately transfused. Comparisons with other such patients fully transfused show clinical improvement in the latter group.

5. The improved clinical state is reflected also in biochemical findings showing little evidence of water or sodium retention in fully transfused patients. Nitrogen excretion does rise in both groups, but nitrogen balances are more easily corrected in transfused patients. It is concluded that the major clinical need is still for early recognition and treatment of blood loss. If this is achieved, most of the symptoms are relieved with minimal general disturbance.

References

CLARKE, R., E. TOPLEY, and C. T. G. FLEAR: Lancet (G.B.) **1955/I**, 629. — COURNAND, A., R. L. RILEY, S. E. BRADLEY, E. S. BREED, R. P. NOBLE, H. D. LAWSON, M. I. GREGERSEN, and D. W. J. RICHARDS: Surgery (U.S.A.) **13**, 964 (1943). — DAVIES, J. W. L., and E. TOPLEY: J. Clin. Path. (U.S.A.) **12**, 289 (1959).   FISHER, M. R.: Clin. Sc. (U.S.A.) **17**, 181 (1958). — FLEAR, C. T. G., and R. CLARKE: Clin. Sc. (U.S.A.) **14**, 575 (1955). — GRABER, I. G.: In: Modern Trends in Accident Surgery and Medicine, p. 39. Ed. Clarke, Badger & Sevitt. London: Butterworth 1960. — GRANT, R. T., and E. B. REEVE: Spec. Rep. Ser. Med. Res. Counc. (G.B.) No. 277 (1951). — NOBLE, R. P., and M. I. GREGERSEN: J. Clin. Invest. (U.S.A.) **25**, 172 (1946). — PRENTICE, T. C., J. M. OLNEY, C. P. ARTZ, and J. M. HOWARD: Surg. Gyn. Obstetr. (U.S.A.) **99**, 542 (1954). — TOPLEY, E.: Proc. 7th Cong. Int. Soc. Blood Transfusion, p. 453 (1958).

Discussion

FINE: I find it difficult to restrain my admiration for this excellent presentation by Dr. BULL. We now have a convenient tool for frequent and repeated determinations of blood volume, accurately and semi-automatically. In any large operating theatre one can observe every day some of the phenomena Dr. BULL has described. It is not the surgeon's fault that he has not been determining blood volume to see how close he is to replacing the true deficit. With this tool, the surgeon's ability to estimate blood loss has been revealed to be wholly unreliable. Except for those that Dr. BULL has described, the conventional methods in use — such as estimating the amount of blood in sponges, on the floor, and in the tissues as distinct from the circulation — result in guessing that is often very wide of the mark. When the surgeon, having assured himself of adequate replacement, finds the patient in a precarious state after operation, he will invoke such hazy concepts as "surgical trauma", anaesthesia, drugs, marginal reserves, etc. that he doesn't try to explain further. And when the patient the next day continues to look haggard and listless, with a gross nitrogen imbalance, fever, and perhaps infection, he is told that this is only to be expected. Too often the trouble is not enough blood. Let me give you an example. We removed a large carcinomatous mass from the abdominal and chest wall. We knew in advance that this would be a long and hazardous procedure. It took 4 hours to complete the operation. During that operation, we were careful to return all the blood we thought this man had lost. By the end of the operation, we had given him 2,000 ml., considering this to be enough, especially since he had had a myocardial infarct some time ago. He had a normal blood pressure and not a very fast pulse, but he looked drawn and vasoconstricted. Seen by someone fresh on the scene, he would have been judged to be on the verge of shock. Dr. BULL has described these marginal people who still have a good blood pressure and a pulse below 90; but it only requires a little further loss of blood or a little anaesthesia, and down they go into the kind of deep shock I described yesterday. So we asked the blood volume machine to tell us how close we were in replacement in this case; we were off by 1,500 ml.! We therefore gave the man 1,600 ml., and the next day he was pink and bright and able to walk a bit. We have repeated this experience time and again. In any large hospital doing 25 or 30 operations a day, some 5 or 10 patients go through the experience Dr. BULL has described in traumatic cases for the simple reason that their blood volume is insufficient. I am delighted to see how beautifully he has demonstrated that it is the loss of blood volume not fully made up, rather than other obscure phenomena, that accounts for persisting illness after supposedly effective surgical therapy. The mysterious post-operative phenomena that are so difficult to understand, such as obligatory nitrogen imbalance, can now be viewed in a fresh light. May I again compliment Dr. BULL on an admirable presentation.

GREGERSEN: I cannot help admiring the reports of the two clinical studies we have just heard, in which clinical signs and symptoms and the appearance of the patients were presented as important evidence. Sometimes I almost wish that doctors did not have a convenient means of measuring blood pressure when it becomes a substitute for observing so much else which can be seen, felt, and heard and which may be of more value than a precise blood-pressure measurement. Am I correct, Dr. FINE?

FINE: Yes, you are.

GREGERSEN: In our studies on trauma patients, Dr. NOBLE and I[1] were interested in the relation between the reduction in blood volume and the severity of the injury. From our results we concluded that a fairly good idea of the extent of the blood loss and volume reduction could be had from information on the number and types of fractures and from the appearance and clinical condition of the patient. Do you agree ?

FINE: Yes

GREGERSEN: In patients with a pelvic fracture, blood volume reduction was nearly always very large. In these cases, the amount of blood found at the fracture site by the surgeon was enough ($1^1/_2$—2 litres) to account for the reduction. I wonder if the surgeons here consider that the chart Dr. NOBLE constructed is in fact a practical guide and a reasonably valid basis for estimating the blood loss when a blood volume determination cannot be had quickly or at all.

FINE: You mention a figure of $1^1/_2$—2 litres of blood, but sometimes it is even more.

GREGERSEN: Yes, more. You can get enormous quantities of blood collected in the pelvis. So there are certain very practical things that serve as guides to the amounts of blood to be replaced, without going through the volume measurement procedure — which anyway is too slow. Dr. FINE has some improvement that enables you to do it quickly; but you do need an apparatus for the purpose, Dr. FINE, and the injured patient is not always near to the apparatus which you need for measuring volume.

FINE: It can be near now.

GREGERSEN: It can be near now, *perhaps*.

FINE: Not perhaps, but for sure. It's not easy, but one can move the apparatus to the scene of trauma.

GREGERSEN Another practical question is to what extent the choice of the normal value assumed for the patient may affect the estimate of loss and hence treatment. What practical parameters are found most reliable ? The lean body mass introduced by BEHNKE seems best, but is impractical for the injured, even when estimated from fluid volume measurements[2]. Would skinfold measurements be useful to estimate lean body mass[3] ? Standard deviations in blood volume are fairly large ($\pm$ 10%) with the other parameters.

Furthermore, in calculating total blood volume by either the cell or the plasma method, it cannot be assumed that the ratio

$$\frac{\text{overall cell percentage}}{\text{venous cell percentage}} \left(\text{or, as some prefer, } \frac{\text{body haematocrit}}{\text{venous haematocrit}} \right),$$

which we call the F_{cells} factor, is always a constant. The F_{cells} factor is known, for example, to change during pregnancy, and we have observed a marked decrease in this ratio in splenectomised dogs given large infusions following blood-letting and in histamine shock. Other shock-like states may also change it, and this would be interesting to know.

Fortunately, in most of the cases that you deal with in the clinic, you have a low or normal haematocrit, and there the distortion of the blood volume value as calculated either by the plasma volume-haematocrit method

[1] J. Clin. Invest. (U.S.A.) **25**, 172 (1946).
[2] MULDOWNEY: Clin. Sc. (U.S.A.) **16**, 163 (1957).
[3] ALLEN et al.: Metabolism (U.S.A.) **5**, 328 (1956).

or by the cell volume-haematocrit method is not too bad. And we are also fortunate in the fact that, as far as we know, severe haemorrhage does not alter this distribution of cells in the circulation as measured by the F_{cells} value. At least we have never been able to find it with double measurements of plasma and cell values. But I would like to hear comments from the surgeons on these questions of measurements of blood volume and the problem of parameters.

NICKERSON: I, too, would like to second almost everything that Dr. BULL has said. In our experience, there is no substitute for an adequate amount of blood or other fluid therapy given early. However, I should like to comment on the blood-pressure measurements mentioned by Dr. BULL and Dr. FINE, and, in a different sense, by Dr. GREGERSEN. I gathered from Dr. BULL's correlation that he was putting major emphasis on the systolic blood pressure. Dr. FINE, when referring to a patient in incipient shock, was, I believe, also referring to systolic pressure. I cannot quite agree with Dr. GREGERSEN that the sphygmomanometer should be thrown away, but in our experience determination of systolic pressure is not its most useful function. We feel that pulse pressure, which reflects pulse volume, is much more important. The ease with which the pressure can be determined also is important. An "unobtainable" pressure is not necessarily very low, but it is an indication of a very inadequate circulation.

BULL: Our work, I would say again, is a continuation and a confirmation of the work that has been done before. We didn't know about the work in Korea until we were already launched on our own programme; obviously we are observing the same thing and are coming to very much the same conclusions. I was trying to say exactly what Dr. GREGERSEN was saying concerning the clinical appearance of the undertransfused patient. It's very difficult to define; I have slides which go some way towards showing what we mean. Recognition of this appearance is a matter of experience — one just needs to look for it. I did already hint that blood volume determinations were not necessary in our hands in a great many injuries, but there are still difficult cases, and I indicated which were the ones for which blood volume estimation is still very valuable. The main source of error in practical use is the estimate of what is normal, exactly as Dr. GREGERSEN says. We tried to check back on this by doing convalescent values of some of our patients, and they were close to the estimate that we had used, which was based mainly on height. This has a scatter, as he says, of about 10%, and our method has a scatter of about 10%. This may total as much as 20%, which is about 1 litre in an adult. But 1 litre is not too bad a margin, and serial blood volume measurements will show the direction of change and, in relation to haematocrit or haemoglobin, will give you the information you need. Regarding the body/venous haematocrit, we have also been concerned about this and have generally preferred to use red cell mass as the index of blood volume, rather than calculating with the haematocrit to total blood volume. Our correlations worked out better to red cell mass than they did to total blood volume. If you are using a red cell method, then you don't need to worry about the body/venous haematocrit. We have found that 0.9 is a reasonable approximation where we have done double plasma and red cell determinations.

With regard to Dr. NICKERSON's comment on blood pressure, someone has said that the systolic may be difficult to find; I think the diastolic is quite often more difficult. We have, however, tried scatter diagrams against diastolic and pulse pressures as well as systolic. They show rather the same picture. None of the pressures is adequate as a single guide.

Pathogenesis and therapy of shock due to infection: experimental and clinical studies

By

W. W. SPINK

The problem of shock due to infection received only random interest by investigators prior to World War II. This is in contrast to the more intensive studies carried out on shock caused by hemorrhage, trauma and burns. Research on shock and infection should be expanded for at least two reasons. First, although the advances in surgical techniques and the availability of blood and blood substitutes have contributed to a better treatment of shock, simultaneously the factor of infection has been brought into sharper focus. Second, while the management of infections has been greatly benefited by the introduction of the sulfonamides and antibiotics, these drugs in turn have led to additional problems in this field. The widespread use of chemotherapeutic agents has resulted in the emergence of antibiotic-resistant strains of staphylococci, often complicating the treatment of patients with shock. In addition, antibiotic-susceptible invasive bacteria have frequently been eliminated from the tissues, leaving the less virulent and resistant species, such as the gram-negative coliform bacilli, to multiply and to cause serious disease. The increasing importance of sepsis due to these gram-negative organisms became apparent during World War II (*1, 2, 3, 4, 5, 6, 7*). This report is largely concerned with sepsis and shock due to gram-negative coliform bacteria.

General considerations of shock and infection

Largely because of the lack of knowledge at the present time, it is generally assumed that there are basic differences in the pathogenesis of different types of shock. Nevertheless, a complicating infection can alter the course of shock unfavorably, regardless of how it was initiated. Peripheral vascular collapse and death can occur during the acute phase of infectious diseases of viral, rickettsial, bacterial, and protozoal origin, as illustrated by influenza, typhus, pneumococcal lobar pneumonia and malaria. Improved methods of control and specific therapy have markedly reduced the incidence of shock in many of these diseases. There are some bacterial infections which persistently pose the threat of a fatal outcome due to shock, including instances of sepsis caused by grampositive organisms that produce exotoxins. Surgery of the biliary tract and abortions are not uncommonly associated with sepsis due to *Clostridium perfringens*, and occasionally to *Clostridium tetani*, in which a focal area of necrosis and suppuration is the source of exotoxin causing vascular collapse and renal failure (*8, 9, 10, 11, 12*). Likewise, staphylococcal sepsis can originate with strains producing lethal exotoxin. The role of endotoxins from gramnegative organisms in the production of shock will be discussed shortly.

Burns and toxins

The advent of sulfonamide and antibiotic therapy, along with the demands of World War II, resulted in outstanding achievements in the understanding and management of severe burns. COLEBROOK and his associates (*13*) effectively concentrated on the problem of cross-infection and the elimination of secondary streptococcal sepsis. In 1951 a Symposium on Bruns, sponsored by the Defense Department and the National Academy of Sciences National Research Council in Washington, reviewed the burn problem, pointed out the many advances in treatment, and at the same time cited some of the unsolved aspects, including secondary infections.

The most outstanding accomplishments in the management of burns in the last decade or two include the prompt administration of fluids, the correction of electrolyte imbalance, and the control and elimination of infection. One of the most disturbing features in severely burned patients does not appear at first, but at a later period, when infection may become superimposed upon a toxic state. Invasion of the burned areas by coliform organisms, particularly by *Pseudomonas aeruginosa*, commonly occurs (*14, 15, 16, 17*). Patients dying of shock and renal failure as a result of bacteremia caused by gram-negative bacilli represent instances of endotoxin shock.

In recent years there has been a re-evaluation of the delayed deaths occurring in burned patients as a result of non-bacterial toxemia (*18*). An old concept has been revived, expressing the view that toxemia and death result from absorption of products formed and concentrated in the burned tissue. Russian investigators have extended this hypothesis to include the role of autoimmunization, in which different antigenic products, presumably absorbed from the burned area, result in sensitization. According to this viewpoint, hypersensitivity may result in illness. However, the appearance of antibodies may also participate in recovery. On this basis, experimental and clinical studies have suggested the use of convalescent human serum from burned patients for the treatment of other severely burned patients. Further carefully controlled clinical studies are desirable before this form of therapy can be properly evaluated.

Clinical observations on patients with shock due to infection at the University hospitals, 1950—1960

During the decade 1950—1960, detailed clinical studies have been made on over 150 patients with shock due to infection at the University of Minnesota Medical Center. The observations have been the subject of several reports (3, 5, 19, 20). Briefly, the outstanding features are the large number of patients, chiefly males of advanced age, whose sepsis and shock were due to the coliform group of gram-negative organisms, especially *Escherichia coli*. The management of these patients has been a most challenging and distressing aspect of the studies, because the mortality rate has approximated 60 per cent, a feature that has stimulated experimental studies on the pathogenesis and therapy of endotoxin shock. Bacterial shock has not been a serious concern in the pediatric age group, excluding infants in the neonatal period.

Table 1. *Age, sex and outcome of 29 patients with shock and renal failure*

Age (years)	Sex		Total number	Number died
	Males	Females		
0—10	3	0	3	2
11—50	2	0	2	1
51—60	4	1	5	3
61—70	6	2	8	7
71—80	4	0	4	4
81—90	7	0	7	4
	26	3	29	21

One of the major complications of endotoxin shock is death due to renal failure. During the 5-year period 1955 through 1959, 29 patients with bacterial shock and renal failure were studied. Pertinent data concerning the age and sex of these patients are presented in Table 1. Twenty-six of the 29 patients, or 90 per cent,

15*

were males, and the mortality rate was 70 per cent. The bacteriologic data on these patients are shown in Table 2, and emphasize
the significance of infection by the coliform group of organisms
and of secondary invasion by staphylococci. The presence of two
or more species of organisms in the blood of some of the patients
reflects the poor defense mechanism in the elderly patient with

Table 2. *Bacteriologic data on 29 patients with shock and renal failure*
(demonstrable bacteremia in 26 of 29 patients)

E. coli	9
+ Staph.	1
+ Klebsiella + Pseudomonas + Strep. fecalis	1
Klebsiella (A. aerogenes)	4
+ Proteus	1
+ Proteus + Pseudomonas + Staph.	1
Proteus	2
+ Pseudomonas	1
+ Staph.	2
Pseudomonas	2
+ Paracolon	1
+ Staph. + α Strept.	1
Neisseria intracellularis	2
Diplococcus pneumoniae	1
	29

shock. Three of the patients had extensive burns, complicated by
infection due to *Pseudomonas*. Malignancy, extensive surgical
procedures, and infections of the urinary or biliary tracts were
precipitating factors in the remaining patients. The problems of
therapy in these patients will be discussed shortly.

Experimental studies on the pathogenesis of endotoxin shock

It is generally accepted that the major cause of shock in sepsis
due to gram-negative organisms is endotoxin, which is a somatic
lipo-carbohydrate complex. The extensive pharmacologic and
physiologic changes induced by endotoxins have been reviewed by
BENNETT and CLUFF (21) and by GILBERT (22).

Our efforts have been directed toward investigations on the
nature of the immediate hemodynamic effects initiated by endotoxin. Recognizing that variable endotoxic effects may be anticipated in different animal species, the majority of the experiments
have been carried out in dogs.

The pertinent results of our investigations in this area can be
summarized as follows: 1. Within seconds after the intravenous

injection of a standardized dose of *E. coli* endotoxin, there is a
marked drop in systemic blood pressure and constriction of smaller
peripheral vessels, resulting in a reduction of blood flow through
some organs, including the kidneys (*23, 24, 25*). This initial constricting effect of endotoxin confirms the observations of DELAUNEY
and his group (*26*) and simulates those described by HADDY (*27*)
for histamine. Depending upon the dose, venous constriction is
prominent following the administration of histamine or endotoxin.
In the dog, hypotension, venous pooling, reduced cardiac output,
and decreased blood flow are associated with hemoconcentration,
acidosis, and oliguria. In the early stages, peripheral resistance is
maintained, but with the larger doses of endotoxin a gradual fall
occurs later.

2. In man and in lower animals, endotoxin results in renal
insufficiency, and death is frequently caused by renal failure.
Decreased renal function is due to diminished blood flow, which
is related to the hypotension and reduced cardiac output and to
the vasoconstriction of renal vessels. There is no evidence that endotoxin has a direct effect upon the renal parenchyma. Whether or
not the renal failure is reversible depends largely upon the duration
of the anoxia that is maintained by reduced blood flow. Clearance
studies have emphasized that the effect of endotoxin on renal
function is related to the amount of circulating endotoxin presented
to the kidneys. Small concentrations cause an increase in renal
blood flow, while larger amounts result in hypotension and vasoconstriction with a marked decrease in renal clearance (*25*). Dogs
dying of endotoxin shock within 24 to 48 hours display no significant morphologic alterations in the kidneys. However, within a
few hours, seriously disturbed renal function can be correlated with
a sharp reduction in the concentration of phosphatase in the
kidney (*28*).

3. The immediate effect of endotoxin upon peripheral small
vessels is not due to direct action on the vessel walls. In this
respect, endotoxin differs from the direct constricting action of
bacterial exotoxins (*29*). The vascular activity of endotoxin is
mediated through a component of blood. Studies on the intact
dog and with isolated vessel strips have demonstrated that histamine is liberated through the intermediary action of endotoxin
and a heat-labile plasma or serum factor (*30*). Other humoral
factors are rapidly involved, including the catechol amines, serotonin, and possibly acetylcholine (*31*). Neurogenic factors have
also been implicated in the vascular activity induced by endotoxin
(*32, 33, 34*). While the sympathetic nervous system and epinephrine

do participate in the complex mechanism of endotoxin shock, histamine appears to be a major humoral factor during the *initial* phase of shock (*35, 36*).

In brief, vasoconstriction of the peripheral venous vessels is a primary and immediate effect of endotoxin, and this action is mediated through the liberation of histamine. Hypotension, decreased cardiac output, and vasoconstriction result in decreased blood flow through the tissues, and the deleterious metabolic effects of anoxia result. Progressive changes occur, leading to irreversible collapse, which is reflected in a decline in peripheral resistance, vasodilation, and a failure to respond to endogenous epinephrine and norepinephrine. Renal failure is an outstanding feature of the end stage of endotoxin shock in the dog.

Clinical and experimental studies on the prevention and reversal of endotoxin shock

Critical evaluation of the management of patients with shock due to infection is difficult because many procedures are carried out simultaneously. On the basis of present knowledge some of these therapeutic steps are justified; others may be open to question (*19, 20*). In general, the management of these patients calls for the administration of the most appropriate antibacterial drug; the infusion of fluids and blood for the correction of hemoconcentration, anemia, and electrolyte imbalance; the use of oxygen, although pallor rather than cyanosis is prominent; the administration of vasopressor agents; and the use of large doses of adrenocortical steroids. Because it has been so difficult to evaluate these procedures, various experimental models have been designed for this purpose. Again the following discussion is concerned primarily with endotoxin shock.

Since shock is such a complex and rapidly changing process resulting in extensive hemodynamic and metabolic alterations, the evaluation of any procedure or drug depends upon the stage of shock at which such an evaluation is made. It has been clearly demonstrated in studies on endotoxin shock that pre-treatment of experimental animals yields results different from those observed in animals whose treatment is instituted when the shock approaches a stage of irreversibility. A review of the experimental data shows that pre-treatment of animals with antihistaminics, adrenolytic agents, serotonin antagonists, adrenocorticosteroids, or an antiproteolytic agent protects them against lethal endotoxin shock (*37, 38, 39*).

Because pre-treated animals do not simulate the problem of shock in human patients, therapeutic agents were evaluated in an experimental model *after* the onset of shock and at a stage when irreversibility appeared imminent. The adult mongrel male dog, anesthetized with sodium pentobarbital, and injected with a standardized lethal dose of *E. coli* endotoxin, was used as the experimental model. Within a few seconds after the injection of endotoxin an abrupt decline in systemic blood pressure occurred (Fig. 1). Fifteen to 30 minutes later the blood pressure usually

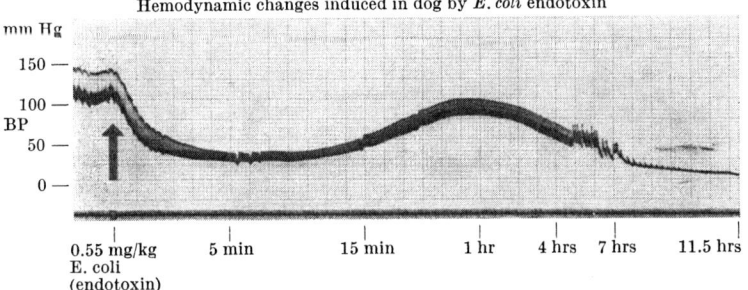

Fig. 1. Composite of original tracing of femoral arterial pressure in a dog given lethal dose of endotoxin

approached the pre-endotoxin level, followed shortly by the stage of irreversible shock, in which there was hypotension, oliguria, hemoconcentration and acidosis. Since several variables could be measured, it was at this later stage that different therapeutic agents were evaluated, either alone or in combination.

Plasma. Using the experimental model as described above, a group of dogs were given large infusions of canine plasma. The shock was not reversed, and the mortality rate was essentially the same as in untreated animals (*37*). The problem of blood volume in canine endotoxin shock is not the extravascular loss of blood but an inadequate circulating blood volume that is due to hepatic and intestinal pooling. Under these circumstances, it is understandable why the administration of plasma would be of doubtful value.

Vasopressor drugs. Two vasopressor agents have been evaluated. Metaraminol[1] was selected for study because it was established in the human subject that the drug could be administered subcutaneously, as well as intravenously. Although the infusion of this agent

---

[1] Supplied as Aramine Bitartrate 10% by the Research Division of Merck Sharp and Dohme, Philadelphia, Pa.

to dogs in shock did elevate the systemic pressure, the animals continued to exhibit acidosis and renal failure and died (40). More recently, preliminary studies have been carried out in canine endotoxin shock with synthetic angiotensin II[1] (Table 3). In the first group of animals the drug was infused intravenously. The hypotension was corrected, but because of pulmonary edema the dogs survived for a shorter period of time than did the control animals. Subsequently, smaller amounts of angiotensin II were

Table 3. *Hypertensin in canine endotoxin shock*
(each animal given 0.55 mg. per kg. of *E. coli* endotoxin)

Dog. No.	Weight (kg.)	Dose of Hypertensin (γ)		Outcome
		Intravenous	Subcutaneous	
1	10.5	1,500		Died 18 hr
2	12.3	2,000		Died 3 hr
3	11.0	1,000		Died 10 hr
4	11.0		300	Survived
5	10.5		500	Died 18 hr
6	9.1		200	Survived
7	10.0		75	Survived
8	11.0		350	Died 7 hr
9	15.0		150	Survived
10	12.0		250	Survived

slowly administered subcutaneously in total doses that approximated 250 γ. Under these circumstances the blood pressure was stabilized, the acidosis was corrected and, although renal function remained depressed, recovery occurred in 2 of 7 dogs. Angiotensin II has a potent vasopressor effect in the dog, as in man, and must be used cautiously (41).

Adrenocorticosteroids. In 1954, we observed that exogenous cortisone protected mice against lethal doses of endotoxin (42). Protection was dependent either upon pre-treatment with the steroid or upon simultaneous administration of the steroid and the endotoxin. Subsequently, it was found that the injection of large doses of hydrocortisone offered no significant degree of protection in canine endotoxin shock when the steroid was given *after* the onset of shock (40).

Turning from the glucocorticoids to the mineralocorticoids, a small amount of aldosterone became available in 1955. Aldosterone was compared with the protective effect of 9 α-fluorohydocortisone,

---

[1] Supplied as Hypertensin by the Research Dept., CIBA Pharmaceutical Products, Inc., Summit, N. J.

cortisone, and hydrocortisone in adrenalectomized mice given endotoxin. In all the groups of mice pre-treated with the steroids, including aldosterone, survival time was prolonged (43).

Synthetic d-aldosterone[1] has been evaluated in canine endotoxin shock. Ten control dogs given endotoxin died, with an average post-endotoxin survival time of 4.0 hours. Eight dogs were given a lethal dose of endotoxin followed by 2 mg. of aldosterone. All of these animals died. Continuous ECG tracings and femoral

Endotoxin control ECG and femoral pulse. Dog # 1, ♂, wt 6.1 kg, 2-28-61

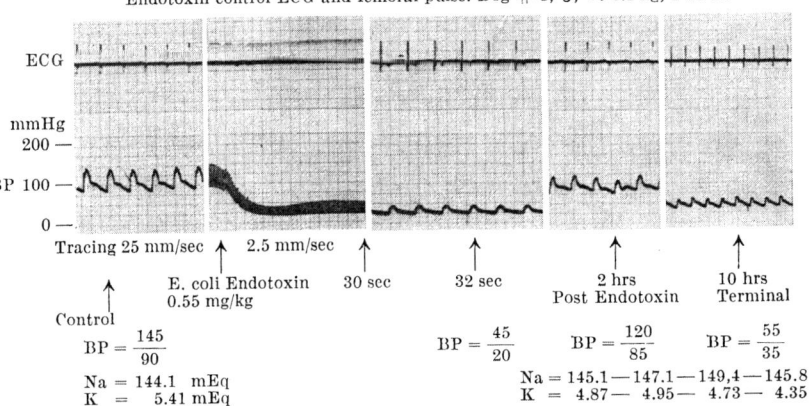

ECG

mmHg
200 —

BP 100 —

0 —

Tracing 25 mm/sec ↑   2.5 mm/sec ↑   ↑   ↑   ↑   ↑

↑   E. coli Endotoxin   30 sec   32 sec   2 hrs   10 hrs
          0.55 mg/kg   Post Endotoxin   Terminal
Control

$BP = \dfrac{145}{90}$ $BP = \dfrac{45}{20}$ $BP = \dfrac{120}{85}$ $BP = \dfrac{55}{35}$

Na = 144.1 mEq   Na = 145.1 — 147.1 — 149,4 — 145.8
K =   5.41 mEq   K =   4.87 — 4.95 — 4.73 — 4.35

Fig. 2. Composite of original ECG and femoral arterial pulse tracings of dog given lethal dose of endotoxin. Note the decline in femoral pressure immediately after the injection of endotoxin, and also the change in the pattern of the pulse wave. Except for a transient inversion of the T waves there was no significant change in the ECG pattern. A decrease in serum K occurred

arterial pressure tracings were made over a period of several hours, including control measurements before and after the injection of endotoxin and after aldosterone. In addition, a series of serum sodium and potassium determinations were obtained on each of the animals. Fig. 2 is a composite of the original tracings in a control dog given a lethal dose of endotoxin. An immediate decline in blood pressure is observed with a marked change in the pattern of the pulse wave. The ECG changes are not remarkable. A decrease in serum potassium was detected.

Figs 3 and 4 are composite tracings of two animals given endotoxin, followed by 2 mg. of aldosterone, which is considered a large dose of steroid. Three significant features were observed in dog 7 (Fig. 3 a and b). First, 4.5 hr post-endotoxin, the pulse pattern was

---

[1] Obtained from the Research Dept. of CIBA Pharmaceutical Products, Inc., Summit, N. J.

that of pulsus alternans. Second, 5 hr post-endotoxin, marked
hypotension was present with a small pulse pressure, and the ECG
tracing resembled the pattern of an acute infarction, which was
probably due to coronary insufficiency and myocardial ischemia.

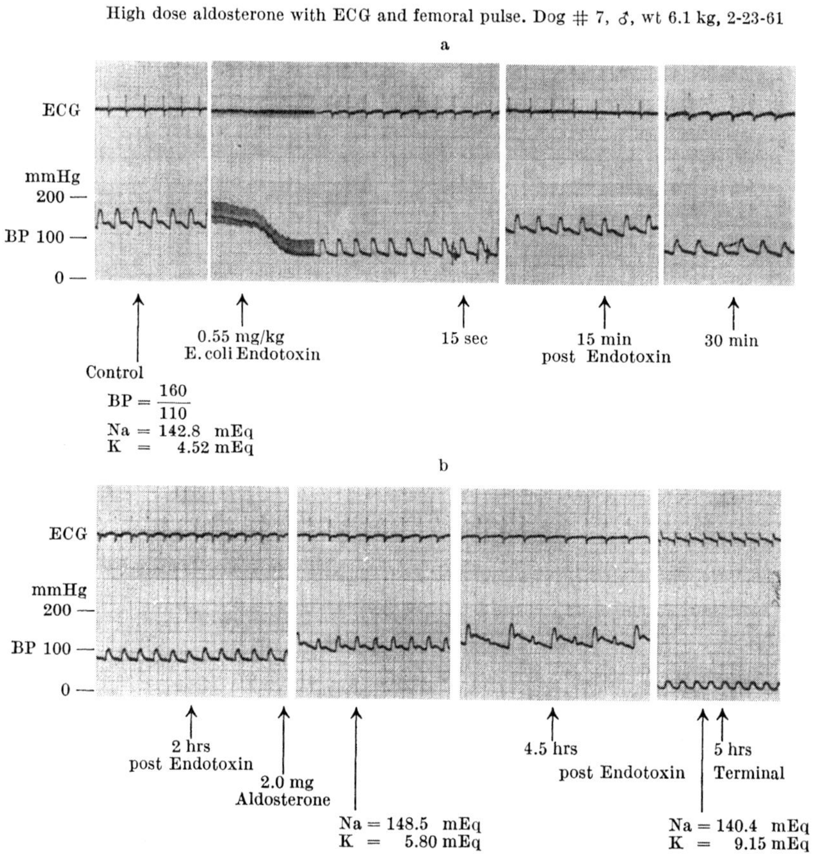

High dose aldosterone with ECG and femoral pulse. Dog # 7, ♂, wt 6.1 kg, 2-23-61

a

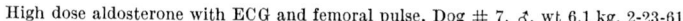

ECG

mmHg
200 —

BP 100 —

0 —

           0.55 mg/kg   15 sec   15 min   30 min
           E. coli Endotoxin   post Endotoxin
Control
BP = $\dfrac{160}{110}$
Na = 142.8 mEq
K =   4.52 mEq

b

ECG

mmHg
200 —

BP 100 —

0 —

     2 hrs   4.5 hrs   5 hrs
post Endotoxin   post Endotoxin Terminal
            2.0 mg
        Aldosterone
            Na = 148.5 mEq   Na = 140.4 mEq
            K =   5.80 mEq   K =   9.15 mEq

Fig. 3a and b. Composite of original ECG and femoral arterial pulse tracings of dog given endotoxin, followed by 2 mg. aldosterone. After the injection of aldosterone note three features:
1. Pulsus alternans 4.5 hr post-endotoxin. 2. At 5 hr post-endotoxin, hypotension with small
pressure, and the ECG pattern of coronary insufficiency. 3. The rise in serum K terminally

And third, a significant rise in serum potassium occurred termin-
ally. Dog 10 (Fig. 4a and b) showed slightly different patterns.
Prominent features were arrhythmia and reduced cardiac output.
There was also a significant rise in serum potassium terminally.

In summary, when a large dose of aldosterone (2 mg.) was given to dogs approaching the irreversible stage of endotoxin shock, changes occurred in cardiac function and in concentrations of serum potassium that were not demonstrated in animals given

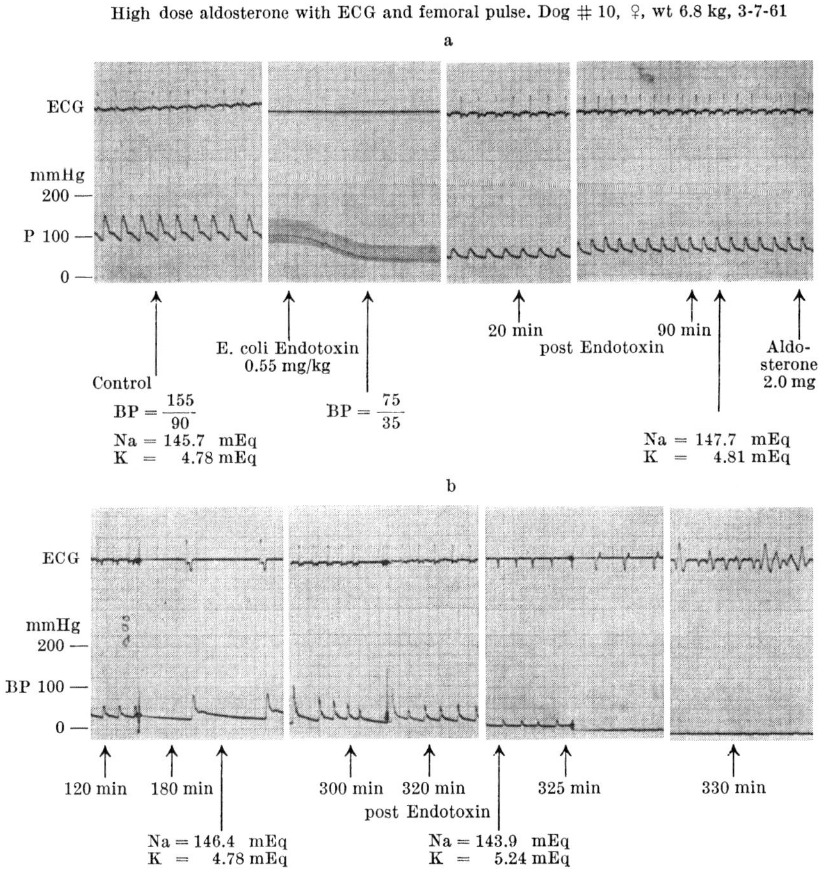

High dose aldosterone with ECG and femoral pulse. Dog # 10, ♀, wt 6.8 kg, 3-7-61

a

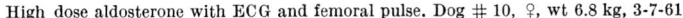

ECG

mmHg
200 —

P 100 —

0 —

Control
E. coli Endotoxin
0.55 mg/kg

$BP = \dfrac{155}{90}$ $BP = \dfrac{75}{35}$

Na = 145.7 mEq
K =   4.78 mEq

20 min   90 min
post Endotoxin

Aldo-
sterone
2.0 mg

Na = 147.7 mEq
K =   4.81 mEq

b

ECG

mmHg
200 —

BP 100 —

0 —

120 min   180 min   300 min   320 min   325 min   330 min
post Endotoxin

Na = 146.4 mEq
K =   4.78 mEq

Na = 143.9 mEq
K =   5.24 mEq

Fig. 4 a and b. Composite of original ECG and femoral arterial pulse tracings of dog given endotoxin, followed by 2 mg. aldosterone. Note the hyperkalemia and the changes in the femoral pulse and ECG

endotoxin alone, or given endotoxin followed by smaller doses of aldosterone. The ECG tracings revealed the pattern consistent with coronary insufficiency and myocardial ischemia. These features of myocardial incompetence were consistent with reduced cardiac output, which was reflected in tracings of the femoral artery, revealing hypotension, a diminished pulse pressure, and pulsus alternans. A consistent finding was the elevation of serum potassium, which was usually detected terminally. This increase occurred at a time when a state of acidosis, hemoconcentration, hypotension and oliguria was present. It is possible that the rise in serum potassium was associated with a decrease in intracellular potassium of the myocardium and that this in turn was related to the myocardial incompetence.

In view of the undesirable effects of the larger doses of aldosterone, a group of animals was given a lethal dose of endotoxin followed by an injection of aldosterone not exceeding 0.3 mg. Continuous ECG and femoral pressure tracings were obtained in a manner already described. Although only one animal survived, this combination of endotoxin and aldosterone did not result in the arrhythmias and in the other ECG changes that occurred with the larger dose of steroid, and hyperkalemia was not detected.

Adrenocorticosteroids and vasopressor agents given simultaneously. Although neither hydrocortisone nor the vasopressor drug metaraminol favorably affected dogs with endotoxin shock when either was given alone, a significant number of dogs survived when the combination was used, providing the steroid was administered prior to the pressor agent (*40*). Comparing dogs given metaraminol alone to those also given hydrocortisone, one-eighth the dose of metaraminol was sufficient to maintain the systemic pressure around 90 to 100 mm. Hg when the two agents were given together. The presence of a large amount of exogenous steroid appeared to "sensitize" the peripheral vessels to the pressor action of metaraminol.

A group of 25 dogs with endotoxin shock received aldosterone and metaraminol. Ten untreated control animals died, whereas there were 18 permanent survivors among the 25 animals that were treated. The remarkable feature in the latter group was the relatively small doses of the vasopressor agent which supported the systolic blood pressure at about 100 mm. Hg when the dogs had been given 0.1 mg. of aldosterone prior to the injection of the pressor drug. The average total amount of metaraminol necessary to support systolic pressure was only 0.8 mg., which compares with doses of 25—30 mg. when metaraminol was used alone (*40*).

Hydralazine and renal failure in endotoxin shock. Although a combination of hydrocortisone and metaraminol successfully sustained the blood pressure of a significant number of dogs given a lethal dose of endotoxin, depressed renal function still posed a serious problem. Hydralazine[1], used as an anti-hypertensive agent, has the property of increasing renal blood flow. In a series of experiments in dogs with endotoxin shock, the administration of hydralazine alone increased the flow of urine, although the hypotension was more severe than in the untreated group of animals (44). When hydralazine was administered in conjunction with hydrocortisone and metaraminol, the number of dogs surviving endotoxin shock was slightly greater than that of the group receiving only hydrocortisone and metaraminol. These treated animals all exhibited an excellent output of urine during the course of the experiment.

Use of organic acid buffer (THAM) in endotoxin shock. Since acidosis is a characteristic alteration in canine endotoxin shock, an organic acid buffer, 2-amino-2-hydroxymethyl-1, 3-propanediol (THAM)[2], was evaluated in several groups of dogs (45). An infusion of THAM into animals with endotoxin shock corrected the acidosis and caused a marked increase in the output of urine. However, the hypotension persisted, and none of the animals survived. When THAM was used in conjunction with hydrocortisone or metaraminol, or both, the acidosis was also eliminated and there was a good secretion of urine. Although dogs did survive when THAM was used in combination with these drugs, the results were inferior to those obtained with hydrocortisone and metaraminol alone.

Concluding remarks

Many clinical and experimental studies have emphasized the complex nature of shock. Rapidly changing hemodynamic and metabolic alterations occur. Adequate quantitative functional and chemical studies in the human subject are not easily obtained, and for this reason investigations have been carried out in an experimental model involving the lower animal species.

This report is concerned with shock due to infection, especially that form due to sepsis caused by gram-negative coliform bacteria. This type of peripheral vascular collapse has been designated as endotoxin shock. The present study has employed largely the adult mongrel dog as the experimental model and a standardized preparation of *E. coli* endotoxin.

Although canine endotoxin shock cannot be considered the precise prototype of human endotoxin shock, the experimental

---

[1] Supplied as Hydralazine HCl by the Research Dept. of CIBA Pharmaceutical Products, Inc., Summit, N. J.

[2] Supplied by Scientific Divisions, Abbott Laboratories, North Chicago, Ill.

investigations have not been unfruitful. In an attempt to obtain more information on the pathogenesis of endotoxin shock, the initial phase has been studied intensively. Immediately following the injection of endotoxin, vasoconstriction of peripheral vessels occurs. This vascular activity simulates that following the administration of histamine, and a rise in serum histamine can be demonstrated. However, other humoral vasoconstrictors are also quickly involved, as well as neurogenic factors. Anoxia, caused by the vasoconstriction and reduced blood flow, contributes to the rapid deterioration of bodily function. The stage of irreversible shock in the dog is marked by hypotensison, myocardial incompetence, reduced cardiac output, hemoconcentration, acidosis and oliguria.

Intensive studies have also been carried out on dogs at the stage when irreversible shock appeared imminent. Correction of the hypotension with vasopressor agents, or with generous amounts of plasma, did not reverse the course of lethal endotoxin shock. Elimination of the acidosis with a buffering agent was without effect. Increasing renal blood flow and, simultaneously, the flow of urine, did not reverse the shock. Adrenocortical failure is often suspected of contributing to the severity of shock, but it was observed that neither the administration of glucocorticoid nor of mineralocorticoid reversed the shock. However, canine endotoxin shock was successfully reversed by the administration of either hydrocortisone or aldosterone, when immediately followed by a pressor agent. The steroid, in a manner unknown, "sensitized" the peripheral vessels to the action of the pressor drugs. It is possible that sodium, and possibly potassium, are involved in the steroid-pressor activity.

Since one must be most cautious in transposing the results observed in the experimental model of canine shock to the problem of human shock, it is desirable to seek out a model which most closely simulates the course of shock in human subjects. Preliminary observations on a primate indicate that it would be worthwhile to continue the present studies in monkeys, and such experiments are under way.

References

1. Batterell, E. H., and D. Magner: Lancet (G.B.) 1945/I, 112. — 2. Florey, M. E., R. W. N. L. Ross, and E. C. Turton: Lancet (G.B.) 1947/I, 855. — 3. Waisbren, B. A.: Arch. Int. Med. (U.S.A.) 88, 467 (1951). — 4. Yow, E. M.: J. Amer. Med. Ass. 149, 1184 (1952). — 5. Weil, M. H., and W. W. Spink: Arch. Int. Med. (U.S.A.) 101, 184 (1958). — 6. Forkner, C. E. Jr., E. Frei III, J. H. Edgcomb, and J. P. Utz: Amer. J. Med.

25, 877 (1958). — 7. FINLAND, M., W. F. JONES, and M. W. BARNES: J. Amer. Med. Ass. 170, 2188 (1959). — 8. AUB, J. C., P. C. ZAMECNIK, and I. T. NATHASON: J. Clin. Invest. (U.S.A.) 26, 394 (1947). — 9. BERG, M., S. A. LEVINSON, and K. J. WANG: Arch. Path. (U.S.A.) 51, 137 (1951). — 10. BRADFORD, W. Z. Jr., and C. BACHMAN: Amer. J. Med. Sc. 237, 785 (1959). — 11. ADAMS, R. H., and J. A. PRITCHARD: J. Obstetr. Gynaec. (Ind.) 16, 387 (1960). — 12. DEANE, R. M., and K. P. RUSSELL: Amer. J. Obstetr. Gynec. 79, 528 (1961). — 13. COLEBROOK, L.: A New Approach to the Treatment of Burns and Scalds, Fine Tech. Pub., London 1950. — 14. LIEDBERG, N. C. F., E. REISS, and C. P. ARTZ: Surg. Gyn. Obstetr. (U.S.A.) 99, 151 (1954). — 15. LOWBURY, E. J. L., D. J. CROCKETT, and D. M. JACKSON: Lancet (G.B.) 1954/II, 1151. — 16. TUMBUSCH, W. T., E. H. VOGEL Jr., J. V. BUTKIEWICZ, C. D. GRABER, D. L. LARSON, and E. T. MITCHELL: Septicemia in Burn Injury, U. S. Army Surgical Research Unit, Brooke Army Medical Center, Fort Sam Houston, Texas, MEDEW-RS-6-60, October 1960. — 17. ROSENTHAL, S. M.: In: The Biochemical Response to Injury, p. 397. Ed. by H. B. Stoner, Oxford; Blackwell Scientific Publications 1960. — 18. Editorial: Toxaemia of Burns. Lancet (G.B.) 1960/I, 153. — 19. SPINK, W. W.: Arch. Int. Med. (U.S.A.) 106, 433 (1960). — 20. SPINK, W. W.: Ann. Int. Med. (U.S.A.) 53, 1 (1960). — 21. BENNETT, I. L. Jr., and L. E. CLUFF: Pharmacol. Rev. (U.S.A.) 40, 245 (1960). — 22. GILBERT, R. B.: Physiol. Rev. (U.S.A.) 40, 245 (1960). — 23. HALBERG, F., and W. W. SPINK: Laborat. Invest. (U.S.A.) 5, 283 (1956). — 24. WEIL, M. H., L. D. MacLEAN, M. B. VISSCHER, and W. W. SPINK: J. Clin. Invest. (U.S.A.) 35, 1191 (1956). — 25. HINSHAW, L., W. W. SPINK, J. A. VICK, B. MALLET, and J. FINSTAD: Amer. J. Physiol. (in press). — 26. DELAUNEY, A., P. BOUQUET, J. LEBRUM, Y. LEHOULT, and M. DELAUNEY: J. physiol. (Fr.) 40, 89 (1948). — 27. HADDY, F. J.: Amer. J. Physiol. 198, 161 (1960). — 28. SPINK, W. W., and M. J. LANDERYOU: J. Clin. Invest. (U.S.A.) 39, 302 (1960). — 29. THAL, A. P., and W. EGNER: J. Exper. Med. 113, 67 (1961). — 30. VICK, J.: J. Laborat. Clin. Med. (U.S.A.) 56, 953 (1960). — 31. HEIFFER, M. H., R. L. MUNDY, and B. MEHLMAN: Amer. J. Physiol. 198, 1307 (1960). — 32. PENNER, A., and S. H. KLEIN: J. Exper. Med. (U.S.A.) 96, 59 (1952). — 33. PENNER, A., and A. I. BERHEIM: J. Exper. Med. (U.S.A.) 111, 145 (1960). — 34. WEIL, M. H., L. D. MacLEAN, W. W. SPINK, and M. B. VISSCHER: J. Laborat. Clin. Med. (U.S.A.) 48, 661 (1956). — 35. WEIL, M. H., and W. W. SPINK: J. Laborat. Clin. Med. (U.S.A.) 50, 501 (1957). — 36. HINSHAW, L. B., J. A. VICK, C. H. CARLSON, and Y. L. FAN: Proc. Soc. Exper. Biol. Med. (U.S.A.) 104, 379 (1960). — 37. SPINK, W. W.: Yale J. Biol. Med. 30, 355 (1958). — 38. SPINK, W. W.: In: The Biochemical Response to Injury, pp. 361—376. Ed. by H. B. Stoner, Oxford; Blackwell Scientific Publications 1960. — 39. SPINK, W. W., and J. VICK: Proc. Soc. Exper. Biol. Med. (U.S.A.) 106, 242 (1961). — 40. SPINK, W. W., and J. VICK: Circulation Res. (U.S.A.) 9, 184 (1961). — 41. McQUEEN, E. G., and R. B. I. MORRISON: Brit. Heart J. 23, 1 (1961). — 42. SPINK, W. W., and D. ANDERSON: J. Clin. Invest. (U.S.A.) 33, 540 (1954). — 43. HALBERG, F., W. W. SPINK, and J. J. BITTNER: Endocrinology (U.S.A.) 59, 380 (1956). — 44. VICK, J., and W. W. SPINK: Proc. Soc. Exper. Biol. Med. (U.S.A.) 106, 280 (1961). — 45. VICK, J. A., L. B. HINSHAW, and W. W. SPINK: Ann. N. Y. Acad. Sc. 92, 662 (1961).

Toxic factors in shock (with special reference to burns)*

By

M. ALLGÖWER

I have been invited to discuss Dr. SPINK's paper and to say a few words on burn toxins as well.

First, I was very interested in Dr. SPINK's obvious success in treating the shocked animal at the beginning of the irreversible stage. In 1956, my collaborator LAVER (1956) obtained similar results in fatally burned rats. He observed a significant prolongation of the survival time in rats treated with acemethonium or hexamethonium bromide. SCHWALB (1959) and later VERAGUT (1961) reported similar responses with isoindoline (Fig. 1). This successful "after-treatment" is in keeping with the observations of INGLIS

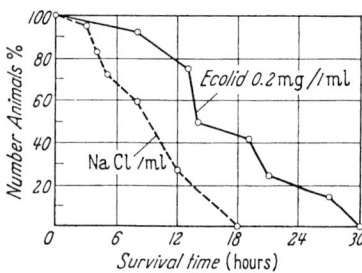

Fig. 1. Comparison of survival times of scalded rats (15 sec. at 90°C) treated with isoindoline and NaCl (VERAGUT 1961)

et al. (1959) and has a clinical parallel in septic shock, where combination of hydrocortisone with vasopressor agents yields good results provided the patient is receiving adequate antibacterial therapy as well as sufficient blood volume replacement.

Turning to the "endotoxin model of shock" I must confess that I am confused. There is no doubt in my mind that endotoxin is capable of provoking circulatory failure with all the accompanying signs of shock. But in the past, many other substances have enjoyed a notoriety similar to that of endotoxin at present, and the treatment of shock was based on such analogies (like histamine and antihistamines). Admittedly some clinical cases with gram-negative sepsis may show signs of endotoxin present in the circulation. Even here, I would be happier if accurate figures were available for

---

* The experimental work, unless otherwise indicated, was carried out together with E. FREI and Dr. U. F. GRUBER at the Laboratorium für experimentelle Chirurgie, Forschungsinstitut, Davos.

the concentrations of endotoxin in the blood or if autopsies were to yield the classical findings of experimental endotoxin administration, as for example the generalised Shwartzman reaction. Dr. SPINK tells us that the generalised Shwartzman reaction occurs only in the rabbit. As we have heard at this symposium, there are some people who like rabbits and others who don't. Those who don't will not even allow these poor animals to participate in our efforts to analyse the mechanisms of shock. Now, if the rabbit is the only animal that shows the generalised Shwartzman reaction and if we are otherwise at a loss to detect small quantities of endotoxin, I think we cannot refuse to use the rabbit as a "test tube" in which to detect the possible presence of endotoxins, McCLUSKEY and ZWEIFACH et al. (1960) have recently pointed out that no repeated shock, other than repeated endotoxin administration or Thorotrast administration followed by endotoxin, will cause histological alterations corresponding to those observed when endotoxin is given experimentally. Now I do not know how sensitive this rabbit test is as regards the detection of endotoxin. According to McCLUSKEY and ZWEIFACH the test is an extremely sensitive one. Probably somebody can give us quantitative data on this point, especially in comparison with the chick-embryo test or the vein-strip technique mentioned earlier in this symposium (see papers by Dr. FINE and by Dr. SPINK).

Histamine has been related to shock in various ways. While it is known that in shock the blood histamine concentration in the later phases does not parallel the clinical course, it is often considered crucial during the first hours after tissue damage. On clinical grounds the histaminase "Torantil" has recently been claimed to be highly beneficial in the early treatment of burns (SCHREUS, 1959).

In the paper just presented, histamine is considered to act as a mediator between endotoxin and the vascular wall. Now obviously this in no way links Dr. SPINK's work with the experiments we have been performing on burned rats in order to determine the influence of histaminase. It may nevertheless be of interest to note that the survival time was not affected at all by the administration of histaminase in large quantities. Assuming that endotoxin depends on histamine as a mediator, histamine does not at all events seem to be instrumental in acute fatal scald injury. However, it might be interesting to determine the influence of such histaminase preparations on endotoxin shock.

Regarding the question of burn toxins, I should like to begin with a few general remarks, or "platitudes" as you might say. The in some respects privileged research workers of the last century were in the habit of seeking *"veritas"* by deductive meditation based on a few careful observations. That is how much of the framework of modern medical science was established. Much the same holds true for our knowledge of cellular defence mechanisms, such as diapedesis and phagocytosis, as well as for the reticulo-endothelial system (RES). Had we placed a large burn with all its destroyed tissue in front of those pioneers and had we told them that we could find no evidence that such extensive tissue necrosis had a deleterious effect, they might well have laughed at us as people who could not see the wood for the trees.

All of us who have endeavoured to pin-point the toxic effects of tissue burns may have been impelled by similar motives, namely, to analyse the almost obvious in order to find some clue to enable us to cope with the clinical situation if not in burn shock, then at least in so-called "burn disease". Though it may be true that all our efforts to date have been largely unavailing, this does not mean that we need do no more.

Time does not permit me to survey the many efforts that have been made in this connection; but in reviewing my own work, which was stimulated by the more recent publications in this field, I hope to show that much further research remains to be done (reference is made to the recent survey by O. Malm, 1961). Experiments carried out together with E. Schwalb (1959) on the survival time of rats scalded with water at 85°, 90°, and 95°C showed significantly decreased survival times with increasing burn temperatures without any evidence of greater fluid loss at higher temperatures. This seems to suggest that some toxic factors may play a part at higher temperatures.

Table 1

	+ 48 h.	+ 8 d.	>8 d.
80°C	—	1	10
~98°C	8	5	13

Survival of rabbits after administration of a depot of heated whole blood (100 ml. per rabbit of approximately 2,500 g. body-weight) into the peritoneal cavity.

The animals are listed as follows: death within 48 hours; death within 8 days; survivors.

Simonart has repeatedly pointed out that heating various plasma proteins above 80°C makes them toxic to frogs, rabbits, and mice. We have administered such heated proteins, especially blood constituents, intraperitoneally (Allgöwer and Siegrist, 1956; Allgöwer, Aschieri, and Hulliger, 1961). Testing the toxic activity of heated proteins by intraperitoneal administration involves certain snags, such as fluid loss into the abdomen, etc., but on the other hand it offers many advantages, e. g. a large surface and, if rapid absorption is rendered impossible, prolonged contact between the absorption surface and the test substance.

Table 1 shows the mortality we observed when introducing heated total blood into the peritoneal cavity. (An intraperitoneal depot of 100 g. heated rabbit blood was employed in rabbits of a mean weight of 2,500 g.) Table 2 gives more detailed information as to how the various groups of animals reacted. While the difference in mortality of the groups receiving blood heated to 80° C as opposed

Table 2. *Haemoglobin and blood urea determination of animals listed in Table 1*

		Hb (N = 35) 73 ± 1.4%				Urea (N = 35) 32 ± 1.6 mg.%			
		N	24 h.	p	90 h.	p	N	24 h.	p	90 h.	ν
80°C	+48h.	0	—		—		0	—		—	
	+ 8d.	1	87		62		1	57		86	
	> 8d.	10	78+4.6	>0.05	61+2.3	0.01	10	51+2.8	0.01	50+6.0	0.01
98°C	+48h.	8	88+8.6	0.01	—		8	63+8.0	0.01	—	
	+ 8d.	5	82+5.3	0.05	67+2.9	0.05	5	55+10.0	0.01	83+10.0	0.01
	> 8d.	13	78+3.1	0.05	58+2.3	0.01	13	41+3.3	0.01	46+2.9	0.01

to 96° C is significant, the mortality in both groups is closely related to the signs of blood-volume shock, despite the fact that the haemoconcentration was in no case as high as could be expected in a severe clinical burn. In more recent experiments we did our best to apply the heated proteins in a more "physiological" form. The heated blood was homogenised and diluted to 2.5 times its original volume with balanced salt solutions. Haemoconcentration can thus be avoided. Here again, the aim of the experiments was to demonstrate possible toxic factors by heating rabbit plasma and erythrocyte stroma to different temperatures over different periods of time. These substances were injected into healthy rabbits and mice s. c. and i. p. in large amounts, though so far without producing much of a deleterious effect.

Several authors have shown burn oedema to be highly toxic, and both SIMONART (1958) and GODFRAIND (1958) have reported similar findings in the case of peptone oedema. We tried to repeat these experiments ourselves. As reported earlier (ALLGÖWER, ASCHIERI, and HULLIGER, 1961), we could reproduce the results of SIMONART and GODFRAIND only with infected peptone oedema. There was no effect if the peptone oedema was rendered sterile by membrane filtration.

Since it is very difficult to produce sufficient quantities of burn oedema in rabbits, we combined scalding with peptone injection in

16*

an attempt to collect the possible toxic factor in the large quantities of oedema thus formed. The experimental procedure was as shown in Table 3: 8 animals were scalded for 15 seconds in a hot-water

Table 3. *Production of burn and peptone oedema*

T	Immersion	6 g. Peptone kg./B.W.			Total rabbits used
		10 h. p.b.	36 h. p.b.	Peptone alone	
80°C	15"	8	13	—	21
97°C	15"	8	13	—	21
—	—	—	—	17	17

bath at either 80° or 97°C. Ten hours afterwards, they received 6 g. of 10% peptone/kg. body-weight under the scalded surface. In 13 animals scalded in this way, the peptone was not administered until 36 hours after scalding. A control group of 17 animals was not scalded and received peptone only. In all three groups, the peptone was injected subcutaneously 14 hours before sacrificing the animals, and the subcutaneous oedema formed was collected by excision, centrifuged, and then sterilised through membrane filters. Bacteriological tests for the presence of aerobic and anaerobic bacteria were carried out as soon as the animals had been sacrificed, i. e. just after opening up of the skin and before collection of the oedema. This oedema was tested in mice (i. p.) and rabbits (i. v.) for possible toxic effects, using 20 ml./kg. body-weight. Table 4 gives our very

Table 4. *Survival after burn and peptone oedema injection. 2% B. W.*

	79 MICE S. C. & I. P.			62 RABBITS I. V.				
	80°C	97°C		80°C		97°C		
	Peptone injected 10 h. p. b.	Peptone injected 10 h. p. b.	Peptone oedema alone	Peptone injected		Peptone injected		Peptone oedema alone
				10h. p.b.	36h. p.b.	10h. p.b.	36h. p.b.	
Number of animals injected	25	24	30	9	18	9	16	20
Death	0	1	0	1	1	0	10	2
Survival after 14 days	25	23	30	8	17	9	6	18

Group	Number	Weight g.	Surface burned %	Survival time min.	t	p
Ecolid	12	194±27	24.8±1.1	1079±454	4.465	<0.001
NaCl	26	214±18	25.4±1.6	561±267		

rough mortality data, other parameters of the oedema effect await-
ing more careful analysis. Peptone oedema, peptone oedema after
scalding at 80°C induced 10 and 36 hours after scalding, as well as
peptone oedema after scalding at 97°C induced 10 hours after scalding do not provoke any deaths within 2 weeks after administration,
whereas peptone oedema induced 36 hours after scalding at 97°C
causes a 50% mortality in the animals. These findings bear a strong
resemblance to those of WILSON (1937), who did not detect toxic
substances in aseptically burned muscles until 36 hours after burning.

In our experiments it was very difficult to avoid infection of the
oedema, even by using sterile solutions and instruments and by
carefully cleansing the peptone injection site. Fig. 2 shows the
bacteriological controls (on agar) of a typical experiment in which
oedema formation was induced 36 hours after burning. Seven animals served to produce oedema fluid after burning at 97° C, while
5 animals were used to produce oedema after burning at 80°C.
Five animals served to produce control oedema. In this experiment
the oedema produced in the animals burned at 97°C showed only
moderate bacterial contamination, whereas the peptone oedema
and the oedema of the 80°C animals were quite heavily infected.
Even so, after filtration of the exudate, only the animals injected
with the high-temperature oedema showed a mortality of over 50%,
whereas in the other two groups there were no deaths. We are not
yet prepared to venture a definite opinion on these findings, as more
experiments will have to be carried out. The crucial point in all this
work seems to be that the bacteriological factor must be considered
very carefully in all experiments on burn toxins, whether they be
acute experiments lasting a matter of hours or experiments on so-
called "burn disease". Nevertheless, it does appear likely that some
time and temperature factor is involved in the damaging effect
exerted by burned tissue.

It has been claimed that the effect of burning is characterised by
alterations in protein metabolism and more specifically by an
increase in proteolytic activity in the tissues. Either the enzymes
or the resulting metabolites are considered to be the toxic agent. If
this were true, enzyme inhibitors could be expected to prove effective in treating burns. To test this possibility, we have used a
kallikrein inhibitor (Trasylol-Bayer) in our standardised scalding
tests on rats. Trasylol inhibits trypsin and plasmin-like enzymes. In
our short-term experiments this enzyme inhibitor did not prolong
the survival time of the scalded animals. This suggests that it is very
questionable whether these enzymes have any decisive importance
in acute fatal scalding.

Time does not permit me to enter into the immunological aspect of "burn toxins". Here again it has been a difficult task to separate bacterial factors from "pure tissue toxins". This holds true for the antigen as well as for the immune sera advocated by certain authors for clinical use.

Burning-and-peptone oedema

97° C

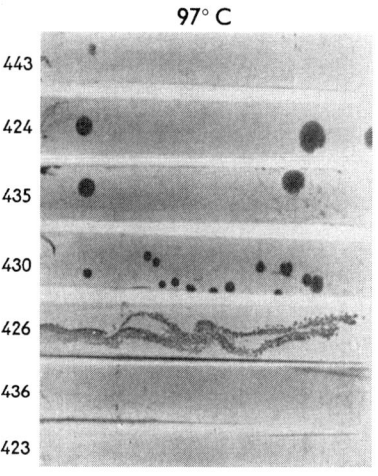

a

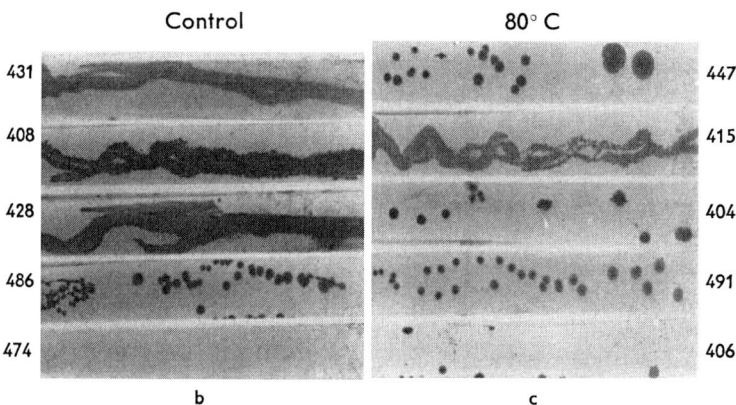

b   c

Fig. 2. Bacteriological controls (on agar) of oedema induced by subcutaneous injection of peptone (6 g./kg. body-weight) 36 hours after burning at 97°C and 80°C. Each number represents oedema of one individual rabbit. These tests were made at sacrifice of animals, 14 hours after the peptone injection, before sterilisation of the oedema by membrane filtration. While there were no deaths with control oedema and oedema produced by 80°C burning, the oedema produced by 97°C burning caused a 50% mortality despite the less marked infection in the initial material

When we consider the many approaches used by us and others, we must admit that we have precious little on hand by which to prove and analyse the "obviously" damaging effect of burned tissue, but we are far from having ruled out such a possibility.

Summary

Dr. SPINK's successful "after-treatment" of endotoxin-shocked animals finds a certain parallel in the observations made by our group with ganglionic blocking agents in burned rats.

Whether or not endotoxin is involved in the irreversible stage of various forms of shock should be verified by measuring the amount of endotoxin present in the blood of shocked animals. No such direct proof has been published to date.

Burn toxins have remained a most controversial subject during the last decade. The experimental analysis of such hypothetical toxins presents two main difficulties: 1. Bacterial infection and intoxication are extremely difficult to differentiate from the effect of "pure tissue toxins". 2. If heated and sterilised tissues are introduced into healthy animals at some local site (thus eliminating bacterial contamination) inflammatory reaction with fluid loss is bound to complicate the picture. There is suggestive evidence, however, that — apart from infection — there is a time as well as a temperature factor involved in the damaging effect exerted by the heat-destroyed tissue.

References

ALLGÖWER, M., and J. SIEGRIST: Verbrennungen. Berlin-Göttingen-Heidelberg: Springer-Verlag 1957. — ALLGÖWER, M., R. ASCHIERI, and L. HULLIGER: Ann. chir. plast. (Fr.) (in press). — GODFRAIND, T.: L'autointoxication après brûlure. Brussels: Editions Arscia S. A. 1958. — INGLIS, F. G., L. G. HAMPSON, and F. N. GURD: Ann. Surg. (U.S.A.) **149**, 43 (1959). — LAVER, M. B.: Surgery (U.S.A.) **40**, 520 (1956). — MALM, O. J.: Proc. 1st Internat. Cong. Research on Burns, published by Amer. Inst. of Biol. Sci. 1961. — McCLUSKEY, R. T., B. W. ZWEIFACH, W. ANTOPOL, B. BENACERRAF, and A. L. NAGLER: Amer. J. Path. **37**, 245 (1960). — SCHREUS, H. T.: Berufsdermatosen (G.) **7**, 158 (1959). — SCHWALB, E.: Surgery (U.S.A.) **46**, 383 (1959). — SIMONART, A.: Sem. hôp Paris **34**, 777 (1958). — VERAGUT, U. P.: Helvet. chir. acta (in press). — WILSON, W. C., J. S. JEFFREY, A. N. ROXBURGH, and C. P. STEWART: Brit. J. Surg. **24**, 601 (1937).

On the pathogenetic therapy of shock

By

B. K. Ossipov

First of all, I should like to thank Professor von Euler for kindly inviting me to take part in this meeting. Having worked as a surgeon now for a number of years, I am most interested in the reports of so many famous scientists from leading countries. And now, I want to say a few words about the pathogenetic therapy of shock.

In spite of the fact that scientists all over the world began to investigate shock as far back as the first half of the 19th century, it is impossible to consider the problem as completely solved even today.

A thorough study of the development of shock due to various causes is of great practical importance for the surgeon. The principal types of shock which he encounters are as follows: traumatic and surgical shock, shock due to burns, shock caused by the compression of soft tissue, and, finally, shock developing as a sequel to a combination of traumata — i.e. mechanical trauma and ionising radiation, or thermal shock associated with ionising radiation.

Evidently, therefore, it is impossible at the present time to speak just of shock in general without qualifying the term.

An examination of the work of both Russian (J. P. Pavlov, A. A. Bogomoletz, N. N. Burdenko, J. R. Petrov, and others) and foreign (Stedman, Rott, Dorland, Bickham, Wright, Sherrington, etc.) authors reveals that it is not easy to define accurately and completely the concept of shock. The reason for this, we believe, is that many authors still lack a definite starting point from which they could proceed to assess all the various manifestations of this complex pathological process.

According to A. V. Vishnevsky, and from our own observations, shock is an intricate dystrophic complex linked with overstimulation of the nervous system. All disorders of tone, as well as tissular and humoral disturbances, should in this connection be classified together under the heading of metabolic disorders and regarded as secondary phenomena.

J. R. PETROV has shown that the reflex theory of shock is the one generally accepted nowadays and that this theory is still worth studying in detail. Functional changes developing in the central nervous system in cases of shock may influence the whole organism both neurogenically and neurohumorally — in particular, via the endocrine system.

J. D. KUDRIN (Chair of Pathological Physiology at the Military Academy of Medicine directed by Prof. J. R. PETROV) observed that in the majority of cases of pulmonary and pleural trauma the opening of the thoracic cage was very quickly followed by the development of marked eosinophilia, indicating a decrease in pituitary and adrenocortical function which is probably connected with the rapid occurrence of hypoxaemia and hypercapnia.

The results of investigations performed in J. R. PETROV's laboratories have shown that in cases of shock the functional changes in the nervous system are primary, and those in the endocrine glands secondary. It is important, however, to stress the fact that the functional endocrine changes exert a significant influence on central nervous function.

It follows, therefore, that the reflex theory of shock, with particular reference to endocrine influences, still requires further investigation.

Another topical question concerns the mechanism by which central nervous exhaustion develops in cases of shock.

It is a well-known fact that contemporary achievements in cardiovascular and pulmonary surgery are closely linked with the use of modern methods of general anaesthesia. However, reflex reactivity is still maintained to some extent in the presence of prolonged surgical trauma, even in the case of operations on the heart or main blood vessels performed under artificial hypothermia. Moreover, a number of unfavourable factors may sometimes combine to produce surgical shock which is often extremely difficult to diagnose in good time.

Prof. V. A. IVANOV and E. M. YUKHTINA point out quite rightly that at the present time anaesthesiologists have a leading part to play in the treatment and prevention of shock. But this, we are firmly convinced, does not in any way mean that the surgeon's role is limited merely to that of an observer. Under certain circumstances it is the surgeon first of all who must take the necessary countermeasures to control shock.

In spite of the fact that a large amount of experimental and clinical data on the pathogenesis of shock are available, these data are at times contradictory, and it is still not always easy to assess them correctly. Nevertheless, a correct assessment is essential if we are to devise a rational and differentiated therapy for shock.

Great progress has been made in the prevention and treatment of shock in recent years,but there is still no universally applicable method of controlling the phenomenon — particularly since it occurs in widely differing phases and degrees.

The treatment of shock must be complex, directed at combating the disturbances affecting the nervous system, circulatory organs, respiratory system, metabolism, and the endocrine system.

I do not intend here to discuss at length the various measures widely employed today for the control of shock. They are sufficiently well known and include the use of morphine, immobilisation, neuroplegic drugs, intra-arterial or intravenous blood transfusions, of anti-shock hypertonic solutions, muscle relaxants in the event of respiratory disorders, nitrous oxide anaesthesia, artificial respiration using a pulmotor, tracheotomy, etc.

In this paper I should like to deal with only one of the measures commonly employed by us in combination with other ways and means of preventing and treating shock. It consists of applying a Novocaine block using the method of Prof. A. V. VISHNEVSKY, which has been further developed by his collaborators (A. A. VISHNEVSKY, N. N. ELANSKY, B. K. OSSIPOV, G. A. RICHTER, etc.). Since we define shock as an intricate neurodystrophic complex due to overstimulation of the nervous system, we regard toxaemia as a secondary phenomenon which develops as a result of widespread metabolic changes caused by this overstimulation of the nervous system. Thus, the syndrome of shock should be defined as a synthesis of two basic theories of shock — reflex and toxic.

A. V. VISHNEVSKY and other Russian scientists believe that the pathogenesis of shock is always the same — i.e. neurodystrophic — but that its aetiology may differ. Whatever the cause of the shock (trauma, burns, operation, transfusion, etc.), the mechanism of its development begins from a primary nervous reaction. Under these conditions, the treatment of shock, like that of any other disease, must be causal, pathogenetic, and symptomatic. In line with our views on the mechanism of the development of shock, our method of treatment is designed chiefly to combat the pathogenetic factors. Of all the available ways and means of promptly decreasing overstimulation of the nervous system, we prefer the Novocaine method devised by A. V. VISHNEVSKY, consisting of a vago-sympathetic, paranephric, or skeletal muscle block.

The vago-sympathetic block is used in cases of pleuro-pulmonary shock and is considered by us to be of both prophylactic and therapeutic importance. We employ it on a wide scale at the beginning of operations performed under local anaesthesia on the lungs, mediastinum, etc. We, and many other surgeons, have also made frequent and equally successful use of it in cases of open traumatic pneumothorax. Its application is as a rule accompanied by a rise in arterial pressure.

Our experience with the vago-sympathetic block in pulmonary operations carried out under local anaesthesia has been recorded in a paper published in the journal "Anaesthesia and Analgesia" in 1960 and entitled "Local Anaesthesia in Thoracic Surgery: 20 Years' Experience with 3,265 Cases".

The lumbar paranephric Novocaine block is also widely used by us in shock of varying aetiology. Paranephric block elicits a prompt response in cases of post-transfusional shock, the signs of shock disappearing in 2—3 minutes. We believe the explanation to be as follows: The condition of the nervous system induced in this case by albumin incompatibility is modified by the stimulation of a new sector of the nervous system. The block produces the same effect in cases of anaphylactic shock developing after repeated administration of serum.

Skeletal muscle block with Novocaine is used in shock caused by trauma of the extremities and developing after removal of the tourniquet. It should be emphasised that prompt application of the skeletal muscle block with Novocaine in cases of severe injury to a limb often helps, by relieving the pain and eliminating overstimulation of the nervous system, not only to prevent shock, but also to reduce those symptoms of shock which are already present.

In conclusion, I should like to point out that in the earlier stages of its use the Novocaine block (0.25% Novocaine solution) was considered important only as a method of chemical neurotomy, but with the passage of time it was found to exert a great variety of effects on the course of a number of pathological processes. In particular, the Novocaine block produces a beneficial effect in various forms of shock.

Summary

A thorough study of the development of shock due to various causes is of great practical importance for the surgeon.

In our opinion, shock is a dystrophic complex connected with overstimulation of the nervous system. Hence, all disorders of tone, as well as tissular and humoral disturbances should be classified together under the heading of metabolic disorders and regarded as secondary phenomena.

Defining shock as a neurodystrophic complex originating from overstimulation of the nervous system, we regard toxaemia as a secondary phenomenon which develops as a result of widespread metabolic changes.

Whatever the cause of shock may be (trauma, burns, operation, blood transfusion, etc.), the mechanism of its development always begins from a primary nervous reaction. This being the case, the treatment of shock must be causal, pathogenetic, and symptomatic.

Great progress has been achieved in the prevention and treatment of shock, but there is still no universally applicable method of controlling the phenomenon — particularly since it occurs in widely differing phases and degrees.

The treatment of shock must be complex, directed at combating the disturbances affecting the nervous system, circulatory organs, respiratory system, metabolism, and the endocrine system.

One of the techniques widely employed in my clinic in combination with other measures for the prevention and treatment of shock is the use of a Novocaine block as advocated by Dr. A. V. Vishnevsky. This technique involves vago-sympathetic block of the neck, paranephric, or skeletal muscle block, and we find it preferable to all other ways and means of promptly decreasing overstimulation of the nervous system. Vago-sympathetic block is used in pleuro-pulmonary shock and is considered by us to be of both prophylactic and therapeutic importance.

A report on the use of vago-sympathetic block was published in my article entitled "Local Anaesthesia in Thoracic Surgery: 20 Years' Experience with 3,265 Cases," which appeared in the journal "Anaesthesia and Analgesia" (July-August 1960).

Paranephric block is also widely employed by us in shock of varying aetiology; it elicits a prompt response in cases of post-transfusional shock, the signs of shock disappearing in 2—3 minutes. Skeletal muscle block is resorted to in cases of shock due to trauma of the extremities and developing after removal of the tourniquet. In such cases, it often helps not only to prevent shock, but also to reduce those symptoms of shock which are already present.

In the earlier stages of its use, the Novocaine block (0.25 % Novocaine solution) was considered important only as a method of chemical neurotomy, but it has since been found to exert a great variety of effects on the course of a number of pathological processes. In particular, the Novocaine block produces a beneficial effect in various forms of shock.

Myocardial shock

By

K. MATTHES

Cardiogenic shock, meaning shock due to acute heart failure, may occur in a variety of conditions, such as myocardial infarction, peracute myocarditis, extreme paroxysmal tachycardia or extreme slowing of the heart, and tamponade of the heart due to heart rupture, as well as in the terminal phase of chronic cardiac failure. The clinical picture of cardiogenic shock may be similar to the picture of shock due to loss of blood volume or to acute arrest of the circulation as in pulmonary embolism.

The condition common to these different clinical pictures is the sudden reduction in cardiac output, which instantly endangers the oxygen supply to the tissues. That such a condition may be cardiogenic will be accepted without further argument in cases of shock due to acute disturbances of cardiac rhythm, such as extreme slowing or acceleration of the heart.

In the case of myocardial infarction or acute myocarditis, the similarity of the clinical picture to peripheral shock has induced many authors to suspect — in addition to the damage to the heart muscle and its contractile power — other important causes of shock, such as failure of the peripheral arteriolar vessels to adapt total peripheral resistance to the diminished cardiac output and failure of the low pressure system, including especially the systemic veins, to provide a degree of vascular tone sufficient to ensure adequate venous return to the heart.

Experiments performed by our Heidelberg group, Dr. MEES-MANN, Dr. SCHMIER, and Dr. BRAASCH (21—27, 32, 6), which are well in keeping with similar work done in other laboratories, e.g. by ORIAS (28) (1932) and SARNOFF (31, 8) (1955), seem to indicate that shock occurring after interference with the coronary circulation in the dog is due almost exclusively to failure of the damaged part of the heart to maintain an adequate stroke volume (Fig. 1).

A narrowing of a branch of the coronary artery supplying part of the left ventricle will result in a reduced aortic blood flow and a reduced systemic blood pressure; the left auricular pressure is enhanced, while the right auricular pressure remains unchanged, and pulmonary arterial pressure shows a somewhat belated and less conspicuous reduction.

If the right coronary artery supplying the right ventricle in the dog is obstructed, the right auricular pressure as well as the pulmonary pressure and blood flow will show the primary reaction. This sequence of events will occur in the same way both in the heart-lung preparation and in the intact animal.

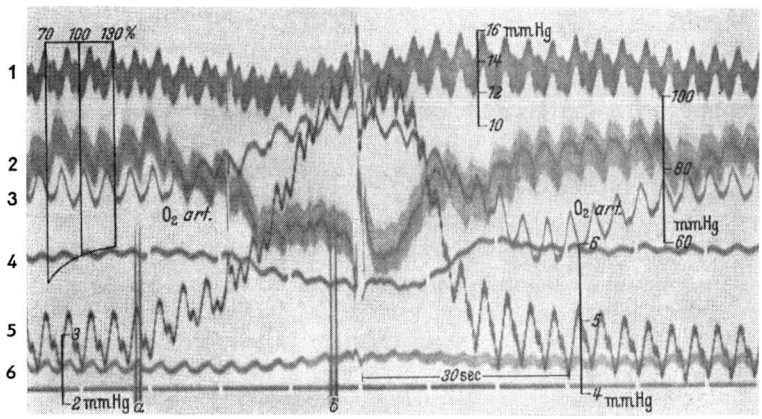

Fig. 1. Overcritical narrowing (a—b) of the ramus circumflexus of the left coronary artery, a branch which supplies parts of the left ventricle only. Artificial respiration of the dog with open thorax. Recordings: *1* pulmonary artery pressure; *2* brachial artery pressure; *3* oxygen saturation of arterial blood (O_2 art.) (increase = upward deflection); *4* blood flow femoral vein; *5* left atrial pressure; *6* right atrial pressure. MEESMANN and SCHMIER, 1955

As myocardial infarction in man, with rare exceptions, affects only the left ventricle, severe damage to the contractile power of the left heart results in a combination of shock and pulmonary congestion. In cases of myocarditis, both ventricles may be damaged, and in children in particular acute systemic congestion accompanying shock may be observed.

When the systemic blood pressure falls in shock, the increase in total peripheral resistance is as a rule greater than that due to elastic recoil. But the net effect will not be proportional to the fall in the systemic pressure. The reciprocal value of total peripheral resistance represents the sum of the reciprocal values of the resistances of different vascular beds, which may react differently depending on initial local conditions, on local metabolic needs, and on the extent of the fall in blood pressure.

The fact that total peripheral resistance may sometimes not rise appreciably in severe shock does not therefore prove the existence of a special reflex which counteracts the presso-receptor-induced vasoconstriction that accompanies the fall in blood pressure in shock.

In the dog is has been shown that peripheral vascular resistance in the limbs (skin and muscle vessels) always increases considerably after occlusion of a coronary artery. This local effect as well as the general effect of coronary occlusion on total peripheral resistance will not, however, be maximal. Occlusion of both carotid arteries (carotid sinus), cooling of the vagi, and infusion of noradrenaline may further increase total peripheral resistance and stabilise the blood pressure.

On the other hand, such extra vasoconstriction induced by artificial means may override the limits imposed on local reduction of the blood flow by metabolic needs and may therefore in the end do more harm than good.

Occlusion of both carotid arteries as well as vagotomy in the dog,

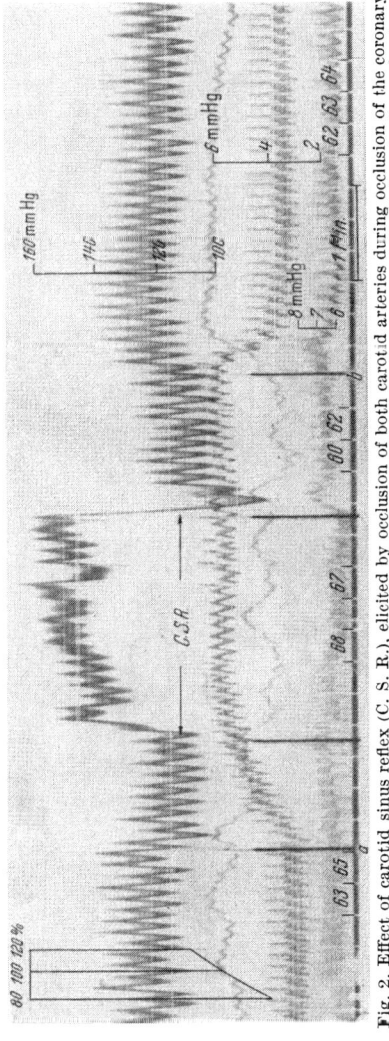

Fig. 2. Effect of carotid sinus reflex (C. S. R.), elicited by occlusion of both carotid arteries during occlusion of the coronary artery (occlusion art. cor. dextr., between marks a—b), on: 1 brachial arterial pressure: 2 blood flow in femoral artery; and pressure in (3) the right and (4) left atrium. (BRAASCH et al. 1961)

though exerting an effect on the systemic blood pressure and resistance vessels, has no demonstrable influence on the general pattern of changes in pressure in the auricles elicited by coronary occlusion (Fig. 2). This may be taken to indicate that the increase in sympathetic tone on the venous side of the circulation caused by coronary artery occlusion is already near maximal, so that a further carotid-sinus block can-

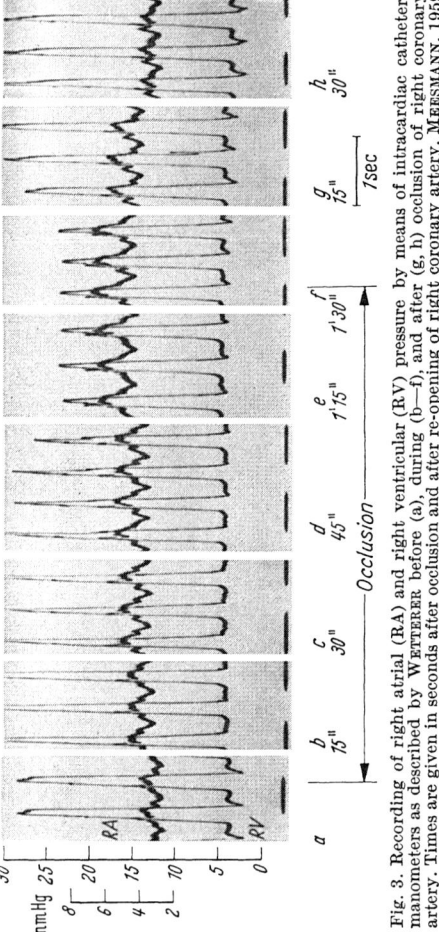

Fig. 3. Recording of right atrial (RA) and right ventricular (RV) pressure by means of intracardiac catheter-manometers as described by WETTERER before (a), during (b—f), and after (g, h) occlusion of right coronary artery. Times are given in seconds after occlusion and after re-opening of right coronary artery. MEESMANN, 1959

not increase the effect. This excludes a primary decrease in the venous return to the heart as one of the major causes of cardiogenic shock.

Fig. 3 illustrates an experiment by MEES-MANN (24) showing right auricular and intraventricular pressures, recorded with intracardiac catheter-manometers in the dog during occlusion of the right coronary artery. After 1 min. 15 sec. the ventricular pressure pulse becomes definitely hypodynamic. Already immediately after coronary occlusion one can observe that the proto-diastolic drop in intraventricular pressure, which normally brings about a clearly negative pressure gradient with a suction effect across the atrioventricular valve, is eliminated. This may be due to a change in the mechanism of ventricular contraction. After myo-cardial infarction the heart chamber involved may dilate slightly. There may therefore be less shortening of individual muscle fibres and hence less systolic change in interfascicular tension, the reversal of which is responsible for the suction occurring at the start of the diastole. The systolic force, as well as the suction effect, may be further impaired by the buffering action of the anaemic, noncontractile portion of the ventricular wall, whose elasticity does not decrease when the ventricle contracts and which may thus even distend during the systole.

As already shown by ORIAS (28) (1932) and confirmed by MEES-MANN (24), the speed of systolic contraction as well as of diastolic relaxation is reduced after coronary occlusion. This, in addition to the diminished systolic force, may also help to reduce diastolic suction.

A left-ventricular infarction may also interfere with the systolic shift of the valve ring, which causes systolic acceleration of the blood towards the heart. As valve-ring movement in the heart as a whole is primarily determined by the left ventricle, the corresponding mechanism of the right heart, which is haemodynamically more important, may also be impaired. Accordingly, quite apart from the loss of contractile power of the part of the muscle actually affected by the infarction, there are plenty of other factors which may lead to a diminuton in cardiac output and to cardiogenic shock. They may be partially offset by the inotropic effect of baroreceptor-induced sympathetic stimulation of the surviving muscle and by cardiac acceleration.

The clinician has every reason to regard the shock occurring in myocardial infarction or acute myocarditis as being of purely cardiogenic origin. There is no evidence of any primary insufficiency of resistance or capacitance vessels to which the cause of the shock could be attributed. Nor in either experimental animals or man is there any conclusive evidence of a reflex which could aggravate or provoke shock by influencing the peripheral vessels. The conclusion to be drawn from this as regards treatment is that, in addition to sedation of the patient, repeated small doses of strophanthin or digitalis, designed to act on the surviving muscle, are probably a very appropriate means of treating myocardial shock. If the blood pressure can no longer be measured and fails to rise, recourse must be had to intravenous drip infusion of noradrenaline or synthetic hypertensin.

If shock in myocardial infarction is brought about by acute insufficiency of the left ventricle, it is conceivable that this may result in a combination of forward and backward failure, i. e. in cardiogenic shock combined with pulmonary congestion. The fact that frank pulmonary oedema is a rare occurrence in comparison with the incidence of acute episodes of left-ventricular failure in cases of chronic left-ventricular strain, may be attributed to the co-existing state of shock, in which venous return is reduced along with cardiac output.

In view of the possibility of a combination of shock and pulmonary oedema, the dangers of treating the one without due regard to the other are obvious. An attempt to treat shock with some kind of blood volume replacement — a procedure which may well be adopted if myocardial infarction is not suspected as the cause of the shock — may bring about pulmonary oedema, whereas on the other hand an attempt to treat pulmonary congestion and a suspected tendency to pulmonary oedema with, for instance, ganglionic-blocking substances, may easily provoke a full shock syndrome in a case where shock had hitherto been merely latent. One major therapeutic problem, to which I will not allude in detail here, is the regulation of cardiac arrhythmias in cases of myocardial infarction, which may seriously aggravate cardiogenic shock.

Unfortunately, cases of severe myocardial shock in which it proves necessary to resort to intravenous drip infusion of noradrenaline have a very high mortality, even when treated with extreme care. One reason for this may be that damage to the heart is so extensive that its contractile power cannot be restored. Another reason may be that, if the shock cannot be overcome quickly, secondary damage may supervene, which tends to make the shock irreversible. This is essentially true of other types of shock as well.

Our observations of shock in myocardial infarction have led us to become interested in the question as to what causes infusions of noradrenaline or synthetic hypertensin often to become less and less effective, so that the dose per minute has to be steadily increased in order to maintain a certain level of blood pressure.

In the light of clinical experience, we have come to prefer hypertensin — which is about five times more active than noradrenaline — chiefly because it is far less likely to induce cardiac arrhythmias [BOCK (2), MEESMANN (26)]. However, one also encounters cases in which hypertensin becomes less and less effective whereas noradrenaline continues to exert some effect, albeit reduced. In such cases we suspect metabolic acidosis; if this suspicion can be confirmed, the response to hypertensin may be partially restored by infusing 5% NaH CO_3 (27).

In a case of severe post-traumatic shock with oliguria (N.P.N. 160 mg.), it was necessary to give 120—220 μg./min. hypertensin or 56 μg./min. noradrenaline in order to stabilise the blood pressure at 100/85 mm. Hg. The arterial serum pH was 7.3 and the arterial p CO_2 12.8 mm. Hg.

After an infusion of 500 cc. 5% $NaHCO_3$ the arterial serum pH rose to 7.46 and the arterial pCO_2 to 25.4, whereupon the dose necessary to maintain the blood pressure at 100/80 mm. Hg was

found to be 15 μg./min. hypertensin or 27 μg./min. noradrenaline
[MEESMANN et al. (27)]. When respiratory acidosis is induced
experimentally in dogs, the same decrease in sensitivity to synthetic
hypertensin — and, to a lesser degree, to noradrenaline as well — is
observed [MEESMANN et al. (26)].

Another reason for loss of reactivity to noradrenaline and
hypertensin in cardiogenic shock may be an alteration in the blood-
coagulation-fibrinolysin system.

In certain cases of cardiogenic shock, extreme local slowing of
the circulation may induce microthrombus formation in the peripheral arteriolar vessels, which in turn may completely arrest the
circulation and lead to local extravasation of blood (20).

We recently observed a woman who, owing to paroxysmal
tachycardia lasting for 7 days, suffered an extreme cardiogenic
shock with complete loss of consciousness and blood-pressure levels
too low to measure [FRIESE et al. (11)]. As a result of extreme cen-
tralisation, the blood flow in the hands virtually ceased; this led to
microthrombus formation and haemorrhagic diathesis in the
fingers, followed by necrosis of the finger-tips. When we had an
opportunity of examining the patient, we found that she had
thrombopenia and a marked deficiency of fibrinogen and certain
blood-coagulation factors (11).

This type of case reminds one of MOSCHKOWITZ's thrombotic
thrombocytopenic purpura and, if the condition is generalised, of
the generalised Sanarelli-Shwartzman phenomenon. I should perhaps
mention here that BOHLE and KRECKE (3, 4) have described a case
in which — following multiple Adams-Stokes attacks accompanied
by cardiogenic shock — the typical histological picture of a generalised Sanarelli-Shwartzman phenomenon was discovered at autopsy,
i. e. fibrin thrombi in the minute vessels of almost all the organs
and bilateral necrosis of the renal cortex (Figs. 4a and 4b).

BOHLE and KRECKE (3) have described from our material 9
further cases which showed at autopsy a similar picture closely
resembling the anatomical findings characteristic of a generalised
Sanarelli-Shwartzman phenomenen. These patients had died in
shock or in acute renal failure. The underlying diseases had been
infectious conditions, consisting chiefly of meningococcal meningitis
(4 cases) and post-abortive states (3 cases).

During life such patients often show a haemorrhagic diathesis
and a characteristic complex disorder of the blood-coagulation
system (14, 15). An initial shortening of the coagulation time as
measured in the thrombelastogram occurs, followed by a marked
prolongation at a later stage. In this second phase there is a

17*

diminution in the fibrinogen and prothrombin concentration, loss of activity of factors V and VIII (*12*), and marked thrombocytopenia with loss of activity of thrombocyte factors 1 and 3 (*14*). Consequently the maximal amplitude of the thrombelastogram is greatly

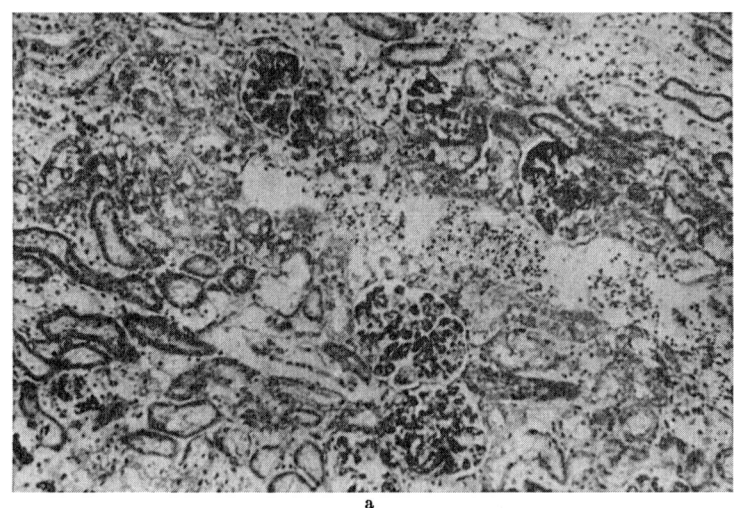

a

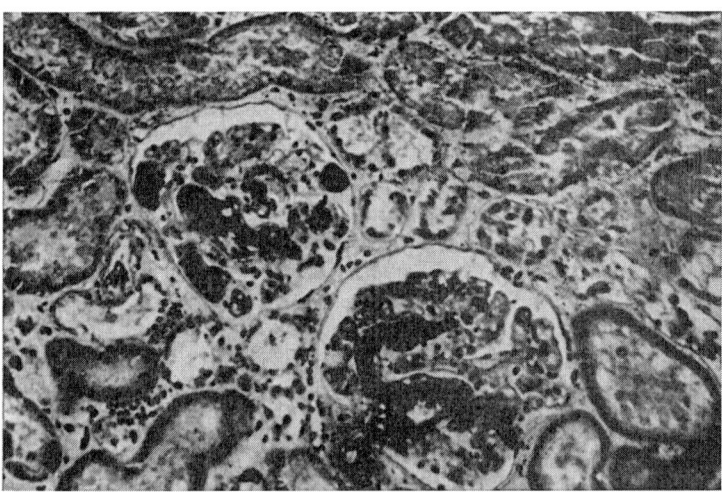

b

Fig. 4. Fibrin precipitates in the glomerular capillaries and patchy tubular necrosis: a) in a patient who died after severe Adams-Stokes attacks; b) in a rabbit with a typical Sanarelli-Shwartzman reaction. Goldner-trichrom staining. BOHLE and KRECKE, 1959

reduced. This condition is apparently due to a speeding up of the normally latent turnover of coagulation factors in the blood, which ultimately results in the appearence of thrombin in the blood in sufficient amounts to cause widespread blood coagulation leading to intravascular fibrin deposition as well as to an increasing consumption of fibrinogen and other coagulation factors and to the disappearance of platelets (14).

As pointed out by DEUTSCH (10), KOLLER (13), and MARX (19), endogenous fibrinolysis may also be increased under these circumstances.

In such cases, despite the general tendency to haemorrhage, heparin should be used in order to combat accelerated intravascular coagulation and thus to reduce the consumption of platelets, fibrinogen, and other coagulation factors (15).

We recently observed a 25-year-old woman with post-abortion *E. coli* septicaemia who was in profound shock and semiconscious. She had multiple haemorrhagic lesions on the cheeks and especially on the nose (Fig. 5). She had

hardly any fibrinogen left in her blood (0.08 g. %) and the prothrombin and factors V and VIII were between 65 and 50% of normal. Platelets 32,000; platelet factor 1 and 3 under 50%. Threefold increase in coagulation time. Maximal amplitude of thrombelastogram only half the normal. She recovered completely after treatment with heparin, noradrenaline infusions, and chloramphenicol (15).

Lately we came across 2 cases of very severe traumatic shock with fat embolism. Both made a dramatic recovery from shock in response to treatment with human plasmin and streptokinase, designed to induce fibrinolysis, followed by heparin therapy. Unfortunately, both patients died a few days later from acute renal failure.

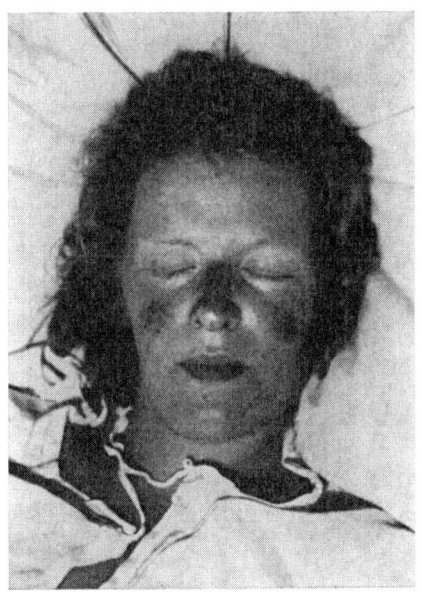

Fig. 5

In one of these cases the dose of intravenous noradrenaline had to be increased to 150 μg./min. in order to maintain the blood pressure at 90/60 mm. Hg (pulse rate: 140/min.). After fibrinolysis and subsequent heparinisation, it was possible to reduce the noradrenaline to 45 µg./min. in the following 90 min., although in the next 6 hours the dose had to be increased again to 130 µg./min. Two hours after a second dose of plasmin+streptokinase, the noradrenaline needed was only 20 µg./min.; finally, no further noradrenaline was required at all.

We have studied this problem experimentally in the rabbit by injecting olive oil intravenously. When a large dose (more than 0.7 cc./kg.) was administered, the animals died within 2 hours in shock with colourless pulmonary oedema. In the thrombelasto-gram the coagulation time was much reduced, while factors V, VIII, and IX showed a reduction in activity, sometimes after a transient initial rise (34).

When a smaller dose was injected, some animals survived, whereas others died in shock after 1 or 2 days. The oedema fluid in the lungs was tinged with blood and a general haemorrhagic diathesis was observed [SESSNER et al. (34)].

Fig. 7 shows the results of blood-coagulation analyses. In the animals which died, there was a decrease in fibrinogen as well as in the platelet count. The maximal amplitude of the thromb-elastogram was correspondingly reduced. Neither the surviving animals nor the controls showed these changes (Fig. 6).

As long ago as 1953, CAMMERMEYER (7) demonstrated that intra-vascular fibrin deposits occur along with fat embolism.

In many cases of clinical shock due to various causes, including cardiogenic shock, our coagulation analyses have revealed traces of this syndrome, which is a mixture of thrombopathy and coag-ulopathy, and which we refer to as Verbrauchskoagulopathie, i. e. "consumption coagulopathy" (15).

According to LASCH, MECHELKE, and NUSSER (16), the normal turnover of coagulation proteins in the blood, leading to a slow break-down of prothrombin and to the appearence of accelerator factors, may be considerably enhanced if the blood flows very slowly and takes too long to return to the liver for prothrombin regeneration. This is precisely what happens in vasoconstrictive shock. The entry of depot-blood into the general circulation may aggravate this tendency. Hence in shock the stage is set for the appearance of thrombin in the blood in such large amounts as to cause either local or generalised clinical symptoms.

If an additional factor supervenes, such as an endotoxin in septicaemia, fat emboli (which per se accelerate coagulation), thromboplastic substances from the placenta, or even a very low temperature, the full syndrome resembling the Sanarelli-Shwartz-man phenomenon may appear. According to our experience, this in

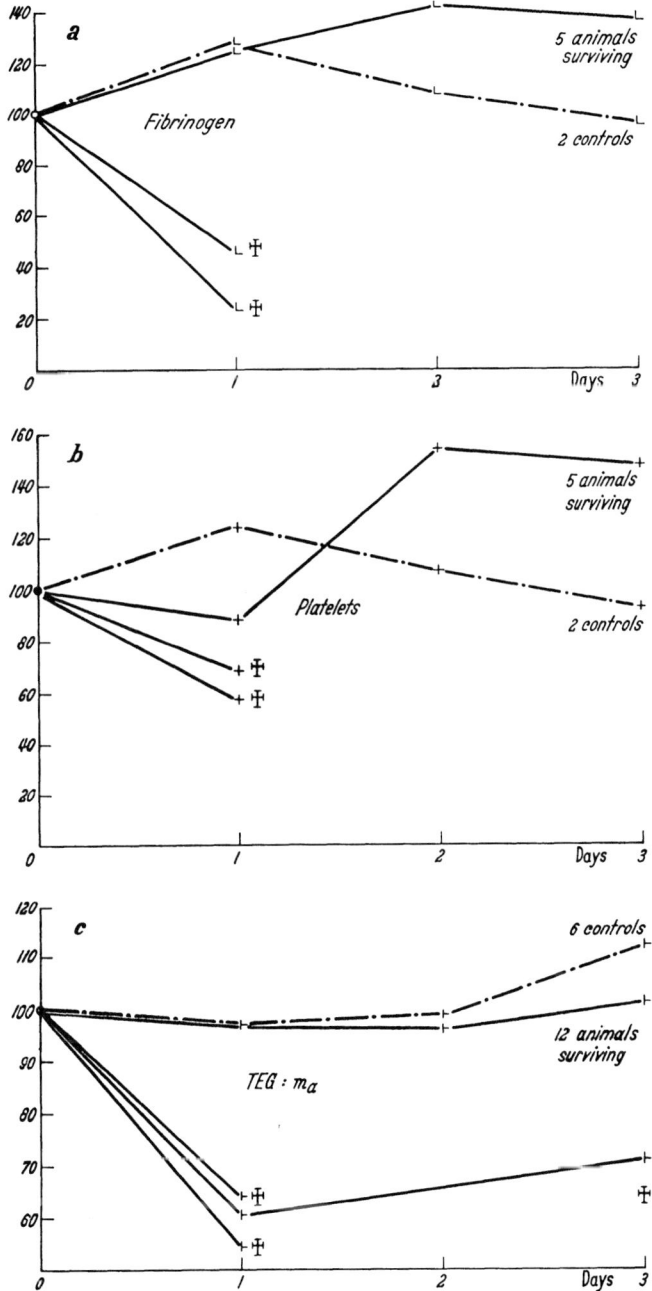

Fig. 6. Fibrinogen (above), platelets (middle) and maximal amplitude of thrombelastogram (below) after intravenous injection of 0.6—0.63 ml./kg. body-weight of olive oil (rabbit). The animals which died showed a diminution in all three values, whereas the surviving ones behaved more or less like the controls. All values in % of the control values

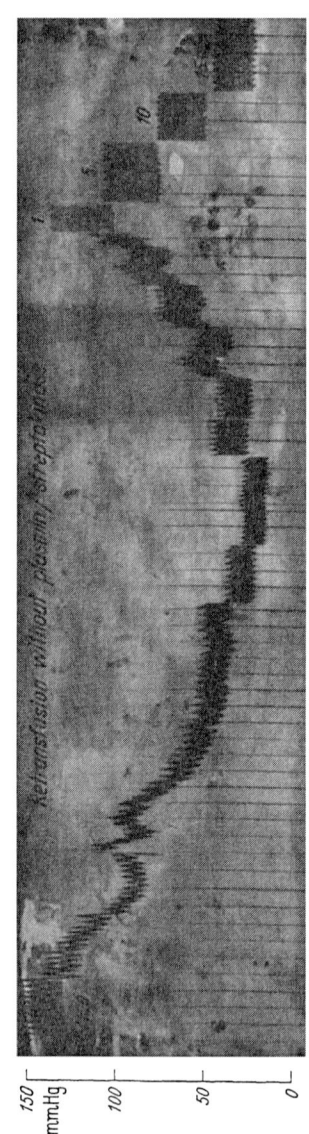
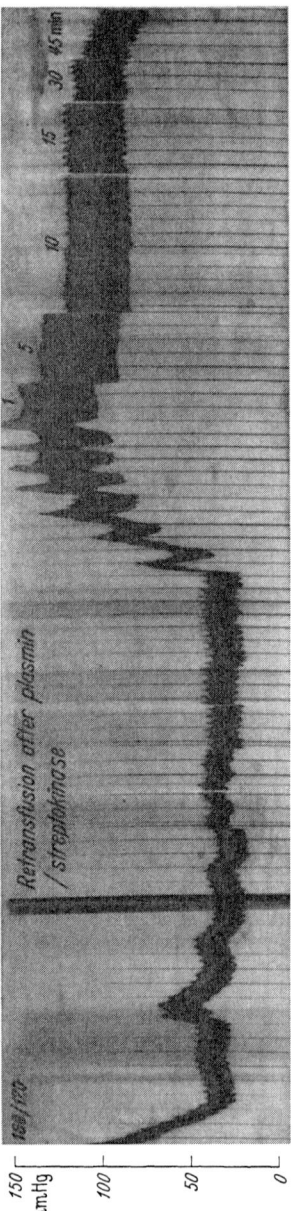

Fig. 7. Blood pressure during haemorrhagic shock in the cat. Above: exsanguination and retransfusion after 40 minutes of hypotension. Below: the same; during the period of hypotension fibrinolysis was induced by injecting plasmin + streptokinase at the point indicated

itself aggravates the shock and makes it almost completely refractory to conventional methods of treatment. Therapy in such cases therefore has to be supplemented by heparinisation or by inducing fibrinolysis and then administering heparin.

LASCH et al. have meanwhile studied the influence of fibrinolysis on haemorrhagic shock in the cat (17). Fig. 7 shows the results of a typical haemorrhagic-shock experiment with retransfusion. When fibrinolysis was induced at the beginning of haemorrhagic shock, the animal survived, whereas the control died. Only five experiments of each type have so far been performed, but on the whole they support the conclusion that fibrinolysis has a beneficial effect on haemorrhagic shock in cats. It is interesting to note that if ε-aminocaproic acid, a strong inhibitor of fibrinolysis, was given together with the fibrinolysin, the animals died in the same way as the controls (17).

It was also demonstrated that fibrinolysis increases the effect of noradrenaline in haemorrhagic shock in the cat. This effect, too, can be inhibited with ε-aminocaproic acid. These results are rather difficult to explain, as in ordinary haemorrhagic shock no widespread fibrin deposition occurs in the minute vessels, nor is there any marked tendency to bleeding But it can be shown that there may already be some depletion of the coagulation proteins and sometimes a shortening of the coagulation time.

It is conceivable that the contractility of the pre-capillary vessels may depend in some fashion upon the latent prothrombin turnover, a minute film of fibrinogen derivatives being possibly formed on the inner surface of such vessels [ROKA (29), COPLEY (9), ROOS (30), LÜSCHER (18), and ASTRUP (1)]. An increase of blood coagulation in shock may influence the catecholamine sensitivity of the vessels, and this might also tend to make the shock irreversible. Fibrinolysis may interfere with this process.

Fibrinolysis has been used with some success by BOYLES et al. (5) (1961) to treat myocardial infarction, the idea being to dissolve the thrombi in the coronary arteries. It is possible that fibrinolysis may indeed have this effect; we would also suggest that, in cases of myocardial infarction with severe shock, fibrinolysis should be resorted to in an attempt to overcome irreversibility of shock in instances where hypertensin and noradrenaline have failed. However, we have not yet had enough clinical experience of this method to be able to report on it.

Although I have stressed the conviction that myocardial shock is initiated and brought about by acute insufficiency of the damaged heart and that the origin of shock has nothing to do with reflexes of any kind or with insufficiency of either the resistance or the capacitance vessels, it should be added that in any kind of shock, as it progresses to irreversibility, secondary cardiac insufficiency may supervene as well as secondary insufficiency of the resistance and capacitance vessels. This can of course also happen in primary cardiogenic shock.

In clinical practice, a reduced response to noradrenaline and hypertensin is a sign of such insufficiency. In some cases, however, the effectiveness of noradrenaline and hypertensin can be restored by correct adjustment of the blood pH and perhaps by fibrinolysis and subsequent heparinisation.

References

1. ASTRUP, T.: Blood (U.S.A.) 11, 781 (1956). — 2. BOCK, K. D.: Zschr. Kreisl.forsch. (G.) 49, 890 (1960). — 3. BOHLE, A., and H. J. KRECKE: Klin. Wschr. (G.) 1959,803. — 4. BOHLE, A., H. J. KRECKE, H. SITTE, and F. MIL-LER: Ist. Internat. Symp. on Immunopathology. p. 339. Basle: Schwabe 1959. — 5. BOYLES, P. W.: J. Amer. Med. Ass. 175, 279 (1961). — 6. BRAASCH, W., B. v. ISSEKUTZ, and J. SCHMIER: Klin. Wschr. (G). 39, 120 (1961). — 7. CAMMERMEYER, J.: Arch. Path. (U.S.A.) 56, 254 (1953). — 8. CASE, R. B., E. BERGLUND, and S. J. SARNOFF: Amer. J. Med. 18, 397 (1955).— 9. COPLEY, A. L.: Amer. J. Physiol. 137, 178 (1942). — 10. DEUTSCH, E.: Schweiz. med. Wschr. 90, 1252 (1960). — 11. FRIESE, G., and D. WITTE-KIND: Medizinische (G.) 1959, 828. — 12. KLEINMAIER, H., K. GOERGEN, H. G. LASCH, J. H. KRECKE, and A. BOHLE: Zschr. exper. Med. (G.) 132, 275 (1959). — 13. KOLLER, F.: Schweiz. med. Wschr. 90, 1233 (1960). — 14. LASCH, H. G., F. RODRIGUEZ-ERDMANN, and H. J. KRECKE: Verh. Dtsch. Ges. inn. Med. 66, 992 (1960). — 15. LASCH, H. G., H. J. KRECKE, F. RO-DRIGUEZ-ERDMANN, H. H. SESSNER, and G. SCHÜTTERLE: VII. Verh. Dtsch. Ges. Hämatol. Wiesbaden (1961). Fol. haemat. (G.) (1961) (in press). — 16. LASCH, H. G., K. MECHELKE, and H. H. SESSNER: In: Thromboembo-lytische Erkrankungen. p. 140. Stuttgart: Schattauer 1960. — 17. LASCH, H. G., K. MECHELKE, E. NUSSER, and F. DAOUD: Klin. Wschr. (G). 1961 (in preparation). — 18. LÜSCHER, E. F.: Schweiz. med. Wschr. 86, 345 (1956). — 19. MARX, R.: 11. Tagung Dtsch. Ges. Blutgerinnungsforsch. Heidelberg (1956). — Thromb. Diath. haem. Suppl. (G.) 1957. — 20. MATTHES, K.: Cardiologia (Switz.) 35, 324 (1959). — 21. MEESMANN, W., and J. SCHMIER: Pflügers Arch. Physiol. (G.) 261, 41 (1955). — 22. MEES-MANN, W., and J. SCHMIER: Pflügers Arch. Physiol. (G.) 261, 48 (1955). — 23. MEESMANN, W., and J. SCHMIER: Zschr. Kreisl.forsch. (G.) 44, 304 (1955). — 24. MEESMANN, W.: Zschr. exper. Med. (G). 131, 200 (1959). — 25. MEESMANN, W.: Arch. Kreislaufforsch. (G.) (in press). — 26. MEES-MANN, W., W. BRAASCH, and R. D. HERBERG: Verh. Dtsch. Ges. Kreisl.-forsch. 27 (1961) (in press). — 27. MEESMANN, W., W. BRAASCH, and R. D. HERBERG: Klin. Wschr. (G.) (in preparation). — 28. ORIAS, O.: Amer. J. Physiol. 100, 629 (1932). — 29. RÓKA, L.: IV. Tagung. Dtsch. Ges. Blutgerinnungsforsch. Bonn (1959). — 30. ROOS, J.: Thromb. Diath. haem. (G.) 1, 471 (1957). — 31. SARNOFF, S. J.: Physiol. Rev. (U.S.A.) 35, 107 (1955). — 32. SCHMIER, J.: Probleme der Coronardurchblutung. II. Bad Oeynhauser Gespräche. Berlin-Göttingen-Heidelberg: Springer 1958. — 33. SEEGERS, W. H.: Angiology (U.S.A.) 7, 436 (1956); Coll. papers 1938—1957. — 34. SESSNER, H. H., G. SCHÜTTERLE, and D. STUMMEYER: Dtsch. Arch. klin. Med. 207, 177 (1961).

Discussion

BIÖRCK: Most of this meeting has been devoted to haemorrhagic shock. However, Dr. MATTHES has rendered an invaluable service in giving us such a masterly presentation of the problems of cardiogenic shock, because this is the kind of shock that about half of us here are likely to experience ourselves. And I think that this risk is far greater than the risk of a patient's developing haemorrhagic shock. Unfortunately, the treatment of cardiogenic shock is not so easy as the treatment of haemorrhagic shock, where the problem is simply that of proper replacement, as we have heard from Dr. FINE and Dr. BULL. The "replacement" of the bad heart is a problem about which perhaps Dr. SENNING is going to talk later on this afternoon. The use of extracorporeal circulation in cardiogenic shock is today a well-nigh practical possibility. But apart from this, I think it would be very useful here at this meeting, where we have so many eminent physiologists gathered together, to enlist their aid in the fight against cardiogenic shock.

I would like to mention just a few figures. Medical wards in our country seem to show a mortality rate which is three times as high as that in surgical wards. Furthermore, 5% of the patients in our medical department have myocardial infarcts, but these are responsible for 33% of our total mortality. Of the total mortality rate for myocardial infarction, three-quarters are accounted for by only one-quarter of such patients, i.e. by those who arrive in, or develop, shock. Thus, one-quarter is responsible for three-quarters of the mortality. I agree completely with Dr. MATTHES that the size of the infarct seems to be one of the factors that determine mortality, because, as judged from transaminase and other enzymatic tests of myocardial necrosis, there exists a good correlation between the magnitude of the muscle necrosis and the mortality rate. However, there is also an almost linear relationship between the age of the patient and the mortality, except for the younger ages, below fifty, which appear to have a higher mortality rate than they should have if there were an absolutely linear relationship between age and mortality. Another fact that should be stressed is: "once a coronary, always a coronary"; 90% of people who have had a myocardial infarct and survived will die from another infarct or from related cardiac causes. We have been struck by the fact that our therapy is very meagre and insufficient. Looking back over records covering 25 years of myocardial infarcts in a university hospital setting, there has been no apparent improvement in mortality over these 25 years. The average mortality in several thousand myocardial infarcts in Sweden, from three different university hospitals, is 33% and has remained so over the years. The hopes we placed in noradrenaline have not been fulfilled. In our material, we have not found the chances of survival to be significantly better for those treated with noradrenaline than for corresponding patients without such treatment, and this seems to be corroborated by the findings of other workers presented at this meeting.

To my mind, a great number of patients with myocardial infarction should be kept in the emergency ward for one week or more. The internists have to be even more vigorous and alert than the surgeons, because of this higher average mortality rate with which we have to contend. We try to keep the patients who arrive in shock or pre-shock under 24-hour observation with

an oscilloscope attached and an indwelling catheter inserted, so that everything can be rushed in if the shock increases. I would agree with Dr. BULL
that it is very important to note even minor signs of pre-shock, such as a
certain restlessness or distress, which cannot be measured in figures but
which is nevertheless an important danger signal. However, in connection
with Dr. MATTHES's paper I would like to stress that a number of patients
who *arrive* in shock *do not die* from shock. They may die from pulmonary
oedema or from sudden arrhythmias, which of course can be precipitated by
a state of "shock". I agree with Dr. RUSHMER that "shock" is not a very
good phrase to use here, but it is about "shock" that we have been asked
to talk.

For acute left heart failure (pulmonary oedema) and in certain instances
of arrhythmia, we do have some treatment. I agree completely with Dr.
MATTHES that digitalis should be given for the failing myocardium; and all
kinds of drugs suitable for use in combating arrhythmias should be immediately to hand. A prerequisite for early and effective treatment of arrhythmias
is monitoring of the electrocardiogram on the oscilloscope, because you must
get at the arrhythmias at the very moment they appear — otherwise you
don't know about them until it's too late. But apart from that, we are faced
with the question as to what *more* we can do over and above combating pulmonary oedema and arrhythmias. And this is the area, the big area, in which
we now have to turn to the physiologists and other experimenters to help us.

I was glad to hear the other day about results obtained with chlorpromazine
because, with very little background information, we have started to put our
myocardial infarcts on chlorpromazine. We have been struck by the fact that
we do not actually get dangerous hypotension, but rather a controllable
hypotension, and this seems to relieve the heart of some work; furthermore,
even if the patients' blood pressure is a little on the low side, they are nevertheless dry and warm. We may also try hydrocortisone once again. We have
abandoned noradrenaline in favour of Aramine, and our impression is that
Aramine may be a little better, but it is hard to judge. Finally, I have been
very much impressed by the data presented here on the possible role of endotoxins and other products from the gut and from the liver, and I am sure that
this is an area which has been neglected by cardiologists. We would like to
have practical advice on this. Incidentally, some of the questions that I have
dealt with here have been discussed in more detail in two recent papers[1]
from our department.

MATTHES: I would like to add that I completely agree with what Dr.
BIÖRCK has said. We should try hydrocortisone, especially in cases with
arrhythmias, i. e. in addition to the usual treatment for arrhythmia. I have no
personal experience concerning the use of chlorpromazine in myocardial shock.

VON EULER: I propose that we now proceed to the part of the discussion
which we did not have time to complete on previous days, and that we have
a free discussion on the foregoing papers.

RUSHMER: As a participant in this symposium with little previous
experience on shock, I should like to present a summary of my reaction to the
problem of shock as it exists today. As I see it, the term shock undoubtedly
served a useful purpose in the past by identifying a group of clinical states
with a few common characteristics. Given the restricted quantity of basic
physiological information available at that time, it was not possible to
explain these clinical syndromes on the basis of sound fundamental prin-

---

[1] BIÖRCK, G.: Acta med. Scand. **168**, 245 (1960); BIÖRCK, G., H. ELIASCH,
R. O. MALMBORG, and F. WAHLBERG: Minerva med. (It.) **52**, 2232 (1961).

ciples. The available tools for clinical research were inadequate to provide concise and quantitative descriptions of the different clinical states. So long as therapeutic procedures were limited, the diversity of causative mechanisms made little difference.

Faced with patients who desperately needed immediate care, clinicians were required to initiate treatment without waiting for an elucidation of the basic physiological mechanisms. And for this purpose they used sound clinical judgment and experimental models which to them appeared reasonable. Note that the validity of these models as substitutes for the specific clinical states cannot be tested until complete and quantitative descriptions are available regarding both the clinical states and the experimental models.

Modern methods of clinical research have been developed to the point that a much more complete picture of the various kinds of shock-like states could and should be available now if the techniques were fully utilised. I have listed a few to indicate some of the measurements that are now available on patients.

I. Cardiac output
   a) Indicator dilution techniques
   b) Cardiac catheterisation
II. Total peripheral resistance
   (computed from mean arterial pressure and cardiac output)
III. Regional blood flow
   a) Skin and muscle in extremities
      1. Volume plethysmograph
      2. Variable resistance gauges (WHITNEY) consisting of delicate rubber tubes filled with mercury
      3. Thermocouple needles for muscle flow (HENSEL needle)
      4. Thermocouple discs for skin flow (HENSEL)
      5. Indicator dilution techniques
   b) Splanchnic blood flow by Bromsulphthalein
   c) Renal flow by clearance techniques
IV. Blood volume
   a) Indicator dilution techniques
V. Regional distribution of blood volume
   a) Limb circumference measurements
   b) Local indicator dilution techniques
   c) Regional counting of intravascular radioisotopes
   d) Segmental weighing (FELL technique)
VI. Oxygen consumption
VII. Regional oxygen tensions (determining oxygen content and tension in samples of venous blood from different tissues)
VIII. Respiratory function tests
   a) Lung volumes
   b) Diffusion capacity
IX. Tests for the presence of circulating chemicals
   a) Catecholamines
   b) Electrolytes
   c) Adrenal hormones
   d) Vasodilator principles
   e) Vasoconstrictor principles
   f) Bacteria
   g) Toxins
   h) Etc.

If these measurements are employed individually, a tremendous number of patients will be required to elucidate shock problems. However, relatively few patients studied by comprehensive batteries of tests provide a wealth of data at a much faster rate, and each study has tremendous value. It implies that a few laboratories specifically designed for the study of shock should be equipped and staffed so well that these studies can be instituted promptly and efficiently with little delay in care of the patients.

Similarly, recent developments in physiological research methods provide opportunities for quantitative descriptions of the models; you have heard from Dr. GREGG's laboratory and from my own that comprehensive batteries of research equipment now permit continuous recording of many critical variables simultaneously in intact unanaesthetised animals.

Finally, a great deal of new information about the basic priciples of cardiovascular function and control has accumulated, and this is not really applicable or applied adequately to the problems of shock. A wealth of information has been presented at this meeting in three separate categories, namely clinical syndromes, descriptions of experimental models, and the basic physiological mechanisms of function and control.

Unfortunately, this information tends to flow into three different compartments with very little communication between them. This is partly due to the fact that we still do not know the essential relationships between the information in the different categories. We will never successfully analyse the contents of these compartments as long as each contains an assorted mixture of items. On the other hand, I believe that it should be possible now to select information from this tangled and chaotic mass and to begin to synthesise cohesive and useful concepts regarding certain of these clinical problems. What steps would be required to accomplish this objective ?

1. Each clinical syndrome should be precisely and quantitatively described by modern research techniques.

2. Criteria to provide universal recognition of the syndrome might then be agreed upon.

3. Experimental models could then be based on the essential quantitative criteria and validated using a point-by-point comparison between the models and the clinical syndromes.

4. Finally, more appropriate experimental models could be devised as needed in terms of the demonstrated fundamental mechanisms. Compensatory mechanisms could then be studied, including the physiological control systems and analysis of the sequence of the functional change with time. Of greatest importance would be identification of species differences, which in many cases, I believe, have invalidated the models, as we have heard during this symposium.

Unfortunately, we have not taken the first and essential step, namely the establishment of generally accepted criteria for the various clinical states we call shock. Lacking these criteria we cannot demonstrate the validity of the experimental models or the applicability of basic physiological control.

Future research is likely to be controversial and unrewarding until these essential steps have been taken for each of the different clinical states. I feel it is not now reasonable to search for common aetiological mechanisms, for similarities in compensatory reactions, or for fundamentally sound therapeutic techniques without having essential information of the sort described.

SENNING: I wish to discuss Dr. BIÖRCK's remarks. What I should like to stress in connection with cardiac shock is the picture of extreme peripheral vascular constriction; this is in my opinion mainly due to the fact that in left heart infarctions there is an enormous displacement of the blood volume from the periphery to the pulmonary circulation. When we make a cut-down in the femoral vein, for instance, this is practically empty; you don't have any blood flow in the vein. I think that in left heart infarctions treatment with chlorpromazine is much more promising than with adrenaline or noradrenaline. What we have to do is to stimulate the heart and not the periphery. We have one means of supporting the circulation and preventing pulmonary oedema, and that is to give good artificial respiration. We can also control the venous return. If we raise the pressure against the expiration, we can practically always prevent or successfully treat the pulmonary oedema. And of course it's very important that we follow up the pH; a low pH (at normal pCO_2) is the best indication we have for an inadequate tissue perfusion. Treatment with streptokinase is the most promising we have seen during recent years in severe acute infarctions.

NICKERSON: I would like to comment on the "refractoriness" to the pressor effect of noradrenaline that Dr. MATTHES showed. We have tried in a variety of ways and have been quite unable, within a reasonable dose range, to produce real refractoriness of the vascular system to noradrenaline. It is true that with prolonged infusion the pressor response diminishes. However, the peripheral resistance may continue to increase, and the decline in pressure is due primarily to a decrease in the cardiac output.

GROSS: I was most interested in Dr. SPINK's findings, and I too would like to comment on his observations. First, in your dogs, you found — with rather high doses of aldosterone — not only an unusual toxicity but also a definite increase in the plasma potassium concentration. This is just the opposite from what you would expect if you give a high dose of aldosterone to an intact animal, in which a loss of potassium is observed in response to aldosterone. This effect, however, does not become distinct within the rather short period of about 2 to 3 hours, as you have seen in your dogs. To me, this is especially interesting, since the increase in plasma potassium demonstrates that aldosterone must have an extrarenal action on the distribution of sodium and potassium. The second point I should like to make concerns the doses of angiotensin given by you. Firstly, you gave far too high a dose of angiotensin (1—2 mg.) and observed pulmonary oedema. I feel that in the other dogs you treated you gave too small a dose of angiotensin, as you injected it subcutaneously. We observed that, at least if you take the blood pressure as a parameter, doses of the order of magnitude you have given by subcutaneous injection don't have any action on blood pressure, as the ratio between the effective pressor doses, when administered intravenously as compared with the subcutaneous route, is much greater for angiotensin than, for example, for noradrenaline. Angiotensin is destroyed very rapidly by angiotensinase and other polypeptidases in the tissue; and for this reason we feel that it is preferable not to give angiotensin by the subcutaneous route but that it is much better to administer it in the order of magnitude of 0.25—1 μg./kg. bodyweight per minute in the form of a continuous infusion. As I mentioned already yesterday, the possibility cannot be excluded that even by the continuous infusion of these small doses of angiotensin you may stimulate aldosterone secretion, and for this reason it is conceivable that you have a double effect which is not only due to the blood-pressure elevating action of angiotensin but might well also be mediated through the adrenal cortex.

SPINK: Did I understand you to say, Dr. BIÖRCK, that in the last 25 years you had observed no improvement in the mortality rate of myocardial infarction in Sweden ? We have been informed in the United States that the mortality rate had been reduced following the routine use of anticoagulants in acute myocardial infarction. It would be pretty difficult at this time to treat patients without using anticoagulants. Dr. MATTHES did use heparin in selected cases. The second remark that I would like to make refers to Dr. RUSHMER's suggestion that the human model should be studied more intensively. Some of us clinicians are trying desperately to do this very thing, but it is extremely difficult to get a base line in patients critically ill with shock. In many instances, treatment has been instituted before we see them, and rightly so. The prompt use of morphine for pain, and of blood and oxygen, often prevents quantitative serial observations. However, a team of competent scientific and medical personnel in a large general hospital should and will study the human being in shock in more detail. I am delighted to hear the suggestions made by Dr. RUSHMER.

HALPERN: I wish to comment upon Dr. SPINK's paper on two points. One of the points concerns the potentiation of the effect of the pressor agents by cortisone or hydrocortisone. Ten years ago, evidence was provided in my laboratory that cortisone or hydrocortisone potentiate the effect of adrenaline on peripheral vascular tonus. We used mice, which are very resistant to the angiotoxic action of histamine. And this can be very easily measured by determining the threshold dose of histamine which, when given by intradermal injection, will produce a threshold effect on capillary permeability as evidenced by the local seepage of macromolecular dyes. Removal of the adrenals will render the animal extremely sensitive to any type of shock, including histaminic shock. In adrenalectomised animals, the dose of histamine necessary to produce a minimum effect on capillary permeability is about 100 times lower than in normal animals. Treatment with cortisone did increase the tolerance — but the percentage involved was only about 10—15 %, even when very high doses of cortisone were used. Treatment with quite high doses of adrenaline and noradrenaline produces a similar effect. But when both substances were administered, we were able to normalise the level of resistance of the vessels to the angiotoxic effect of histamine in an adrenalectomised mouse. This shows that cortisone does potentiate the effect of pressor agents on the tone of the capillaries.

The second point is the possible role of complement. Mice are very suitable for this kind of study, because they contain an exceedingly small quantity of complement. They can be more or less completely decomplemented, and the amount of complement can be reduced to a level at which it is no longer measurable. In spite of the fact that the animals have been almost completely decomplemented, the pattern of the anaphylactic shock remains completely unchanged.

FINE: I would like to comment on Dr. LILLEHEI's paper. Dr. LILLEHEI's model of haemorrhagic shock in dogs, as you noted, produces a terminal severe hypovolaemia, a substantial rise in the haematocrit, and a plasma haemoglobinaemia. This is not the same model that I have been talking about. In our hands, our technique does not result in a terminal severe loss of plasma or a rise in haematocrit. On the contrary, there is usually a slight fall in haematocrit, because of mobilised fluid. Haemolysis occurs occasionally, but this is inconsequential. If the hypovolaemia in Dr. LILLEHEI's experiments is caused by bleeding from necrotic intestinal mucosa, one would not expect to find a preferential loss of plasma. One suspects that portal hypertension is playing a significant role in these experiments. In any case, if the leak cannot be sealed, one shouldn't be surprised to find that antibiotics are as useless as blood or plasma, just as is the case in tourniquet shock, for example.

The observation that endotoxins also produce a type of severe shock, in which the hypovolaemia alone is enough to cause death, indicates that here, too, Dr. LILLEHEI has a model in which there is a preferential loss of plasma, a finding which has not been obtained in other species dying of endotoxic shock. Perhaps Dr. LILLEHEI should seek to determine in what way his preparation differs, so as to account for the disparity between his data and the data obtained in other laboratories. It is difficult to see how his data have relevance to the state of haemorrhagic or endotoxic shock in the rat, the rabbit, or man. Dr. LILLEHEI attempts an explanation of species differences by postulating a submucosal rather than a mucosal injury in species other than the dog. Very careful histologic studies (including electron-microscopy) of the gut, undertaken by Dr. LEON WEISS in these two types of shock, do not support this assumption.

The observation that cross-perfusion of the shocked dog's intestine with a normal donor dog's circulation preserves the integrity of the intestine is an interesting one and deserves close study. It has long been known that Dibenamine is able to do this. Hence, one might expect a similar result by supplying better flow from an outside source. Prevention of injury to the gut and death by such cross-perfusion does not demonstrate that the gut injury is the key injury in shock in the dog, for the perfusion may improve flow through the liver as well as the gut. In our hands, an Eck fistula prevents injury to the gut, but does not prevent the development of irreversibility. To exclude better flow through the liver by cross-perfusion of the superior mesenteric artery, as playing a role in preventing death, would require quantitative measurements on the distribution of the donor animal's blood, even in dogs with an Eck fistula. Dr. LILLEHEI believes such a study unnecessary, because direct cross-perfusion of the liver did his dogs no good, a finding which contradicts ours. But this liver perfusion experiment is not comparable with our experiment or with his own superior mesenteric artery perfusion experiment. If he had cross-perfused the liver from the beginning of the shock period, as he cross-perfused the intestine from the beginning of the shock period, he could have made a valid comparison. But in fact he did not start the liver perfusion until after the dog had been in shock for over an hour. In our hands the best results from perfusion of the liver were obtained when it was started with the onset of shock. Those who have used our technique precisely have confirmed our observation that this protects against irreversibility.

Having said all this, I nevertheless believe, as he does, in the great importance of the gut. If the morphologic data are confusing, let us look at the chemistry of this organ no less than that of other organs, and not only at the endotoxins, but at other products of bacterial activity, such as the indoles, the pyrimidines, the volatile tertiary amines, etc., whose suppression by antibiotics may account for their impressive effect in the treatment of hepatic coma.

I agree entirely with Dr. LILLEHEI that the adrenergic compounds are central to the problem of the mechanism of the development of irreversibility. More data are needed on what vital functions they choke off, not only in the gut, but elsewhere.

TROELL: In addition to Dr. RUSHMER's remarks on the necessity for studying the details in the shock picture, I would like to draw attention to the importance, as regards the clinical assessment of acute shock, of knowing the cardiac output and its changes. I should like to ask Dr. BULL for his opinion and to enquire whether he has done any measurements in patients and, if so, by what method.

BIÖRCK: Dr. SPINK has asked me about the effect of anticoagulants on mortality statistics. I think that a large portion of our deaths occur in the early phase of the acute infarct when the effect of anticoagulants is rather limited. I believe that anticoagulants have decreased the number of deaths in pulmonary embolism, which is now responsible for only a minor proportion of the deaths. We are now in the process of finding out whether there has been a change in the characteristics of infarct deaths over these years, because in all clinical material there is a bias in selection, which has to be traced in order to enable one to make a valid interpretation of the observations. As for Dr. SENNING's remarks, I should have added that we believe — as he does — in the usefulness of artificial respiration in certain instances of cardiogenic shock.

BACQ: In spinal dogs which had recovered from spinal shock SHER-RINGTON demonstrated the existence of spinal vasomotor reflexes to sensory — probably pain — stimulation. These segmental reflexes, for some reason which I do not know, have apparently been almost forgotten. It is quite possible that such a spinal segmental reflex can maintain — in the contra-lateral, perfectly intact limb, for instance — a kind of physiological tourniquet by pain stimulation coming from the injured limb. This reflex will persist if the sensation of pain is abolished by an analgesic, but it will be abolished if a Novocaine block is applied as suggested by Dr. OSSIPOV.

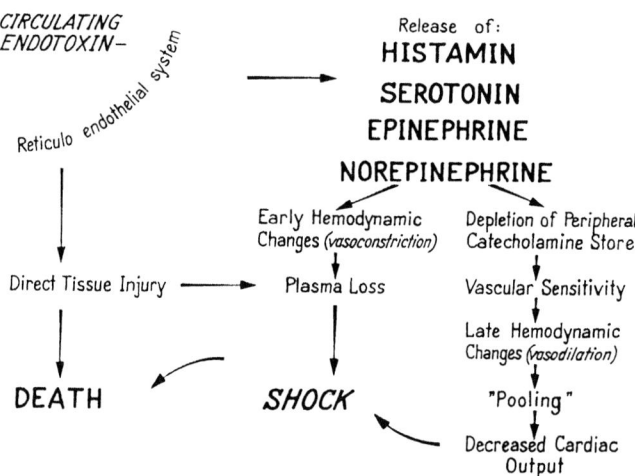

Fig. 1 (to Discussion LILLEHEI)

SELKURT: I should like to know quite a lot more about the renal changes in endotoxic shock, but will summarise my questions very briefly by asking: Is the effect of endotoxin in the kidney a direct action of endotoxin itself on the vasculature or an indirect action by way of histamine or serotonin release? Both of these compounds, I believe, are renal vasoconstrictors, at least when injected directly into the renal artery.

SPINK: In answer to Dr. SELKURT's question, we do not believe that endotoxin has a direct effect on the kidney. Our present concept is that endotoxin causes alterations in renal blood flow by liberating or activating humoral factors that result in vasoconstriction. One of these factors is histamine, but not necessarily the only factor.

LILLEHEI: I would like to thank Dr. FINE for his comments on my presentation. How can these apparent differences be resolved ? At the moment I don't know. There is one point that I should make, however. Dr. FINE is certainly one of the doyens in the study of shock. Through his writings he has been my teacher and I his student. In this regard, I have thought that perhaps a measure of the greatness of a teacher is that his students have learned so effectively from him that they no longer can agree with him. I hope that one day a student of mine might feel the same way. It would reassure me that I had been as effective a teacher as Dr. FINE.

I have one other comment in regard to Dr. SPINK's presentation. I have one slide to show (Fig. 1) which might clear up some of the apparent discrepancies in the various papers heard during the past few days. This slide is somewhat like a political platform; there is something in it to please almost everyone, and thus it should offend no one. I believe it is self-explanatory.

BULL: I was asked what experience we had had with cardiac output. My colleagues have measured a great many cardiac outputs, some of them in the patients whom I described this morning. This work has not yet been published, because we came across a snag in the procedure. We were trying too much, and I suspect that that would be Dr. RUSHMER's trouble if he attempts to do as he proposes. We were trying this four years ago, and one of the aims was to get repeated cardiac-output measurements using I^{132} as a variation on the I^{131} albumin method. We ran into trouble from extraneous counts, so we have had to go back over the data on these cases. Cardiac output certainly can be measured in such cases; it relates to basic changes in shock with and without transfusion and is the most important measure of the circulation further to estimation of blood volume.

Allergic shock

By

B.-N. HALPERN

1. Immunological factors in anaphylactic shock

Allergic shock is conditioned by immunological factors. It is a consequence of the reaction between the sensitised cells and the specific antigen. Opinions still differ concerning the train of reactions which lead from the antigen-antibody union to the release of the chemical agents directly responsible for the clinical manifestations.

Although I have no wish to become involved here in the details of this controversy, I must mention the two main opposing opinions. According to a theory elaborated by Sir HENRY DALE (*1, 2*), it is the union of the antigen with cell-fixed antibody which is the central factor concerned in anaphylactic shock. This phenomenon gives rise to a disturbance of membrane permeability resulting in the diffusion of toxic agents stored in the cell as inactive precursors.

Among the various arguments advanced in favour of this hypothesis, the most pertinent are: 1) that isolated cells or isolated tissues carefully cleared of blood and plasma show a prompt anaphylactic response to the addition of the antigen; 2) that in passively sensitised animals there is an obligatory latent period before anaphylaxis can be induced, this latent period corresponding to the delay required for antibody fixation on the specific cell receptors; 3) that there exists a species specificity in heterologous antibody fixation; thus, for example, the guinea pig can be readily sensitised with rabbit, mouse, or human antibody, but not with horse, beef, or goat antibody.

It is on these facts that the *"cellular theory of anaphylaxis"* is based.

According to the *"humoral theory of anaphylaxis"*, the release of toxic agents from the cells is due to the formation in the circulating blood of a specific factor which acts as a histamine liberator. This hypothesis is based on the old observation made by FRIEDBERGER (*3*) and BORDET (*4*) that incubation of rat serum with certain colloidal substrates such as agar, inulin, or the precipitated antigen-antibody complex renders the serum highly toxic in the guinea-pig. The injection of such a serum may lead to death of the animal with typical anaphylactic-like symptoms.

This view has recently gained substantial support from evidence that soluble antigen-antibody complex isolated from the serum of animals in anaphylactic shock is able to produce typical anaphylactic-type reactions when injected into normal guinea-pigs and to elicit anaphylactic-like contraction of isolated smooth tissues *in vitro* (5).

Whatever the initial mechanism may be, it is becoming more and more evident that the release of the intracellular chemical agents by the antigen-antibody complexes is a complicated phenomenon and is likely to involve several factors including specific enzymes (6). It is extremely doubtful whether complement plays any role in the anaphylactic type of reaction. Recent investigations from my laboratory have shown that in mice, which normally contain an exceedingly small amount of complement, reduction of the complement to non-measurable quantities (less than 10%) causes no change at all in the development of the anaphylactic shock or in the sensitivity to histamine. In the experiments in question, the mice were passively sensitised with homologous antibody and pre-treated with *Hemophilus pertussis* in order to increase their susceptibility to anaphylaxis and to histamine (7). On the other hand, complement probably does play some part in the development of other types of hypersensitivity reaction, such as the Arthus phenomenon, Shwartzman phenomenon, organ-specific sensitivity, etc. But I shall not deal here with these problems, which are beyond my scope.

2. Polymorphic aspects of allergic shock

Since the objective signs of anaphylactic shock in man and various animal species are so well known to all of you, I shall not waste time by describing them again.

In the present paper dealing with shock, the vascular changes occurring in various animal species will be briefly described and the mechanism of these haemodynamic changes analysed.

The changes in the systemic blood pressure result from circulatory impairment in different vascular beds.

One of the most common vascular phenomena encountered in allergic shock is the fall in the systemic blood pressure.

Intravenous injection of the antigen into an animal sensitised, whether actively or passively, causes hypotension in all the mammalian species studied. Although the degree of response varies in different species, it is usually of sufficient severity to justify its description as shock.

It will be seen later that there are great differences in the effects of anaphylactic shock upon the specific vascular beds in different species. There are nevertheless qualitative similarities.

Let us consider now in some detail the vascular changes occurring in certain animal species.

a) Dog. As early as 1902, RICHET and PORTIER (8) observed a sharp fall in the systemic blood pressure of dogs during anaphylactic shock. This vascular collapse is accompanied or preceded by various other severe symptoms, i.e. vomiting, diarrhoea, ataxia, prostration, dyspnoea, and coma. The main changes affecting the blood are: leucopenia, haemoconcentration, and incoagulability. Death may occur from vascular collapse within a matter of hours following injection of the antigen.

The diminution in cardiac output observed in anaphylactic shock in dogs is related neither to myocardial failure nor to impairment of the coronary circulation, as has been proved by electrocardiographic recordings. Instead, it is a direct result of the decreased venous return, a great part of the circulating blood being sequestrated in the portal vascular bed.

The main features of anaphylactic shock in dogs are the vascular changes in the liver and in the portal circulation. There is a sharp rise in the portal venous pressure by some 15 to 20 centimetres of H_2O, accompanied at the same time by a fall in central venous pressure. The congestion and engorgement of the liver occurring in anaphylactic shock was first observed by MANWARING in 1911 (9) and was extensively studied by WEIL in 1912 (10). This author concluded that stagnation of the blood in the portal region was quantitatively sufficient to explain the fall in blood pressure. A quantity as high as 61% of the total blood of a dog suffering from anaphylactic shock may be sequestrated in the portal vascular bed.

Congestion of the liver and stasis in the portal circulatory system are the dominant features of the vascular impairment observed in allergic shock in the dog and may well account for the gastrointestinal congestion and haemorrhages described by RICHET (11).

The steady gain in weight indicates injury to the liver sinusoids, as a result of which transudation, oedema, and stasis occur. Consequently, lymph drainage is considerably increased, the increase being far in excess of that produced by a corresponding rise in blood pressure (12). Similar phenomena occur in the mesenteric circulation.

The increased back-pressure observed in dogs during anaphylactic shock is very probably due to constriction of the hepatic veins caused by liberation of a large amount of histamine (*13, 14, 15*). In dogs, as shown by SIMONDS and AREY (*16*), the hepatic veins — which contain a greater amount of smooth muscle than in any other of the 22 animal species studied — play the role of a genuine sphincter.

May I remind you at this point that a rise in portal pressure and hepatic engorgement have also been observed in dogs in response to endotoxin and have been attributed to the same cause (*17, 18*).

There are only fragmentary published data concerning vascular reactions in other parts of the circulation. Vasodilatation has been observed in the hind limb. A rise in skin temperature marks the first stage of the anaphylactic reaction, indicating dilatation of the small cutaneous arterioles. It is therefore likely that general arteriolar and capillary dilatation is the main vascular feature of anaphylactic shock in dogs.

Blood volume. There is evidence that the blood volume is reduced in anaphylactic shock, and this phenomenon is probably a contributory factor in severe and fatal forms.

The changes in the hematocrit observed in dogs in my laboratory indicate a considerable alteration in capillary permeability (*19*). The same phenomenon has been noted following injection of polyvinylpyrrolidone, which acts as a histamine liberator in dogs (*20*).

The rate of water and protein filtration through the capillary wall is considerably increased, as is also the protein concentration in the capillary filtrate. The increase in the permeability of the capillary wall has also been confirmed by measuring the rate of diffusion of macromolecular dyes.

The diminishing plasma volume observed in anaphylactic shock in dogs may result either from dehydration caused by vomiting and diarrhoea or from loss into interstitial space, or both.

The fact that the symptoms are of the same severity or even aggravated in anaesthetised dogs, in which gastro-intestinal disorders are more or less absent, suggests that the increase in capillary permeability is the main reason for the reduction in blood volume.

On the whole, the vascular disturbances observed in severe anaphylactic shock in dogs bear a surprising resemblance to the haemodynamic effects of endotoxins. This resemblance will also be found under other circumstances.

b) Rabbit. The vascular changes encountered in anaphylactic shock in rabbits are of a complex nature.

The main characteristic of this syndrome is a fall in the systemic pressure, usually preceded by transient hypertension (21). Analytical haemodynamic studies nevertheless indicate that other vascular modifications occur simultaneously: a) pallor and coldness of the tegument suggest peripheral arterial constriction; b) the steady rise in the P.A.P. accompanying the fall in systemic pressure results from intense constriction of the pulmonary arterioles (22); c) electrocardiographic studies made recently in my department (23) indicate right-ventricular congestion and coronary ischaemia.

Peripheral vascular constriction has been clearly evidenced by VALLERY-RADOT and his co-workers (24) by means of arteriographs taken after intra-arterial injections of Thorotrast.

On the other hand, FRIEDBERGER and SEIDENBER (25), in an extensive series of perfusion experiments with various blood-vessel preparations of the limbs and ears, have demonstrated that the vessels from previously sensitised animals show strong arterial constriction when perfused with antigen.

As for the pulmonary hypertension, this is related to increased vascular resistance, since it also occurs in the isolated and perfused lung (26), as shown by studies undertaken in my department.

Direct observation of the vascular changes in the rabbit's ear, using transparent chambers (27, 28), showed transient obliterative constriction of the arterioles and stasis. The capillaries and venules were unaffected.

The pulmonary vasoconstriction characteristic of anaphylactic shock in rabbits is more or less the equivalent of hepatic congestion in dogs and is responsible for the fall in arterial blood pressure and for right ventricular failure. In this connection, attention should also be drawn to the highly developed smooth muscle of the pulmonary arteries in rabbits and guinea-pigs, which is much the same as the sphincter-like structures observed in the hepatic veins of dogs.

When the antigen is given intravenously there is no evidence of hepato-splanchnic blood pooling and the changes in portal pressure are insignificant.

Blood. One of the characteristic features of anaphylactic shock in rabbits is the steady decrease of the circulating leucocytes and platelets. The blood elements are found aggregated in the pulmonary bed (29). In the rabbit, the leucocytes and particularly the platelets contain a considerable amount of histamine and serotonin (30). There is probably a correlation between the disaggregation of the blood elements in the pulmonary bed and the violent constriction of the pulmonary vessels in anaphylactic shock.

May I emphasise again the resemblance between the haemo-dynamic changes occurring in anaphylactic shock and endotoxin shock in this animal species (*31*).

c) **Guinea-pig.** The main feature of anaphylactic shock in this animal species is the violent bronchial constriction which leads to death by asphyxia.

The vascular changes are dominated by signs of acute hyper-capnia. When the haemodynamic disorders were analysed in sudden forms of shock, they appeared to resemble those observed in rabbits.

It should nevertheless be stressed that typical anaphylactic shock in guinea-pigs, which culminates in asphyxia due to irrevers-ible bronchial contraction, can only be produced when the antigen is injected intravenously and thus reaches the lungs directly. By contrast, when the antigen is injected intraperitoneally and is therefore first absorbed into the portal circulation, the animal's reaction takes the form of *protracted shock*. In these circumstances, respiratory distress may be slight or even absent, and the main symptoms (vascular collapse and hypothermia) are provoked by severe haemodynamic impairment of the general and portal circulation (*32*).

Accordingly, as emphasised by BURRAGE and IRWIN (*33*), it is an oversimplification to state that death from anaphylactic shock in the guinea-pig is due to bronchial spasm, in the rabbit to con-striction of the pulmonary arteries and to right ventricular failure, and in the dog to spasm of the hepatic veins. These phenomena are rather the results of the techniques used. Many other possibilities exist, and shock and death result, in fact, from a more extensive injury involving probably the whole vascular bed. This is partic-ularly true of mice.

d) **Rat and mouse.** In the older literature, reference is often made to the fact that rats and mice are refractory to anaphylactic shock (*32*). Recent investigations performed in various laboratories, including my own, have shown that this statement is incorrect and that severe anaphylactic shock can be produced regularly in rats (*34*) as well as in mice (*35*).

In rats, anaphylactic shock is characterised by a fall in the arterial blood pressure, by haemoconcentration, and by intense congestion of the splanchnic organs (*34*). The same has been reported in mice (*36*, *37*).

The mouse has proved exceedingly useful for the study of vascular changes occurring in anaphylactic shock, which can be directly observed under the microscope in the vascular beds of certain relatively transparent parts of the body, such as the claws or ears.

McMaster (*36, 37*) reported that a few seconds after the challenging injection, partial constriction of the vessels occurred and clumps of platelets and white cells appeared in the arterioles, occasionally forming emboli in the smaller vessels. Usually the arteries constricted first but, after a few minutes, spasm of the veins developed as well. Sometimes, in severe forms of shock, the veins constricted before the arteries. Throughout the period of observation the capillaries showed no constriction. They became empty if arterial spasm was intense, or crammed with blood if the veins remained obliterated, but their role appeared to be passive.

e) **Man.** Allergic shock in humans may be very similar to the conditions already described in one of the animal species or may combine features shown by different species.

The clinical picture will depend upon the sensitivity of the individual, on the nature of the antigen, and on the route by which it has been introduced. I have had an opportunity of observing quite a large number of such cases, but fortunately none was fatal. Penicillin, ACTH, procaine, or desensitisation treatment with pollen were mainly responsible for these accidents.

Very severe anaphylactic shock in man bears a close resemblance to that observed in dogs, giving rise to malaise, vomiting, weakness, a dramatic fall in blood pressure, loss of consciousness, and relaxation of sphincters. Death may occur in less than one hour if adequate treatment is not given.

The autopsies usually reveal generalised congestion of the organs, but with no specific or particular organic lesions.

In the majority of cases, the clinical picture is less dramatic, and other signs may develop, such as generalised erythematous rash, violent itching, generalised giant urticaria, congestion of the mucous membranes, oedema and spasm of the bronchi causing severe respiratory difficulties, tachycardia, a fall in blood pressure, decreased blood coagulability, leucopenia and eosinophilia. Although for obvious reasons no detailed studies on the vascular mechanisms of human allergic shock are available, it can be assumed that the reactions are by and large similar to those already considered in the dog.

3. Microscopic observations

As we have already seen, the anaphylactic reaction seems to affect the whole vascular system. The main circulatory changes are due to generalised injury of the small blood vessels. Hence, the vascular reactions of sensitised tissues to antigen, as studied by direct microscopic observation, are of the greatest interest.

We referred above to the observations made by McMASTER (*36, 37*) in mice. Mention should also be made of certain other investigations. LECOMTE and HUGHES (*39*) have studied, by direct examination of the mesenteric vessels in rabbits and guinea-pigs, the effect of an antigen directly applied locally to the tissues in sensitised and non-sensitised animals.

In sensitised animals, the following sequence of phenomena was observed: within a few seconds, leucocytes and platelets stick to the walls of the venules. Ths intravascular agglutination rapidly increases. In about 5 minutes, emboli formed of leucocytes and platelets are visible. Some of them become detached and carried away by the stream. Within roughly the same period, the venules rupture, allowing petechial haemorrhages to occur, and the venous circulation ceases. After about 20 minutes, the whole mesenteric circulation is arrested, starting from the venous side. The arterioles apparently remain undamaged and have a passive role. Antihistamines do not prevent these local alterations.

BURRAGE and IRWIN (*33*) have made similar observations by direct study of the small pulmonary vessels in live guinea-pigs and rabbits during generalised anaphylaxis. Where death occurred rapidly, the arterioles and venules constricted to occlusion, leaving the tissues bloodless. Where the shock was less severe, there was less constriction, clumps of red and white cells formed emboli, and blood-cells escaped from the venules. In the liver, which was also studied directly under the microscope, the sphincters at the junctions of the sinusoids and central veins closed during severe shock, thus filling the sinusoids with blood. Flow ceased in the portal venules and the liver became congested. If death did not occur, emboli and thrombi appeared and blood-cells escaped into the tissues.

The reports of the various workers cited so far are unanimous in concluding that the vascular reactions occurring in anaphylactic shock are a generalised phenomenon. It therefore seems incorrect to refer to "shock organs". If one or another organ seems to play a pre-eminent role in causing the main clinical symptoms, this is probably because of its special anatomical structure, because of the sensitivity of its structural elements to the chemical agents released, or perhaps merely because of the manner in which the antigen first came into contact with the vascular system.

There is a great deal of evidence indicating that the antigen-antibody reaction takes place on the surface of the endothelial cells rather than on that of the smooth muscles. This leads us to conclude that there is really no such thing as a "shock organ", unless we apply this term to the whole vascular bed or to the whole system of tissues formed of smooth muscles.

4. Chemical mediators in allergic shock

As mentioned at the beginning of this report, allergic shock is of an indirect nature and is mediated by the release of endogenous toxic agents. Allergic shock is a typical example of what DALE (40) has referred to as an "autopharmacological syndrome", since it depends on the release or discharge of pharmacologically active substances previously present in an inactive form fixed to the tissue-cell protoplasm or blood elements. One of the main toxic agents responsible for allergic shock is histamine. Histamine has been shown to be released in considerable quantities into the blood of sensitised dogs (41) and guinea-pigs (41) following injection of antigen. The release of histamine into the blood or into the surrounding medium from isolated tissues has also been observed in man in response to addition of antigen (42).

There is a satisfactory correlation – at least in dogs – between the severity of the symptoms of shock and the amount of histamine released. In dogs, the main source of histamine is the liver. By comparing the histamine content before and after anaphylactic shock, OJERS and co-workers found that 2 to 5 mg. of histamine base was liberated (43). Perfused dog liver, in the presence of whole blood (44), and isolated perfused dog skin (45) release a significant portion of histamine. Lung taken from a sensitised guinea-pig and perfused with Locke's solution will release more than 50% of its histamine content upon addition of the antigen (46).

In rabbits, histamine originates mainly from the blood elements and particularly the platelets (40). Addition of antigen to the heparinised whole blood of sensitised rabbits (47) or of washed antigen-antibody mixtures (48) to the blood of normal rabbits results in a considerable release of histamine from the platelets and white cells.

The interdependence of the blood elements on the liberation of histamine in the rabbit has been well established (49, 50). DRAG-STEDT and co-workers (51) calculated from in vitro experiments that the amount of histamine which could be liberated in vivo from rabbit blood cells would work out at about 0.3 mg./kg. of body-weight. This amount is not enough to produce death in a rabbit when injected intravenously, but we must remember that anaphylactic shock in rabbits is seldom fatal and that there is a considerable local concentration of histamine released from the clumps of leucocytes and platelets formed in the small vessels. Therefore even small amounts of histamine may produce considerable pharmacological effects when released in small vascular areas.

A similar release of histamine has been shown to occur from the white-cell layer of human blood, but it is probable that, in this species, blood basophiles rather than platelets are the source of histamine (52).

Time does not permit me to discuss here the problem of the mechanism by which histamine is released. Very recently SCHAYER (53) has provided evidence that histidine-decarboxylase can be activated by stress, antigen-antibody complex, and certain endotoxins. Enzyme activity may increase locally in lymph nodes in response to specific or non-specific agents. This enzyme activation is independent of the nervous regulatory system and of hormonal influences and seems to be a property of the small blood vessels.

5-Hydroxytryptamine. Although 5-HT is present in the platelets of many animal species in widely varying amounts, and although it has been shown to be released with histamine when antigen is incubated *in vitro* with plasma containing antibody and platelets from rabbits, dogs, and guinea-pigs (30), there is no evidence whatsoever to substantiate an hypothesis that this substance plays an essential part in anaphylaxis. It may nevertheless have some local significance at sites where platelets become aggregated, such as in the lung capillaries in rabbits.

Heparin. ARTHUS (54) was the first to draw attention to the incoagulability of the blood during anaphylactic shock. It was definitely proved in 1941 (55) that this phenomenon is due to the release of heparin. The release of heparin is correlated with the release of histamine, i. e. with the severity of the anaphylactic shock. It seems likely that the release of both substances depends upon some analogous mechanism.

Other substances. Other more complex substances such as "slow-reacting substances" (56) and bradykinin (57) may be found either in the blood plasma or in the perfusate of isolated sensitised tissues. The significance and the role of these substances are not yet fully established.

Electrolytic changes may occur in very severe shock. It has been shown in my laboratory (58) that the release of histamine is correlated with the diffusion of a considerable amount of K^+, which may profoundly affect haemodynamics and tissular equilibrium.

5. Antagonists

Sympathomimetic agents. Adrenaline, noradrenaline, and other sympathomimetic agents which are potent antagonists of histamine are also most effective in counteracting allergic shock. Their action is often dramatic and life-saving. They still remain the most valuable for use in emergency cases.

Owing to their effect on the tonus of the arterioles and on capillary permeability and to their action on the smooth muscles, which is exactly the reverse of the effects of histamine, these sympathomimetic agents are able to correct almost perfectly the disorders occurring in anaphylactic shock.

Antihistamines. Synthetic antihistamines have been found to exert a remarkable protective action against anaphylactic shock (19), although there are certain differences in the degree of protection depending on the animal species. The protection afforded is regular and complete in guinea-pigs, dogs, and humans; but it is doubtful in rabbits (59) and rats (34). Antihistamines have also proved effective in mice (60) and in fowls (61).

Some years ago I showed that the antagonism between histamine and antihistamines is of a competitive nature (19). Both probably act as competitors *vis-à-vis* the same receptors. One molecule of antihistamine can neutralise the effect of ten molecules of histamine. The greater affinity of the antihistamines for the cellular receptors and the greater fixity of the receptor-antihistamine complexes may well account for the fact that the antihistamines prevail over the histamine in competitive reactions. Most of the antihistamines, and especially those derived from the phenothiazine ring, are also endowed with anticholinergic and antiserotonin activity and exert depressant effects on the autonomic and central nervous system (62).

Steroids. Adrenal cortical hormones are unable to protect animals against either anaphylactic or histaminic shock, although they do exert a remarkable therapeutic affect in clinical allergic diseases. The reason for this discrepancy may be explained by reference to their action on histamine biogenesis. In a series of investigations performed in my laboratory (63, 64), it has been shown that cortisone and related hormones inhibit histamine synthesis. This is particularly evident where histamine has been previously depleted by administering histamine releasors. The inhibitory action of cortisone on histamine synthesis has been extensively confirmed by SCHAYER (65) using ^{14}C-tagged histidine. The release of histamine is an "explosive" phenomenon, whereas the synthesis of histamine requires several weeks. A short course of treatment with steroids is unable to modify the tissular histamine stock and consequently the rapid histamine release which occurs in anaphylactic shock. Prolonged treatment with cortisone is necessary to decrease the amount of releasable histamine (66).

The mechanism by which cortisone and related hormones affect histamine synthesis is not yet clear.

6. General considerations

As stated by Sir HENRY DALE, the anaphylactic condition is a common and banal syndrome initiated by a highly specific immunological process.

The fundamental disorder results from damage to the smooth muscle cells, including particularly those of the vascular bed. A variety of conspicuous reactions on the part of other smooth-muscle tissues, differing in the various animal species, occur simultaneously with the basic and generalised vascular lesion, constituting the clinical picture of anaphylactic shock characteristic of each animal species.

How far are the signs and symptoms of anaphylactic shock specific ? On several occasions I have emphasised the resemblance between anaphylactic shock and endotoxin shock. This resemblance even involves some conspicuous species differences, such as liver engorgement in the dog and pulmonary arteriolar constriction in rabbits. But in no other animal species is the analogy so striking as in the mouse. The general signs, the vascular reactions, the temperature changes are superposable, if not identical.

Another point should be emphasised here, namely, the ability of certain gram-negative pathogens, i.e. endotoxins, to enhance the sensitivity of mice to anaphylaxis and histamine. This latter phenomenon is rather provocative, although no satisfactory explanation has been suggested for its mechanism. Do these analogies, close as they are, mean that the mechanism of both conditions is the same ?

The possibility that endotoxin shock may be mediated by histamine or 5-HT has been postulated by several authors. WEIL and SPINK (67) found that in rabbits an appreciable increase in the plasma histamine content of blood obtained from hepatic veins occurred after injection of endotoxin. Antihistaminic drugs have been shown to afford some degree of protection against endotoxin (*31*). On the other hand, there are many discrepancies: lack of parallelism between sensitivity to endotoxin and to anaphylaxis; sympathomimetic agents, which are highly effective in anaphylaxis, aggravate the toxicity of endotoxin; antihistamines are of little value in endotoxin shock.

Microscopic observations have shown that endotoxin seems to affect mainly the arterioles — at least in the initial phase — whereas in anaphylaxis the prevailing impact is on the veins.

It is likely that endotoxins and the intrinsic mediators released in anaphylactic shock have certain physiological effects in common, but they are far from being identical. As has been pointed out by DELAUNAY (*68*), ZWEIFACH and THOMAS (*69*), there is a marked similarity between endotoxin shock and trauma, whereas anaphylactic shock bears a much closer resemblance to histamine intoxication.

Summary

Allergic shock is characterised by three main features:
1. It is an indirect form of shock.
2. It is caused by the release of endogenous agents.
3. It can, in most cases, be effectively combated by synthetic agents possessing specific pharmacological activity.

The clinical patterns of allergic shock are polymorphous and vary from one animal species to another. This is bound up with the specific reactivity and sensitivity of certain tissues or vascular beds to the substances released. In most animal species, the result is vascular collapse due to the sequestration of a large portion of the circulating blood mass in certain areas.

In humans, allergic shock seems to be mainly caused by generalised vasodilatation, the individual "bleeding into his own vessels".

Microcirculation studies have also revealed the importance of damage to the small vessels, which seems to be a general phenomenon.

As to the chemical mediators, histamine is undoubtedly the most important factor known at present. The role of 5-HT or other complex polypeptides is far from convincing.

The effectiveness of the various antagonists (pressor agents, antihistamines, and steroids) is reviewed.

While in many respects allergic shock may bear some resemblance to endotoxin shock, analytical evidence suggests that the two forms of shock nevertheless have very different mechanisms.

References

1. DALE, H. H., and P. P. LAIDLAW: J. Physiol. (G.B.) **41**, 318 (1910—1911). — 2. DALE, H. H., and C. H. KELLAWAY: Philos. Transact. Roy. Soc. London **211**, 273 (1922). — 3. FRIEDBERGER, E.: Zschr. Immunit.forsch (G.) **2**, 208 (1909). — 4. BORDET, J.: Compt. rend. Soc. biol. (Fr.) **74**, 877 (1913). — 5. GERMUTH, F.: Fed. Proc. (U.S.A.) **16**, 413 (1957). — 6. MONGAR,

Allergic shock   289

J. L., and H. O. Schild: J. Physiol. (G.B.) 135, 301 (1957). — 7. Parvetjev,
I. A., and M. Goodline: J. Pharmacol. Exper. Therap. (U.S.A.) 92, 41
(1948). — 8. Portier, P., and C. Richet: Compt. rend. Soc. biol. (Fr.) 54,
170 (1902). — 9. Manwaring, W. H.: Z. Immun.forsch. (G.) 7, 598 (1911). —
10. Weil, R.: J. Med. Res. (U.S.A.) 27, 497 (1912). — 11. Richet, C.:
L'Anaphylaxie. Paris: Alcan ed. 1923. — 12. Simonds, J. P., and W. W.
Brandes: J. Immunol. (U.S.A.) 13, 11 (1927). — 13. Dragstedt, C. A., and
E. Gebauer-Fuelnegg: Amer. J. Physiol. 102, 512 (1932). — 14. Code,
C. F.: J. Physiol. (G.B.) 89, 257 (1937). — 15. Rocha e Silva, M., and
A. Grana: Arch. Surg. (U.S.A.) 52, 523 and 713 (1946). — 16. Simonds,
J. P., and L. B. Arey: Anat. Rec. (U.S.A.) 18, 219 (1920). — 17. Freed-
berg, A. S., and M. D. Altschule: N. England J. Med. 233, 560 (1945). —
18. Weil, M. H., L. D. MacLean, M. B. Visscher, and W. W. Spink: J.
Clin. Invest. (U.S.A.) 35, 191 (1956). — 19. Halpern, B. N.: Arch. internat.
Pharmacodyn. thérap. (Belg.) 45, 513 (1942). — 20. Halpern, B. N., G.
Musso, and T. Neveu: Brit. J. Pharmacol. 10, 223 (1955). — 21. Arthus, M.:
De l'anaphylaxie à l'immunité. Paris: Masson ed. 1921. — 22. Airila, Y.:
Scand. Arch. Physiol. 31, 388 (1914). — 23. Halpern, B. N., J. Himbert,
and P. Liacopoulos: Sem. hôp. Paris 6, 677 (1958). — 24. Vallery-Radot,
P.: L'Anaphylaxie humaine et expérimentale: Paris: Masson ed. 1937. —
25. Friedberger, R., and S. Seidenberg: Zschr. Immunit. Forsch. (G.)
51, 276 (1927). — 26. Vallery-Radot, P., B. N. Halpern, and G. Mauric:
Acta allerg. (Den.) 1, 85 (1948). — 27. Abell, R. G., and E. R. Clark: Anat.
Rec. (U.S.A.) 53, 121 (1932). — 28. Abell, R. G., and E. R. Schenck: J.
Immunol. (U.S.A.) 34, 195 (1938). — 29. Rocha e Silva, E.: Ann. N. Y.
Acad. Sc. 50, 1013 (1950). — 30. Humphrey, J. H., and R. Jaques: J.
Physiol. (G.B.) 124, 305 (1954). — 31. Gilbert, R. P.: Physiol. Rev. (U.S.A.)
40, 245 (1960). — 32. Doerr, R.: In: Handbuch der pathogenen Mikro-
organismen. Jena: Urban & Schwarzenberg 1929. — 33. Burrage, W. S.,
and J. W. Irwin: J. Allergy (U.S.A.) 24, 289 (1953). — 34. Halpern, B. N.,
P. Liacopoulos, and G. Perez del Castillo: Compt. rend. Soc. biol. (Fr.)
149, 314 (1955). — 35. Mayer, R. L., and D. Brousseau: Proc. Soc. Exper.
Biol. (U.S.A.) 63, 187 (1956). — 36. McMaster, P. D.: J. Exper. Med.
(U.S.A.) 74, 29 (1941). — 37. McMaster, P. D., and H. Kruse: J. Exper.
Med. (U.S.A.) 89, 583 (1949). — 38. McMaster, P. D.: General and local
vascular reactions in certain states of hypersensitivity. In: Cellular and
humoral aspects of the hypersensitivity states, by H. S. Lawrence, Cassel ed.
London 1959. — 39. Lecomte, J., and J. Hughes: Internat. Arch. Allergy
(Switz.) 8, 72 (1956). — 40. Dale, H. H.: Bull. Johns Hopkins Hosp.
(U.S.A.) 53, 297 (1933). — 41. Code, C. F.: Amer. J. Physiol. 127, 71 (1939). —
42. Schild, H. O., D. F. Hawkins, J. L. Mongar, and H. Herxheimer:
Lancet. (G.B.) 1951/II, 376. — 43. Ojers, G., C. A. Holmes, and C. A.
Dragstedt: J. Pharmacol. Exper. Therap. (U.S.A.) 73, 33 (1941). — 44.
Scroggie, A. E., and L. B. Jacques: J. Immunol. (U.S.A.) 62, 103 (1949). —
45. Feldberg, W., and M. Schachter: J. Physiol. (G.B.) 118, 124 (1952). —
46. Halpern, B. N., P. Liacopoulos, and O. Frick: Unpublished data. —
47. Katz, G.: Science (U.S.A.) 91, 221 (1940). — 48. Code, C. F., and P. B.
Dews: J. Laborat. Clin. Med. (U.S.A.) 38, 798 (1951). — 49. Code, C. F.,
and H. R. Ing: J. Physiol. (G.B.) 90, 501 (1937). — 50. Rose, B., and P
Weil: Proc. Soc. Exper. Biol. Med. (U.S.A.) 24, 494 (1939). — 51. Drag-
stedt, C. A., M. R. Arellano, and A. H. Lawton: Science (U.S.A.) 91,
617 (1940). — 52. Graham, H. T., O. H. Lowry, F. Wheelwright, M. A.
Lenz, and H. H. Parish: Blood (U.S.A.) 10, 967 (1955). — 53. Schayer,
R. W.: Fed. Proc. (U.S.A.) 20, 675 (1961). — 54. Arthus, M.: Arch. internat.

physiol. (Belg.) **7**, 471 (1909). — 55. JAQUES, L. B., and E. T. WATERS: J. Physiol. (G.B.) **99**, 454 (1941). — 56. BROCKELHURST, W. E.: A slow reacting substance in anaphylaxis: S. R. S.-A. In: Ciba Foundation Symposium on Histamine. London: J. & A. Churchill Ltd. 1956. — 57. BERALDO, W. T.: Amer. J. Physiol. **163**, 256 (1950). — 58. HALPERN, B. N., M. BRIOT, D. MOUTON, and J. TRUFFERT: Compt. rend. Soc. (Fr.) **149**, 1223 (1955). — 59. REUSE, J. J.: Arch. internat. pharmacodyn. thérap. (Belg.) **78**, 363 (1949). — 60. MALKIEL, S.: J. Allergy (U.S.A.) **23**, 352 (1952). — 61. LECOMTE, J., and M. L. BEAUMARIAGE: Acta allerg. (Den.) **10**, 31 (1956). — 62. HALPERN, B. N.: Les antihistaminiques de synthèse dérivés de la phénothiazine. In: Proceedings of IInd Intern. Congress of Therapeutics, Brussels, Editions Arscia (1950). — 63. HALPERN, B. N.: Histamine release by long chain molecules. In: Ciba Foundation Symposium on Histamine. London: J. & A. Churchill Ltd. 1956. — 64. NEVEU, T.: J. physiol. (Fr.) Suppl. (1960). — 65. SCHAYER, R.: In: Ciba Foundation Symposium on Histamine. London: J. & A. Churchill Ltd. 1956. — 66. HALPERN, B. N.: Actual. pharmacol. (Fr.) **XIII**, 109 (1960). — 67. WEIL, M. H., and W. W. SPINK: J. Clin. Med. (U.S.A.) **50**, 501 (1957). — 68. DELAUNAY, A., G. LEBRUN, M. DELAUNAY, and E. FOUQUIER: J. physiol. (Fr.) **40**, 89 (1948). — 69. ZWEIFACH, B. W., and L. THOMAS: J. Exper. Med. (U.S.A.) **106**, 385 (1957).

Discussion

SPINK: I enjoyed this presentation of Dr. HALPERN's. A few years ago, Dr. WEIL and I reviewed the subject of anaphylactic and anaphylactoid shock and pointed out that there are almost a hundred different agents that will provoke anaphylactoid shock, which is similar in its manifestations to endotoxin shock. I agree with Dr. HALPERN that we cannot place endotoxaemia and anaphylactic shock in the same category on the basis of the evidence at hand. Anaphylactic shock is specific; it is an antigen-antibody reaction. The reaction depends upon the activation of complement. Recent work in our laboratory suggests that complement may play a role in the initiation of the vascular alteration by endotoxin. In other words, endotoxin is actively dependent upon the presence of an enzyme or enzymes in the blood. Could this enzyme be one of the four components of complement, namely C_1? I would like to ask Dr. HALPERN how complement can be inactivated in the normal experimental animal.

UVNÄS: I was very interested in what you said about the inhibitory effect of γ-globulin on anaphylactic shock in guinea-pigs, because we have found that γ-globulin inhibits histamine release from isolated cells; this applies not only to γ-globulin but also to some other globulin fraction — I think it was α-globulin. Now I would like to know how much you have to inject into a guinea-pig in order to block the anaphylactic reaction. And there is a second point: I agree entirely when you say that the role of serotonin in anaphylactic shock is rather uncertain. It differs in different animals. In the rat, the mast cells contain serotonin, and you can fairly easily show that the release of serotonin and of histamine go hand in hand. The two substances are released by the same mechanism, but the serotonin content is only $1/20$ of that of histamine. So if there is, say, 1 μg. of histamine released, only $1/20$ μg. of serotonin appears.

HALPERN: In answer to Dr. SPINK I want to say that we have chosen mice for this experiment, because mice contain a small quantity of complement (only one unit per ml.), which is very little when we compare it with the guinea-pig which contains about 300. It is easy to obtain a decomplementation by using substances which will absorb the complement. Among such substances are zymosan, the antigen-antibody complex non-related to the antigens that have been used for sensitisation, or, as has recently been shown, γ-globulins aggregated by heating. About 90% of the complement present in the body can be removed by such treatment. Under these conditions, the mortality and the patterns of anaphylactic shock are exactly the same as in normal mice. This casts grave doubt on the role of complement in acute anaphylactic shock, but I am quite sure that in other anaphylactic and allergic conditions — the Arthus phenomenon or specific organ sensitivity — the complement may be an important factor.

Now, in answer to Dr. UVNÄS's question, we have recently shown that it is possible to sensitise normal tissues by a specific antibody *in vitro*. The tissue which is taken from a normal animal and has been sensitised by contact with the immune serum will fix the antibody. You can wash it repeatedly, but the sensitisation does not decrease. The tissues will respond to the antigen, giving rise to an anaphylactic reaction or to the release of histamine, depending upon the tissue which is used. This is of course a very practical method of measuring quantitative factors. A quantity as low as 2 γ of antibody nitrogen is sufficient to produce an anaphylactic contraction. If the same quantity of antibody is added in the presence of the γ-globulins and if the ratio of γ-globulins to the antibodies is 1 : 100, the anaphylactic sensitisation is abolished. Moreover, by using already sensitised preparations, you can displace the antibody if an adequate quantity of γ-globulin is added. I have recently found that these results can also be obtained *in vivo*. In fact, we have to consider the possibility that the γ-globulins circulating in the blood may play a *protective* role. Merely by doubling the quantity of γ-globulins in the body the animal can be completely protected against lethal anaphylactic shock.

Radiation shock

By

Z. M. BACQ

During the development of radiation sickness, various syndromes may appear which present certain features of the shock syndrome.

These syndromes are quite different from one animal species to another; their severity and the moment at which they appear depend on the dose received and on the dose rate. In this paper we have chosen to present the facts from the point of view of the physiopathologist. Further details and a large bibliography are available in a recent book by Z. M. BACQ and P. ALEXANDER (1961).

1. Central nervous system "shock"

When a very large dose (12,000 r or more) of hard X-rays or γ rays is given to a non-anaesthetised mammal at a high dose rate (about 1,000 r per minute), central nervous symptoms are predominant. The following is a quotation from a paper by ALLEN et al. (1960) describing experiments on the monkey (Macaca mulatta): "During irradiation, a few of these animals exhibited hyperirritability and scratching movements at about 3 to 4 minutes (3,000 r). This rapidly subsided, and then all animals entered a period of progressively severe debilitation at about 8 to 10 minutes (7,000 r). A few approached a semicomatose condition without any evidence of ability to support themselves within the cage. Approximately one-third of the animals had salivation, mouthing, or vomiting during irradiation, and a few had watery diarrhea. The incidence of vomiting is related to pre-irradiation feeding, and, since animals were purposely fasted 8 hours prior to irradiation to facilitate their handling, the low incidence of this phenomenon could be expected. Some of the animals demonstrated nystagmus during irradiation and suffered from ataxic movements and convulsive seizures. After irradiation, these animals had progressive symptomatology as described above, with the addition of meningismus as shown by a markedly opisthotonic posture, and tremors which were difficult to distinguish from convulsions and ataxia.

The animals developed the symptoms to a degree and with a rapidity which was dependent on the total dose received. For hours before the heart ceased to beat in these animals, complete loss of consciousness, opisthotonus, spasmodic gasping respiration, persistent tremors, convulsive movements, and often diarrhea were the common clinical observations. This pattern was found in an advanced stage almost universally and solely in the 9,000-r to 40,000-r range. Death occurred in this group within the first 3 days."

Pentobarbital and diphenylhydantoin, two classical anticonvulsive drugs, delay the appearance of convulsions and prolong the mean survival time as much as twelvefold when such high doses are given. The main cause of this CNS disturbance may be the very greatly increased potassium concentration in the plasma; but too little is known about the physiopathology of this interesting syndrome.

When a moderate dose (450 r in the LD_{50} range) is given to monkeys of the same species, the picture is less dramatic, as reported by HUNTER et al. (1957): "The onset of the initial reaction could be readily detected by a quite sudden change in the animal. The monkey would hang heavily from the cage roof, head on chest, or sit dejectedly in a corner and at times lie down on the floor of its cage. Loss of appetite accompanied this change. In most animals these signs would pass off only to return in a few minutes in an exaggerated form, accompanied by retching and vomiting. Waves of the latter signs recurred; but gradually their severity lessened, the interval between them lengthened, and they ceased in 2 hr or so. Appetite then returned, and no further vomiting was observed in the later course of the syndrome."

Vomiting and anorexia in this dose range are prominent in the dog and also in man. Their severity and duration are sufficiently proportional to the dose received to serve as a screening test in the event of an atomic disaster; three categories are usually envisaged:

a) Those who vomit very frequently, who do not stop vomiting two or three hours after irradiation, and who are in a state of shock have received 1,000 r or more and have no chance of survival.

b) Those who vomit only a few times, or experience nausea, during the first few hours after irradiation have not received more than 400 r and are likely to recover in two or three months if they agree to rest and if they receive the classical symptomatic treatment.

c) Those who vomit repeatedly, but experience marked relief two or three hours after irradiation, will have been exposed to an intermediate dose (about 600 to 800 r), which is within the lethal range. Such irradiated humans may have some chance of survival if kept in well-equipped hospitals and treated by experienced clinicians.

Anorexia is also very frequent in the monkey but occurs later (4 or 5 days after irradiation). Rats and mice — even when heavily irradiated — do not vomit, but their stomach and intestinal tract are generally full of fluid.

Loss of fluid and ions due to vomiting give rise to dehydration and shock if it is not carefully controlled.

When anaesthetised dogs are exposed to moderate (400 r) or even large (5,000 r) doses of ionising radiations, the condition of the circulation remains good until agony. The arterial blood pressure and cardiac output are normal. The blood volume is well maintained up to the last day of life in dogs which have been exposed to 1,000 r; cardiovascular changes do not become evident until 12 hours before death. Wide variations in the sensitivity of the vascular bed to adrenaline have been observed in rats following exposure to 600 r, and these variations are said to be due to the substances which can be seen in the blood during any type of shock.

It is indeed surprising to observe how radio-resistant some homeostatic mechanisms are, including especially the peripheral neuro-effector system. During recent unpublished experiments M. L. BEAUMARIAGE and myself observed perfectly normal performances of a nictitating membrane in anaesthetised cats excited by pre-ganglionic stimulation following exposure of the whole system (pre-ganglionic fibres, superior cervical ganglion, post-ganglionic fibres, and effector smooth muscle) to doses ranging from 20,000 to 100,000 r in 4 to 12 hours.

The urinary output is not decreased in any mammalian species by ionising irradiation during the period of normal circulatory conditions; diuresis has been observed by certain authors, but it is irregular in our experience.

It might be mentioned here that a state of marked cortical depression resembling the "typhos" of typhoid fever has been experienced as a delayed symptom by the Yugoslav scientists who in 1958 were accidentally exposed to a mixture of γ rays and neutrons.

2. Exhaustion of the adrenal cortex

There is ample evidence that ionising irradiation stimulates the adenopituitary to discharge ACTH, but careful analysis shows that irradiation is a very special form of stress.

The question has been raised as to the possibility that the adrenal cortex may become exhausted in the final stages of radiation sickness. TONKIKH (1958) has reported histological observations of adrenal cortical damage in the guinea-pig and physiological signs of cortical insufficiency (very rapid muscular fatigue) 4 to 6 days after a total body dose of 800 r; 7 or 8 days following irradiation of the guinea-pig, cortisone injection resulted "in a colossal increase in the efficiency of the gastrocnemius muscle". But such adrenal failure has not been seen in rats, calves, or monkeys following exposure to lethal doses; recent observations on human cases have failed to reveal any important changes in adrenal function. The use of cortisone or cortisone-like substances should be restricted in human cases to very definite indications; for instance, when fever appears and no infection is detectable.

3. Loss of water and electrolytes due to diarrhoea

Diarrhoea is a prominent sign in the rat and monkey and is often seen in man; it appears early if the dose is large; it is a frequent important complication and cause of death during the intermediate stage (3 to 14 days after irradiation). Loss of sodium through the gastro-intestinal tract following severe irradiation (1,500 r on total-body) may be the immediate cause of death in rats. The sodium and chloride losses after total-body exposure (male rats, 700 r of 140 kV X-rays) are strongly influenced by extracellular fluid movements and retention in the gastro-intestinal tract. During the 3—12 hours following irradiation, there is a shift of chloride and water from the body tissues into the gastric secretion. The chloride appearing after 3 hours in the stomach comes mainly from the connective tissues, muscles, and liver. The total-body chloride balance becomes negative. In spite of its small mass, the connective tissue plays a major role by virtue of its capacity to hold water and electrolytes. Many valuable observations on changes in the water and electrolyte balance of different tissues after irradiation have also been made by various authors, but they do not follow any easily describable pattern.

The mean sodium loss in severely irradiated (1,500 r, 250 kV X-rays) rats weighing 200 g. was found to be 1.5 mEq. in excess of that of normal fasting controls. This loss occurs through the gastro-intestinal tract mainly during the third day following irradiation and is due to lack of reabsorption of the sodium normally excreted in the bile. This excessive sodium loss is considered by JACKSON and ENTENMAN (1959) to be the immediate cause of death in the so-called "intestinal syndrome" in the rat because:

a) removal of $1 \cdot 4 - 1 \cdot 54$ mEq. of sodium from fasting non-irradiated rats by means of intraperitoneal dialysis with hypertonic glucose solution causes death within 24 hours; b) ligation of the bile duct immediately before or 24 hours after irradiation (1,500 r) increases the mean survival time very significantly ($5 \cdot 6$ days instead of $3 \cdot 3$ days for sham operated controls).

Recent observations of LUSHBAUGH et al. (1960) do not confirm the occurrence of a large loss of fluid and electrolytes via the intestinal tract except as a terminal phenomenon secondary to denudation of the intestinal mucosa with which it coincides. Food in the stomach of heavily irradiated rats prevents the absorption of orally administered sodium; fasting the animals before irradiation prevents this failure of absorption and allows conservation of Na and K in the body.

The classical chemical protectors (cysteamine and AET[1]) are very effective in diminishing or even completely inhibiting the diarrhoea and its consequences in the rat (J. R. MAISIN and D. G. DOHERTY, 1961).

4. Haemorrhages

Haemorrhages occur in nearly all irradiated dogs (450 r) and human beings; they vary in severity, in location, and in their clinical course, but do not seem to be a frequent cause of death, although they contribute to the incipient anaemia and may accelerate the appearance of circulatory disorders.

Vascular fragility is one of the causes of these haemorrhages. The second cause is undoubtedly the disappearance of the platelets, even after non-lethal doses of radiation. A lethal dose (450 r) reduces the average number of circulating platelets in dogs from 300,000 to 30,000 in 12 days. The coagulation accelerators carried by the platelets become deficient, but the quantity of prothrombin and accelerators in the blood seems to remain normal. Sometimes there is a spectacular increase in the coagulation time, and on other occasions very little. The decrease in coagulability may occasionally be due to the presence of an abnormally large quantity of heparin in the blood; it certainly disappears more or less completely, sometimes even quite completely, after the injection of protamine or toluidine blue, which are specific antagonists of heparin. The effect of toluidine blue, assuming that it exerts any effect at all, is more lasting (24—36 hours) than that of protamine (2 hours). It is suspected that molecular changes in certain proteins which intervene in the process of coagulation may play some part, but no

---

[1] Aminoethylisothiouronium

precise facts are known. Blood transfusion, which is effective
against the anaemia, has no apparent influence on the haemorrhages and does not alter either the thrombopenia or the leucopenia.
A striking increase in urinary and serum fibrinolytic activity has
been observed in irradiated dogs during the three or four days
preceding death. Many authors deny that heparin or heparinoid
substances play any role in the pathogenesis of the incoagulability
of the blood, although the mastocytes, which produce heparin, are
radio-sensitive and seem to disintegrate after irradiation, setting
free their contents. CRONKITE believes that thrombopenia plays a
major role in the haemorrhagic syndrome; his opinion is based on
the experimental observation that platelet transfusion[1] restores
retraction of the clot in irradiated dogs and stops the internal
haemorrhages. Recent human experience has brilliantly confirmed
the observations made on dogs and the important part played by
the platelets. The injection of large amounts (several billions) of
normal platelets has invariably controlled the petechiae and haemorrhages in human cases.

5. Conclusion

Following exposure to ionising irradiation, conditions of shock
may appear in mammals and man at different time intervals and
at different dose levels (Fig. 1).

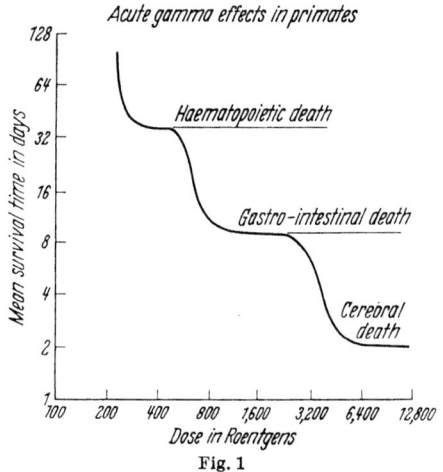

Fig. 1

---

[1] By the use of a chelating agent (disodium-ethylene-diamine-tetra-
acetate) and of silicone-coated flasks, platelets can be separated by fractional
centrifugation without agglutinating.

So far no human case of cerebral death resulting from exposure to very high doses has been published. Gastro-intestinal death is to be feared at the level of about 1,000 r. Careful treatment of humans irradiated at the 400 r level has enabled them to survive and has restored them to an apparently normal condition.

References

ALLEN, R. G., et al.: Radiat. Res. (U.S.A.) **12**, 532 (1960). — BACQ, Z. M., and P. ALEXANDER: Fundamentals of Radiobiology. 2d. ed. Oxford and New York: Pergamon Press 1961. — CRONKITE, E. P., G. J. JACOBS, G. BRECHER, and G. DILLARD: J.Röntgenol. (U.S.A.) **67**, 796 (1952). — HUNTER, C. G., K. L. JACKSON, and C. ENTENMAN: Radiat. Res. (U.S.A.) **10**, 67 (1959). — LUSHBAUGH, C. C., et al.: Radiat. Res. (U.S.A.) **13**, 814 (1960). — MAISIN, J. R., and D. G. DOHERTY: Symposium on Radiations and Milieu. Montreux 1961. — TONKIKH, A.: Second U. N. Intern. Conf. on the Peaceful Uses of Atomic Energy. Geneva 1958. Vol. 22, p. 129. United Nations (1959).

Discussion

BEIN: I would like to make a point of the difference between protection with drugs against X-irradiation and against endotoxin shock, because reserpine was found to be the most powerful agent in affording protection against the lethal effect of X-rays. This was found by JAQUES in our laboratories and confirmed by LANGENDORFF and his co-workers[1] in Freiburg. But reserpine does not afford protection against shock due to endotoxin, as we have heard from Dr. LILLEHEI. I do not know whether protection against X-rays with reserpine is due to a release of serotonin, as LANGENDORFF assumes: he also found protection with high doses of serotonin. On the other hand, Apresoline — which according to Dr. NICKERSON exerts an action in haemorrhagic shock — protects mice against X-ray irradiation as well[2]. In this case, one could assume some connection, whereas a dissociation occurs between shock due to endotoxin and X-ray.

GREGERSEN: I have two slides which illustrate two types of blood volume response to X-irradiation in splenectomised dogs. The first slide has to do with irradiation of the head only. We were fortunate in having the help of Dr. ROBERTS RUGH in the Radiological Research Laboratory immediately adjoining our own laboratory. Dr. RUGH arranged for, and supervised, the radiation exposure for which we used the special 180 kvp 2-tube cross fire X-ray generator designed by Dr. FAILLA many years ago. With the tubes set at 60 cm. apart and the head placed between them, some 20—25,000 r could be given in about 30 minutes. The survival time was of the order of 18 to 24 hours. The measurements shown on the slide (Fig. 1) include blood pressure, heart rate, respiration rate, rectal temperature, circulation time, and tests of carotid sinus reflex. The columns show the blood volume. You will note that in this type of irradiation, there was no change in the blood volume except for a small decrease accounted for by the amount of blood taken out for sampling. Here, then, death occurs without reduction in the blood volume. Until just before death, there were no significant alterations in circulation time, in blood pressure, or for that matter in the pressure rise induced by clamping both common carotid arteries. The course of events clinically and the succession of neurological signs, including dilation of pupils, exophthalmos, decerebrate rigidity, opisthotonus, etc., were as Dr. BACQ has described. Death came when the respiration stopped. It was as though a damaging wave moved gradually from the cortex down through the brain stem, and when the wave hit the respiratory centre, to put it crudely, the animal died. So far that is the best explanation we have. The centres controlling circulation, such as vasomotor centres, involved with the carotid sinus reflex appeared to be unaffected, for it was easily demonstrated that when the respiration stopped, the animal could be kept alive with artificial respiration. In this so-called "CNS death" from radiation, the critical terminal event is failure of the respiration, not of the circulation[3].

---

[1] LANGENDORFF, M., H.-J. MELCHING, H. LANGENDORFF, R. KOCH, and R. JAQUES: Strahlentherapie (G.)104, 338 (1957).
[2] JAQUES, R., and R. MEIER: Experientia (Switz.) 16, 75 (1960).
[3] PENG, M. T., S. CHIEN, and M. I. GREGERSEN: Amer. J. Physiol. 194, 344 (1958).

The next slide (Fig. 2) shows the summary data on splenectomised dogs given 1,000 r total-body radiation and studied rather carefully to determine the premortal changes in volume. These experiments were done by Dr. LUKIN and myself[1]. I should say that in this and other studies we found that the splenectomised dog given 1,000 r total-body radiation is a useful preparation,

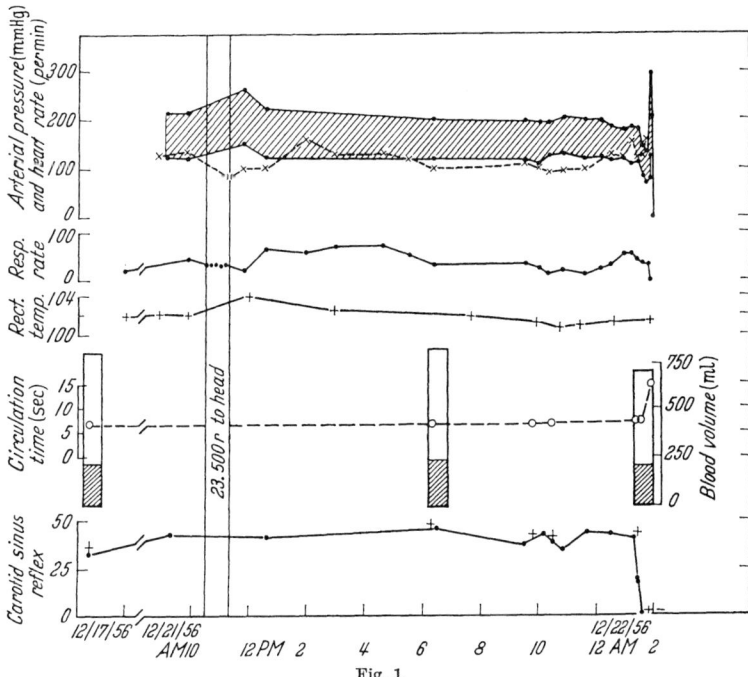

Fig. 1

because the survival time is extraordinarily constant — around 92 hours ± 4 hours, if I recall correctly. For our work we needed a preparation that would give consistent results from animal to animal, and this preparation has fulfilled these requirements.

The gradual fall in the red-cell volume shown in the upper left of the slide is explainable partly by the cessation of the production of red cells in the bone marrow and partly by the loss of red cells from the circulation, as Dr. BACQ stated. In the figure below it may be seen that after irradiation, the plasma volume at first tends to rise, which of course explains why the blood volume is well maintained for the first 2—3 days as shown in the upper right-hand figure. It is interesting that compensatory dilution occurs in this situation where the capillaries are damaged and that the mechanism operates so effectively until the very last day of survival. Directly below, the blood volume data are plotted back from the time of death as zero time. This chart suggests that the precipitous fall in blood volume during the last 12 hours of survival may in itself be sufficient to induce a circulatory state of shock,

---

[1] Radiat. Res. (U.S.A.) **7**, 161 (1957).

stagnant anoxia, and probably death. Yet we cannot be certain that this alone is responsible.

I would like to add that, as I have worked on circulatory shock and on radiation sickness, it has seemed to me that it may be of great interest and rather important to look upon these syndromes also as tools rather than merely pathological states. Radiation is in a sense a wrecking bar that opens doors through which to look at the organism after it has been disturbed by

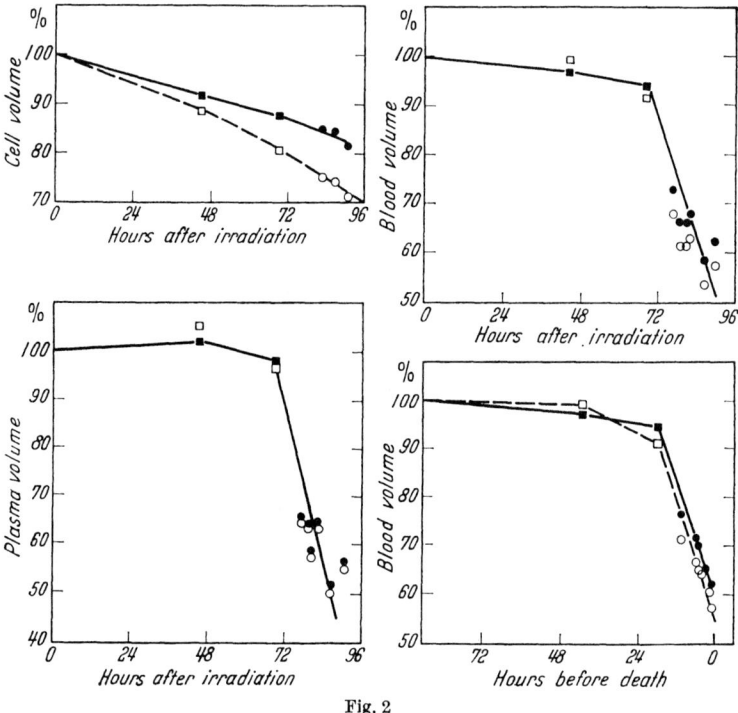

Fig. 2

the insult. The same applies to trauma, haemorrhage, and burns, i.e. various agents that cause shock-like states. All these injuries impinge on homeostatic mechanisms and provide opportunities to study further the responses of the organism or individual cells when the steady state is upset. This idea is by no means original. It goes back to CLAUDE BERNARD and many others. Yet the point of view deserves to be constantly emphasised, if only because it may both broaden and sharpen the attack and make the study of these important clinical problems even more fruitful. Both radiation and shock seem to be particularly useful tools for cellular physiology.

FINE: In connection with Dr. GREGERSEN's remarks I would like to report recent studies by Dr. CHESTER ROSOFF, in which radiation was used as a tool for study of the injured R. E. system. All rats given a dose of 550 r died after 9—30 days. A bacterial cause of death has been excluded, because blood cultures have been negative for the most part. But if the R.E. system is destroyed, death could occur even in the absence of a bacteraemia if an endotoxaemia should occur. On the basis of such a possibility, he pre-treated rats with neomycin orally, and these animals did not develop any of the pathology seen in the control animal. They did not accumulate fluid in the gut, and they survived without loss of weight, and at the end of the 30-day observation period they were healthy and fit.

BACQ: I have no comment on what Dr. GREGERSEN and Dr. FINE have said; but to Dr. BEIN I should like to say that there is unfortunately not the time to discuss the mechanisms of action of the many chemical protectors that have been discovered. There are at least three different mechanisms possible. It has been shown that these mechanisms can operate synergistically and at the same time in one irradiated system, and we have also shown recently that, depending on the various types of systems you are dealing with, these mechanisms may be very different. Anoxia plays an important role in connection with the protection afforded by histamine and 5-hydroxytryptamine for instance. We have confirmed that reserpine provides protection against X-irradiation, but no detailed investigation has been undertaken in order to find out which mechanism is involved.

Shock and extracorporeal circulation

By

Å. SENNING

For several years the great problem in E. C. C. was the immediate fall in blood pressure when total perfusion started. Large
transfusions and noradrenaline were necessary to maintain a satisfactory arterial blood pressure; then, some hours after the perfusions,
most of the experimental animals died in irreversible shock.

Most of the machines were made of plastic materials and were
cleaned with ordinary soap or detergents. The plastic material
absorbed a certain amount of the blood fluid that could not be
washed away. The shock was apparently caused by the large
amounts of toxins and pyrogens in the machine. This problem was
eliminated when the machines were soaked in 10% formaldehyde
or 20% NaOH solution for two hours after each perfusion.

Total body perfusion for open-heart surgery is a rather complicated procedure.

To begin with, the normal high pulsatile flow changes to a low
one. Added to this is the fact that the blood infused is traumatised
when passed through the venous cannula; it has been cooled and
rewarmed and has been stored for several hours. The blood is
further traumatised when it is filled into the heart-lung machine
and recirculated to remove all air and to test flow and the function
of the machine. Finally, its oxygen is partly consumed and it is
slightly acidotic.

The blood which has been circulating in the machine has only
3% CO_2 instead of the normal figure of approx. 5.2%.

There is also often a displacement of the blood volume between
the machine and the body. During the first short period, the machine
does not receive all the venous return until the venae cavae are
strangulated, and during this period the machine is giving the body
a transfusion; it takes some time before this is corrected by the
machine.

In addition, a change takes place in the distribution of the blood
volume in the body. During the open-heart period, the lungs are
practically drained of blood, whereas after closure of the heart
there is a danger of overloading the lungs.

Finally, a change in the systemic flow rate occurs when by-pass starts. If the heart is in poor condition the flow is increased, but more often the flow is more or less diminished. All this tends to make the flow and pressure conditions during the first 3 minutes very unsteady.

Just how a perfect perfusion should be performed is still a moot point. During open-heart surgery in normothermia, some centres are using a low flow of 35—50 ml./kg. body-weight/min., whereas others use a near-normal flow of 100—120 ml./kg. body-weight/min or 1.8—2.2 litres/sq. m./min.

During low-flow perfusion, a clinical picture of shock may be encountered, i. e. low blood pressure and peripheral vasoconstriction with cyanotic pallor. When the flow rate is high, this picture is less pronounced. In our early attempts at perfusion we observed pronounced metabolic acidosis, as was also the case in all other cardiac centres. We noticed that lactic acid formation was inversely proportional to the flow and to the oxygen consumption (1). The Minneapolis group reported the same finding (2). This acidosis is a sign of inadequate perfusion of the tissues.

We therefore undertook an experimental series in order to determine the lowest flow capable of ensuring the same oxygen consumption during perfusion as during the period before. It was assumed that a decrease in oxygen consumption was a sign of incomplete perfusion of the tissues. The flow was varied between 20 and 100 ml./kg. body-weight/min. and the oxygen consumption was calculated from the A—V difference and flow. It was found that the arterial blood pressure and the oxygen consumption were proportional to the flow and that the control level of oxygen consumption was reached at 100 ml./kg./min.

In another series, the oxygen consumption was correlated to the flow before and during E. C. C. (3). The flow rate before by-pass was varied by bleeding or strangulation of the venous return to the heart. The oxygen consumption was measured in a spirometer and the systemic flow rate was calculated according to FICK. We observed the same correlation with or without E. C. C. The O_2 consumption was about 5% higher during circulation without by-pass. This can possibly be explained by the oxygen consumption of the working heart.

According to LILLEHEI, 1.2 litres/sq. m. was sufficient to prevent acidosis. But in the light of our own investigations and findings reported by other cardiac centres, we are of the opinion that a higher flow (75—100 ml./kg. body-weight/min. or 1.8—2.2 litres/sq. m. body-surface area/min.) would be necessary in normothermia. In our clinical perfusions, we have maintained a flow of about 85 ml./kg. in adults in normothermia and a mean arterial pressure of about 70 mm. Hg or higher. It should be pointed out, however, that during a perfusion the flow is never absolutely constant; it varies owing to bleeding or to temporary occlusion of the coronaries, etc.

In order to find out whether E. C. C. as such has a tendency to produce circulatory disorders of the kind seen in shock, we have

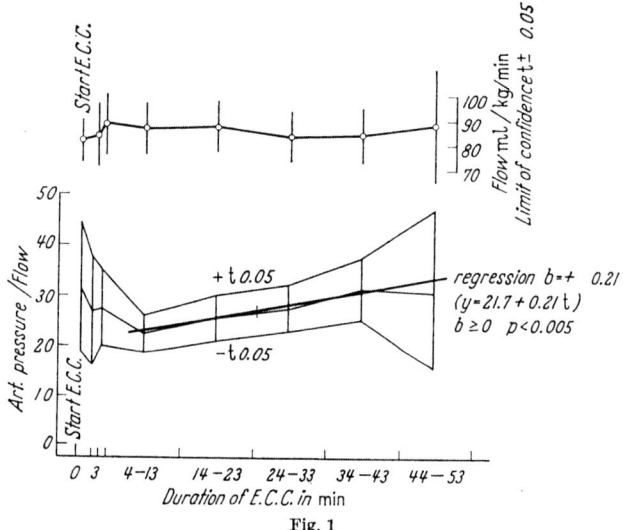

Fig. 1

tried to investigate some of the systemic circulatory reactions on by-pass. The total systemic arterial resistance and the perfusion and function of various organs such as the liver and kidneys were studied during total body perfusion.

The relationship between arterial pressure and flow was calculated in 25 surviving open-heart patients who had a steady-state perfusion for at least 30 min. (Fig. 1). The flow rate is given here in ml./kg. body-weight. The pressure/flow relationship is the mean arterial pressure, expressed in mm. Hg, over the flow expressed in litres/min./sq. m.

The first 3 minutes in normothermia are divided into one-minute periods, as the state is unsteady; the rest of the observations are grouped in 10-minute periods. Comparatively large differences in the flow and the pressure/flow correlation are observed as between one patient and another. This is mainly due to the fact that all

types of heart defect are represented in the group. Patients with
right-to-left shunts generally showed a relatively lower peripheral
total body resistance than patients with left-to-right shunts.

During the first 3 minutes, the relative total peripheral resistance
appears to decline; it then rises continuously during the following
45—50 minutes, by which time it has regained its initial level. In
some cases with a longer perfusion, there seems to have been a
further rise, but the material is too limited to permit of any final
conclusions.

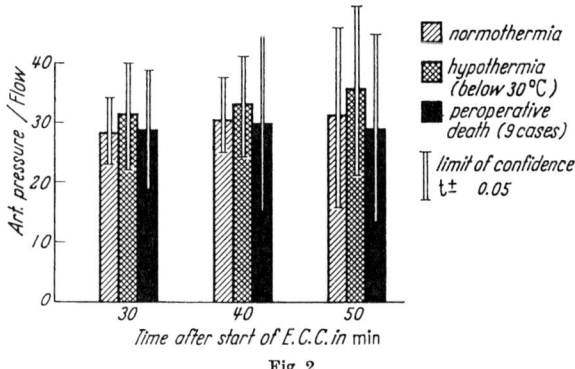

Fig. 2

From previous investigations we had the impression that there
was a difference in the behaviour of the resistance between patients
who survived and those who died within 24 hours after perfusion,
although, in a group of 9 patients who failed to survive, the difference was not statistically significant.

When E. C. C. was combined with hypothermia, the systemic
vascular resistance appeared to be somewhat higher, but here, too,
the difference was not statistically significant (Fig. 2).

As the liver plays an important role in connection with shock,
we also considered it necessary to study hepatic blood perfusion
during E. C. C. In order to separate the hepatic venous blood from
the inferior caval blood, a special cannula was used (4). During the
first period of E. C. C., a rise in portal pressure was observed, as is
often seen in other conditions in dogs. This rise (up to 40 cm. H₂O)
was, however, only temporary. As we were also studying lactic acid
extraction in the liver, we used a comparatively low total body
perfusion of 35—60 ml./kg. body-weight, and this resulted in a
decrease in the liver flow of only 15% as compared with the pre-
perfusion period. This flow, on the other hand, was presumably

20*

somewhat lower than normal because of the surgical trauma. In the lactic acid extraction from the portal blood, no statistical difference was found during perfusion as compared with the pre- and post-perfusion period — and this despite the low total body flow. The Bromsulphalein one-passage extraction from portal to hepatic venous blood was measured and was found to be less during and after E. C. C. than before. This is partly due to the fact that the one-passage extraction of B. S. P. is diminished when repeated doses are given. After labelled B. S. P. has been administered, it reappears in the circulation again when a fresh dose of non-labelled B. S. P. is given.

In view of the well-known sensitivity of the kidney, we felt that an investigation of renal function in connection with E. C. C. was also called for.

Renal function was studied before, during, and after E. C. C., as well as in control dogs which underwent the same surgical trauma but had no E. C. C. (5). The perfusion was performed at a high flow and at a low flow, or at perfusion rates of 100 or 50 ml./kg./min. In some experiments, a period of low flow was followed by high flows, and in others the reverse. The first estimation was made under anaesthesia when cannulas for the withdrawal of samples were inserted, and the next after thoracotomy when all the cannulas for E. C. C. had been inserted. Subsequently, estimations were carried out at half-hour periods during and after E. C. C.

ᶠ During the surgical trauma associated with thoracotomy, there was a decrease in all renal functions measured as well as in the blood pressure. This depression of function was significant in the case of the renal plasma flow, glomerular filtration rate, and mean arterial pressure, but less so in the case of urinary output.

Perfusion at a high flow rate did not produce a significant decrease in arterial pressure compared with control animals in the same periods. Nevertheless, there was a considerable decrease in the renal plasma flow and glomerular filtration rate. There were no significant differences between the first and second half-hour of E. C. C. in dogs which had a high flow rate during both periods.

During perfusion at a low flow rate, a pronounced fall in arterial pressure, clearances, and urine volume was observed as compared with the levels at a high flow rate. The filtration fraction, on the other hand, remained relatively unimpaired. Function during low flow did not differ much in the second half-hour from function during low flow in the first half-hour.

During the periods following completion of one-hour E. C. C., the renal plasma flow and glomerular filtration rate were slightly lower than in the high-flow E. C. C. periods. In comparison with the control animals, there was a significant reduction both in the mean arterial pressure as well as in the urinary output.

The excretion of electrolytes was somewhat depressed by the surgical trauma. In the perfusion period, all electrolyte excretions were reduced. Even with a high flow, a considerable reduction was apparent in the excretion of Na, K, and chlorides — a reduction which was even more pronounced during low-flow periods. But this decrease was more likely to be due to the lower urinary output than to changes in filtration, as a good filtration fraction was maintained even during low flow.

When a high-flow perfusion period followed a low-flow period, the sodium and chloride excretion was higher than usual during perfusion. Otherwise, however, the findings were the same as during other periods of high flow. Whether renal function is impaired during low-flow perfusions lasting longer than one hour in normothermia was not investigated.

Renal function was studied post-operatively in 76 patients who survived E. C. C. The electrolyte excretion and fluid balance followed the same pattern as after other major surgical operations. Similar findings have been reported by other authors (6).

In states of shock certain changes are known to occur in the blood flow through the muscles. Together with GRAF and STRÖM we studied the blood flow through the arm and leg before, during, and after E. C. C. in 13 patients (7). With the exception of two patients who died in connection with the operation, there was no change in resistance in this area, i. e. mainly in the muscular vessels.

The circulation in the brain has also been studied. CLOWES used the brain-tissue pO_2, measured with a Clark electrode, as an index (8). With good perfusion at high flow rates, the blood flow through the brain was found to be normal.

All these studies, however, were undertaken during comparatively short periods (1—2 hour perfusion). We also made a series of 10 experiments with total left-heart by-pass for 24 hours. Without thoracotomy, all the venous return was drained from the left auricle by means of a cannula inserted via the jugular vein, through the superior vena cava and right auricle, passing through the auricular septum via the fossa ovalis. The blood was returned to the systemic arterial circulation with a pump via a femoral artery. Although there was a loss of blood during these 24-hour perfusions, it was possible to maintain the flow at a desired level by means of transfusion, and it was typical that the flow always diminished before changes in blood pressure occurred. In all these dogs the peripheral resistance remained practically stable throughout the 24 hours, and there was no tendency towards a lower or higher systemic vascular resistance at the end. In one dog the urinary output amounted to only 10 ml./kg. body-weight/24 hours, but in the others it worked out at 30—35 ml./kg. body-weight/24 hours. Of the 10 dogs, 9 survived the perfusion.

In cardiac surgery it is, of course, very difficult to separate the cardiac and the vascular factor. From our clinical material it has been impossible to draw any definite conclusions, but there is nothing to suggest that a good 1—2 hour perfusion as such gives rise to a shock syndrome.

In the post-operative course it is extremely important that the circulating blood volume should be kept sufficiently high, and blood has to be given as and when indicated by the usual clinical criteria, including especially the behaviour of the venous pressure and peripheral circulation.

It is also important to keep a check on the pH and standard bicarbonate of the blood post-operatively. If the standard bicarbonate falls, this indicates an inadequate circulation, and either the heart has to be stimulated, as indicated by a high venous pressure, or blood has to be given should the venous pressure be low and the peripheral circulation poor.

If citrated blood is administered, especially with rapid transfusions, it is important that calcium be given in connection with the transfusion.

Provided the heart is working well and the blood volume is adequate, shock does not seem to occur after a good E.C.C.

Summary

The total systemic vascular resistance and the blood flow through the arm and leg were investigated in connection with clinical E.C.C. for open-heart surgery. Hepatic and renal function was studied experimentally before, during, and after E.C.C. No evidence was found to indicate that a good E.C.C. as such causes shock. In the post-operative period a careful control of the circulating blood volume is important. The pH and standard bicarbonate must be checked, since acidosis indicates an inadequate cardiac output.

References

1. SENNING, Å.: Minerva chir. (It.) **13**, 1405 (1958). — 2. DEWALL, R.A., H. E. WARDEN, V. L. GOTT, R. C. READ, R. L. VARCO, and C. W. LILLEHEI: J. Thorac. Surg. (U.S.A.) **32**, 591 (1956). — 3. ANDERSEN, M. N., and Å. SENNING: Ann. Surg. (U.S.A.) **148**, 59 (1958). — 4. ANDERSEN, M. N., B. NORBERG, and Å. SENNING: Surgery (U.S.A.) **43**, 397 (1958). — 5. SENNING, Å., J. ANDRÉS, P. BORNSTEIN,B. NORBERG, and M. N. ANDERSEN: Ann. Surg. (U.S.A.) **151**, 63 (1960). — 6. MORRIS, G. C., W. C. AWE, H. W. BENDER, D. A. COOLEY, and M. E. DEBAKEY: Extr.-Corp. Circ., Springfield: Charles C.Thomas 1958. — 7. GRAF, K., O. NORLANDER, Å. SENNING, and G. STRÖM: Langenbeck's Arch. klin. Chir. (G.) **292**, 671 (1959). — 8. CLOWES, G. H. A.: Personal communication.

Discussion

LILLEHEI: First I wish to congratulate Dr. SENNING on this fine paper. We also have been concerned with the problem of safely prolonging cardiac by-pass so that the more difficult acquired and congenital lesions may be repaired without hurry. In general, when cardiac by-pass and total body perfusions run over an hour, post-operative complications, such as infection, oliguria, and anuria, are more likely to occur. The problem of infection can and is being solved by closer adherence to the principles of aseptic surgery. The problem of the kidney, however, is not so easily overcome, since the underlying causes of the oligurias and anurias have not been clear.

It is my feeling that prolonged cardiac by-pass and total body perfusion is a form of controlled shock. The longer the period of by-pass or "controlled" shock, the more likely are complications to arise following surgery. Moreover, these complications in patients occur despite the fact that so-called "normal" cardiac output is being used for the total body perfusion (75—100 ml./kg.).

Why should certain organs, such as the kidney of man and sometimes the viscera as well, manifest the signs of shock if they are being perfused at "normal" flows with the pump-oxygenator? A clue to unravelling this enigma is found in Dr. SENNING's studies, as well as those of others, in which it is seen that total body resistance rises proportionately to the period of total body perfusion and cardiac by-pass.

In an attempt to explain these findings, my colleagues, Dr. ROBERT REPLOGLE and Dr. MORRIS LEVY, and myself measured plasma catecholamines (epinephrine and norepinephrine) in a number of patients undergoing total body perfusion and cardiac by-pass for repair of congenital and acquired heart defects on the surgical service of my brother, Dr. C. WALTON LILLEHEI. Renal plasma flow and glomerular filtration rates of such patients were also assessed at the same time.

The data obtained from this study are now being analysed and prepared for publication; yet a few provocative generalisations can be made at this time. Patients who are on cardiac by-pass and are receiving total body perfusion for an hour or more have significant increases in the plasma catecholamines, i.e. from levels of less than 1 ug./litre of plasma to levels of 7, 8, and 10 μg./litre. In patients manifesting oliguria and anuria following surgery, levels of 12—15 μg./litre have been measured. Both epinephrine and norepinephrine show such increases. Concomitant with such increases of catecholamines, renal plasma flows and glomerular filtration rates steadily decline to shock levels, and post-operative oliguria or anuria frequently occurs, despite the fact that mean arterial pressure in the large vessels, such as the aorta, may be 100 mm. Hg or more. I should mention here that comparable rises in plasma catecholamines are not seen in major abdominal or thoracic surgery, in which total body perfusion is not used.

More recently, "low" flows (25—50 ml./kg.) have been used for total body perfusion and cardiac by-pass in combination with general body hypothermia to 28—30° C. In these patients, mean pressure in the aorta is often only 50—60 mm. Hg; yet catecholamines in the plasma do not increase to the levels seen using "normal" flows. Moreover, renal plasma flow and glomerular filtration rates do not decrease markedly, and post-operative oligurias or anurias are rare. Before drawing final conclusions, more patients are needed in the study, and we must also evaluate other changes which have been made in the performance of the by-pass and perfusion, such as the use of the patient's own blood and 5% glucose solutions to prime the pump.

SENNING: We have of course also observed anurias — I forgot to say that — anurias after extracorporeal circulation, although we always had them in the group of patients in whom the perfusion had been very prolonged. I think one of the factors is that we get a much more pronounced blood trauma during the long perfusion. We, too, measured the catecholamines in some patients, and we saw that they increased after heart operations carried out under E.C.C., as they also did after other forms of major surgery. So we, too, are today combining practically all — or at any rate all long perfusions — with hypothermia. And it is, as you say, striking how well the urine is secreted. I had, for instance, one patient some months ago, and during the 4-hour perfusion I think she secreted almost 1 litre; and I had another patient down in Zurich, whom we perfused for $2^1/_2$ hours. During the perfusion, she had a very good urinary excretion, but the day after it was only 300 for 24 hours, and the patient came back with a very good excretion again. A trauma certainly seems to be inflicted on the kidney, but in what way, I don't know.

KRAMER: Urinary secretion is not a very good criterion. It is known that the concentrating ability of the kidney is impaired in hypothermia[1], so that a larger urine flow is to be expected. Thus, the increase in urine flow in your hypothermic patients does not mean that their kidney function has improved. I wonder if you have studied the urine-to-plasma osmolarity ratio?

NICKERSON: I should like to direct one question to the by-pass experts. I believe there is some evidence that when blood or plasma is passed repeatedly through a pump mechanism, a non-catechol vasoconstrictor — presumably a peptide — may appear. Has there been any evaluation of the role this material might play in the later complications seen in these patients?

HALPERN: I should like to say to Dr. SENNING — and perhaps this may interest other surgeons — that we have developed, in our department, a new technique for measuring the hepatic blood flow without any catheterisation. I don't want to go into details here of the technique we have used in humans and also in animals, but just to say that, by taking a few blood samples from the cubital vein, it is possible to assess the hepatic blood flow to within a 5% degree of accuracy.

SENNING: What Dr. KRAMER says is true: during the perfusion there is not such a good urinary concentration as afterwards. We have measured the specific weight, and in those patients who have no glucose the specific weight during the perfusion is around 1.012, 1.013 or 1.014 or thereabouts, whereas afterwards it's 1.025 to 1.029, even if there is no glucose. Now, in most of these patients we give a 5% glucose solution, and then the specific weight goes up to 1.033 or even more.

Dr. NICKERSON, I agree with you. We can perfuse a human being for 6 hours, and he doesn't have any trouble at all afterwards from the perfusion if we use a double pump and have his own lungs in the circuit to oxygenate

---

[1] HONG, D., and J. BOYLAN: Amer. J. Physiol. 196, 1150 (1959).

his blood. But if we have an extracorporeal circulation with an artificial lung for 6 hours, I don't think there are many people who survive that in normothermia. In hypothermia, on the other hand, we can go on for at least 4 hours without too much trouble afterwards.

Dr. HALPERN, I know that the system we used to study the hepatic flow is outmoded by modern standards, but this was done many years ago, and I wouldn't use the same method today. But even with these different methods of injecting various types of labelled material, it is very hard to judge the situation during extracorporeal circulation, because the circulation is so changed. It's extremely difficult to determine what is happening to the hepatic circulation if you cannot distinguish clearly between the portal circulation and the hepatic vein circulation.

Humoral and myogenic factors in shock: evaluated by means of isolated arteriolar smooth muscle response

By

D. F. BOHR and P. L. GOULET

An increase in vascular capacity, evidenced by an uptake of reservoir blood, portends the development of irreversibility in hemorrhagic shock. Inquiry is made in the current study as to whether the mechanism responsible for this omen resides in an intrinsic failure of the smooth muscle of the resistance vessels or in a change in circulating humoral agents influencing this muscle. Smooth muscle preparations from resistance vessels rather than the more commonly used ones from large arteries were employed, because of the direct influence of the arterioles on the capacity and the filtration pressure of the capillary bed.

Hemorrhagic shock was produced in dogs anesthetized with sodium pentobarbital (33 mg./kg.) by bleeding the animal into a reservoir bottle at a pressure of (40 mm. Hg. The animal was maintained at this pressure until 7 cc. of blood/kg. had been recovered by the dog from the maximum volume lost to the reservoir. This uptake of blood occurred after a 2 to 5 hour period of hemorrhagic hypotension. At this time the dog was considered to have developed hemorrhagic shock and the mesentery and blood samples were taken.

Arterial blood was obtained through a siliconized polyethylene tube and centrifuged in the cold at high speed in order to remove all of the platelets from the plasma. To obtain dialyzed plasma, exhaustive dialysis was carried out, against Krebs solution, for 48 hours at 4° C.

A semi-micro technique (described in detail in the Proceedings of the Ninth Microcirculatory Conference, Angiology — in press) was used to obtain smooth muscle preparations from resistance vessels of the dog mesentery 200 to 300 microns in diameter. After removing the mesentery from the dog the vessel was dissected free from surrounding tissue under Krebs solution. A fine wire was then threaded through the lumen of the vessel and its two ends were mounted in the chucks of a jeweler's lathe. By pressing the sharp edge of a razor blade against the wire at one end of the resistance vessel, and directing the vessel into the blade, a helical strip was cut from the vessel wall as the lathe rotated slowly. Such a strip, about 100 microns wide and 1 mm. long, was mounted in a 20 cc. bath of Krebs solution and tension was recorded by means of a strain gauge.

Results

The condition of the mesenteric arteriolar smooth muscle following the period of hemorrhagic hypotension was evaluated by recording its responsiveness to epinephrine in the isolated bath. Two parameters of the epinephrine response of the tissue from the shocked animal were compared with those of similar tissue from a normal control. These were the concentration of epinephrine

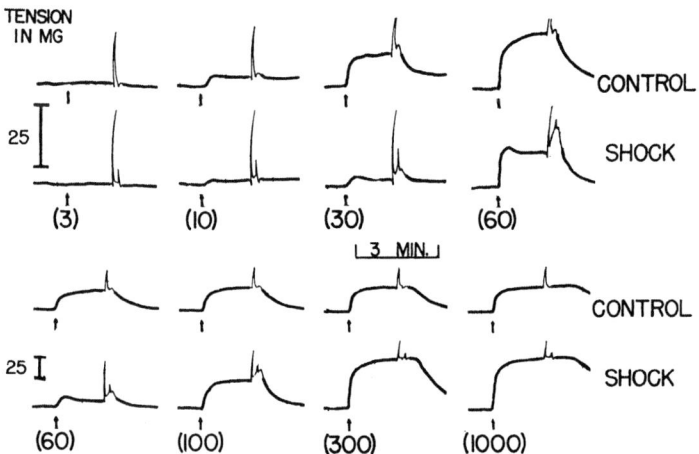

Fig. 1. Responses to epinephrine of mesenteric arteriolar strip from a normal dog (upper tracing of each pair) and from a dog in shock. Spike marks in each tracing are rinse artifacts Both strips responded at 10 μg./l. The lower pair of tracings is a continuation of the upper but with sensitivity of the recording decreased in order to record the "top" of the dose-response curve. This "shocked" strip was apparently capable of greater contraction than the control

required for a threshold response, and the maximum amount of tension that the strip would develop in response to epinephrine. Such a comparative study is illustrated in Fig. 1. It is evident that there is no appreciable difference between the threshold concentration of epinephrine required to produce a response of the arteriolar smooth muscle from normal dogs and that required to produce a response of arteriolar smooth muscle from shocked dogs. In this particular example the maximum tension developed by the arteriolar smooth muscle from the shocked dog is about twice as great as that developed by the preparation from the control animal. In Fig. 2 is a summary of the results of 7 such comparative studies. The degree of variability in each of the parameters measured is great; we attribute much of this to differences in strip width, but there is no suggestion that the responsiveness to epinephrine of the arteriolar smooth muscle from the shocked animal is any less than that from the normal control.

In another comparison the relative influence of dialyzed plasma from control and shocked animals on the magnitude of an arteriolar

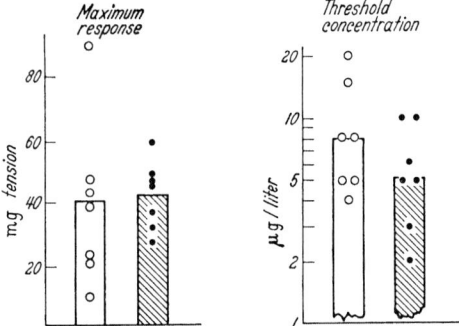

Fig. 2. Comparison of responses to epinephrine of seven pairs of arteriolar strips, one of each pair from a normal *(open column)*, one from a shocked *(cross-hatched column)* dog. Neither in concentration of drug giving a threshold response, nor in maximum amount of tension developed are there recognizable differences between the strips

response to a submaximal concentration of epinephrine was studied. Dialyzed plasma was used in order to circumvent the problems of the direct constrictor effect of whole plasma. In Fig. 3 the tracings

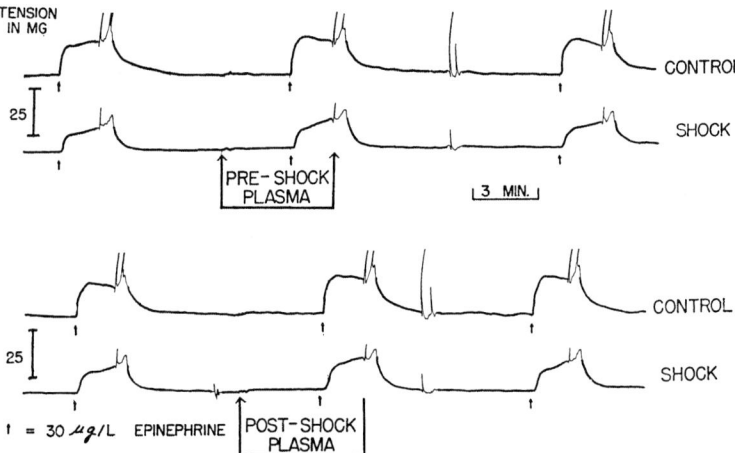

Fig. 3. Effect of dialyzed plasma on responses to epinephrine of an arteriolar strip from a normal dog (upper tracing of each pair) and from a dog in shock. Either pre-shock or post-shock plasma produced a slight potentiation of the response of both strips

made for such a comparison are presented. In this experiment the presence of either pre- or post-shock dialyzed plasma produced a slight potentiation of the epinephrine response in arteriolar preparations from both the control and shocked dogs. Fig. 4 summarizes the results of 7 such comparisons. Here again, although there is marked variability in the quantitative effect of the several dialyzed plasmas studied, there is no suggestion that the dialyzed plasma from the shocked animal depresses the responsiveness of the mesenteric arteriole to epinephrine.

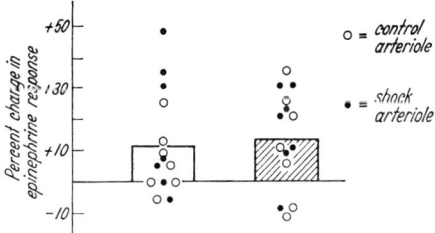

Fig. 4. Comparison of responses to epinephrine of seven pairs of arteriolar strips, one of each pair from a normal *(open column)*, one from a dog in shock *(cross-hatched column)*. There is no recognizable difference between the effects of the two plasmas, or between the responses of the two types of muscle to either plasma

In contrast to the negative results obtained in the search for differences in the shocked animal in, firstly, arteriolar smooth muscle and, secondly, the epinephrine potentiating action of dialyzed plasma, are the consistent alterations observed in preliminary experiments in the vasoactive potency of whole plasma obtained at 3 different stages of the hemorrhagic procedure: 1. control, prior to hemorrhage; 2. early in hemorrhage, as the blood pressure

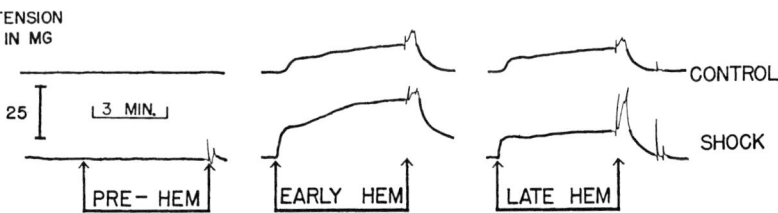

Fig. 5. Response of mesenteric arteriolar strip from normal and from shocked dog to pre-(PRE—HEM), early (EARLY HEM), and late hemorrhagic (LATE HEM) plasma. Plasma collected early in hemorrhage had a much greater constrictor effect than that collected before hemorrhage; this constrictor property was diminished in the plasma collected during shock

approaches its flat trough at 40 mm. Hg (this occurs between 10 and 15 min. after the beginning of hemorrhage); and 3. after the animal has recovered 7 cc./kg. from his maximal bleeding volume. Only 3 such experiments, involving 24 assays for plasma constrictor activity, have been done. Although we do not presume to persuade anybody else of the significance of this limited number of observations, the differences have been so large and so consistent that those of us familiar with the technique are convinced that they will be borne out in further studies. Fig. 5 illustrates one such experiment. The whole plasma obtained early in hemorrhage always had greater vasoactive potency than did the pre-hemorrhage sample. The whole plasma obtained late in hemorrhage was always less effective in causing contraction of arteriolar smooth muscle than was that obtained early in hemorrhage. In one experiment the third sample of plasma showed less than 25% of the contraction potency observed in plasma obtained early in hemorrhage. It is obviously attractive to associate this diminution in compensatory humoral constrictor potency with an increase in capillary vascular capacity and filtration pressure leading to the uptake of blood from the reservoir.

Summary

1. No difference in response to epinephrine was found between isolated mesenteric arteriolar smooth muscle obtained from control dogs and that from shocked dogs.

2. No difference was observed between the effects of dialyzed plasma from normal animals and that from shocked animals, on the epinephrine response of mesenteric arterioles.

3. Whole plasma obtained after the hemorrhaged dog had taken up 7 cc./kg. from the maximum bleeding volume caused less contraction of mesenteric arterioles than did that obtained early in hemorrhage.

Supported by a grant from the American Heart Association.

Hypothermia in shock

By

E. G. Brewin

In the first place, I am not at all sure that we all mean the same thing when we use the term shock. For that reason I will begin with a definition of what I mean by shock. This definition is purely arbitrary and is not necessarily true, but at least it makes the starting point clear.

By shock, I mean a state of circulatory failure which is due to disproportion between the vascular bed and the circulating blood volume, a disproportion brought about by loss of a proportion of the latter.

Loss of part of the circulating blood volume brings about a fall in venous return, and this is followed by a diminution in cardiac output. A reflex vasoconstriction follows and this compensates, more or less, for the loss of circulating blood volume. At this stage, adequate replacement of that loss, if timely, will relax the vasomotor tone whilst restoring the cardiac output, and a normal circulatory status will be resumed. Should the loss not be made good in a reasonable time, the generalised vasoconstriction will persist, and what was primarily a compensatory reaction becomes potentially harmful, producing tissue anoxia through under-perfusion. It is thought that this tissue anoxia brings about the irreversible phase of shock — the phase where circulatory failure persists despite a restored blood volume. The effects of the tissue anoxia may be mediated through entry into the blood stream of toxic factors.

There is no real problem in reversible shock; adequate and timely replacement of the lost circulating volume will restore the patient, as both Dr. Howard and Dr. Bull have already shown so well.

Now clearly, the alternative to improving a failing circulation is to reduce the metabolic requirements of the tissues to a level commensurate with that of the available circulation, and in hypothermia we have a means of achieving this. Equally clearly, the problem is not quite so simple, for there are certain risks attendant on the induction of hypothermia and, moreover, given that the metabolic demands are balanced by the blood supply, the hypothermia may not help more than this and an impasse may be reached from which the patient cannot be retrieved to normality.

A good deal of experimental work has gone into this problem, and it can be divided into two broad groups: one of prophylaxis; the other, therapeusis.

The prophylactic use of hypothermia naturally demands that the body temperature be reduced prior to the insult which will bring about shock, so that foreknowledge of the insult is essential. Hypothermia used in this way has a history rather longer than that of the recent surgical interest in hypothermia, and originates in accidental observations. BLALOCK and MASON (1941) noticed twenty years ago that, when using a standardised technique for the production of experimental shock, survival rates were better in winter than in summer. This observation was confirmed and extended by other workers, body temperature being deliberately reduced in experimental conditions of haemorrhagic, crush and tourniquet shock, with improved survival rates or greater permissible insult.

Such observations seem entirely reasonable, for where insufficient perfusion of tissues follows the reflex vasoconstriction of shock, should these tissues already be cooled to a level at which their metabolic requirements are small, there is less likelihood of tissue anoxia supervening and of dangerous products of anoxia reaching the circulation. I would regard the value of prophylactic hypothermia as well established experimentally.

The trouble is that opportunity to apply this potentially valuable method seldom arises. It is rare indeed to have prior notice of an accident, a sudden haemorrhage or a peritonitis, and the only sphere for prophylaxis lies in planned surgery. It is in such circumstances that shock ought never to be encountered provided that blood loss be made up immediately and completely, as it should be. So here we have a useful manoeuvre but no occasion to use it.

When we come to hypothermia in the therapeusis of established irreversible shock, the ground is less secure, both theoretically and experimentally. Certainly, if shock is established, but not yet irreversible, the picture is similar to that in prophylaxis, and hypothermia should be of value. However, if the irreversible state has already been reached, whatever the toxic products of anoxia may be, they are already in the circulation and hypothermia is unlikely to get them out. Nevertheless, such substances must act metabolically, and hypothermia might interfere with such an action; it should at least retard the production of more. There may be other beneficial effects of hypothermia in established irreversible shock. It is usually said that hypothermia causes generalised vasoconstriction and, to my mind, the evidence for this is by no means conclusive. If the total peripheral resistance of hypothermic experimental animals is computed from the ratio of blood pressure to cardiac output, it is seen to be rather variable compared with that found before cooling. For instance, in seven experiments, it remained more or less unchanged in two, was doubled in two, and in the remaining three was increased by $2^1/_2$ to 3 times. However, in hypothermia of the same order — 26 to 28°C — there is usually a haemoconcentration of $15-20\%$. This would produce an increase in viscosity of $1^1/_2-2$ times; moreover, the fall in temperature alone would increase viscosity by about 20%. These factors together would roughly double the viscosity. This alone could account for the increased peripheral resistance in many instances and in some would imply a vasodilatation. Experimentally, NEIL has shown that there is a diminution in sympathetic outflow in hypothermia.

There is some evidence, then, that hypothermia may help to relax the dangerous vasoconstriction of shock, probably in viscera, for I do not doubt the cutaneous vasoconstriction in hypothermia.

The experimental evidence of the benefit of hypothermia in established irreversible shock is not so convincing as in prophylaxis.

In haemorrhagic shock, for instance, OVERTON and DE BAKEY (1956) showed only a moderate benefit from hypothermia, although POSTEL, REID and HINTON (1957) had more encouraging results, with an 80% survival as opposed to 20% in controls. Experiments of my own lend support to the last-named group. On the other hand, in shock produced by occlusion of the superior mesenteric artery for five hours (uniformly fatal in controls), there is only a slight benefit from hypothermia induced after occlusion, but a convincing benefit from its prophylactic use (MEDINA and LAUFMAN, 1958). There is experimental evidence (FEDOR et al., 1958) that hypothermia retards bacterial proliferation without injury to immune-body and phagocytic responses. This would suggest that, if irreversibility were due to bacterial toxins, hypothermia would be beneficial.

Clinical evidence of the value of therapeutic hypothermia is not easy to obtain. Cases are reported where it is claimed that, but for its use, the patient would have died; this may well be so, but as there can be no control, the evidence is not of the best. Just the same, one might mention as an example the paper of ALLEN and his colleagues (1960) where great benefit was claimed from the induction and maintenance of hypothermia in patients suffering from septic peritonitis with irreversible shock. It is interesting also to find that no evidence of wound healing could be seen during the prolonged hypothermia.

If we are to use hypothermia in shock, there may be a little difficulty in persuading ancillary staff and even colleagues of its value. In a not unrelated field, for instance, there was difficulty in persuading patients, and nursing and even medical staff, that to warm the cold, pre-gangrenous foot in ischaemic arterial disease is to hasten the onset of frank gangrene. It is an automatic reaction to want to warm cold limbs and bodies. I remember, as no doubt do many of you, when such a foot was cooked in a heat cradle. It is now standard practice, and successful practice too, to allow the ischaemic foot to cool at least to room temperature, whilst keeping the rest of the body warm.

I think that hypothermia might well be tried in irreversible shock; at least let us discourage the custom of using hot bottles and drinks to keep the patient warm.

If I am to recommend hypothermia to you, it must be shown that it is unlikely to do the patient harm. Hypothermia might well be harmful, since there is an association between it and ventricular fibrillation. There is a direct relationship between the incidence of fibrillation and the decrement in temperature, the amount of inter- ference with the heart, and the presence of already existing heart disease. The last may be considered as occasion arises; in most cases of shock there is little reason for direct tampering with the heart, and if the temperature is not allowed to fall below 30°C there is not much likelihood of ventricular fibrillation. Again, hypothermia is accompanied by a metabolic acidosis, but it is usually only mild (of the order of 3−4 mEq.) and disappears on rewarming.

On the whole, these considerations need not deter us from the employment of hypothermia in irreversible shock.

Next, is there anything which might encourage us to believe that hypothermia gives protection against anoxia in the human subject? Indeed there is, for although the circulation cannot be arrested with safety for more than three minutes, in the human subject at normal temperature, it can be arrested, by occlusion of the venous inflow to the heart, for up to nine or ten minutes at a body temperature of 30°C without permanent damage. This, of course, is a technique now widely employed in surgery in order to gain access to the interior of the heart. The price paid, as one might expect, is a metabolic acidosis, but if the period of circulatory arrest is kept as short as possible, say only five or six minutes, and if the circulatory status following restoration of the venous return remains satisfactory, the acidosis may not be too severe, and may begin to disappear during rewarming, to have vanished entirely a few hours after rewarming is complete. If the acidosis is really severe, it may require correction.

Now this is a state of affairs very like that of shock itself, for in shock too there is a metabolic acidosis, as has been shown many times. It has been demonstrated in man, by Dr. GREGERSEN and his colleagues at the Bellevue Hospital (Richards, D. W.), and in haemorrhagic, tourniquet and crush shock in animals. In shock, however, unlike circulatory arrest under hypothermia, there is no question of the acidosis being eliminated spontaneously so long as shock persists; it can only get worse.

This metabolic acidosis is seen in shock, in circulatory arrest with moderate or deep hypothermia, and in perfusion operations at normal temperature. There is no doubt but that its prevention, by increasing perfusion rates, or its correction by administration of sodium bicarbonate solution, is attended by better results in surgical patients.

It is interesting that in all these conditions, only 50—60% of the metabolic acidosis is accounted for by lactic acid, as shown by corresponding blood lactate levels. The other fixed acid or acids, accounting for the rest of the acidosis, we do not know the nature of.

Whilst not so exciting as a mysterious substance such as a toxin, it may be that one of the factors determining irreversibility is a much more "normal" substance — a metabolic acid.

Then if we are to employ hypothermia in the treatment of irreversible shock, we must be able to assess and to treat this acidosis. The assessment of metabolic acidosis at body temperatures other than normal is not so straightforward as at 38° C.

This is on account of certain physico-chemical changes which take place with variation of temperature.

Let us consider the carriage of carbon-dioxide by the blood. Carbon-dioxide enters into physical solution in the venous blood plasma; hydration of a little to carbonic acid takes place, but this reaction is very slow and most of the dissolved CO_2 diffuses as such into the red cells. The red cells contain the enzyme carbonic anhydrase which greatly accelerates the hydration reaction. However, the enzyme cannot affect the equilibrium position of the reaction, but only its speed, and the position of equilibrium of the reaction $CO_2 + H_2O \rightleftharpoons H_2CO_3$ lies well to the left. Ionisation of the carbonic acid so formed takes place to give hydrogen and bicarbonate ions, but this reaction too does not proceed to any great extent, since H_2CO_3 is a weak acid. However, there is yet another component in the system, haemoglobin, the most important buffer in the blood,

21*

which acts as a proton acceptor at blood pH, and is therefore able to accept hydrogen ions formed by the dissociation of carbonic acid.

Thus, in the chain of reactions:

$$CO_2 + H_2O \rightleftharpoons H_2CO_3 \rightleftharpoons HCO_3' + H^+ \ldots (Hb)$$

as haemoglobin removes hydrogen ions from the solution, the active masses on the right are diminished, allowing dissociation of carbonic acid to continue and, by the same consideration, more carbon-dioxide to be hydrated. Thus, the whole system moves to the right to form yet more hydrogen ions, which in turn are "mopped up" by the haemoglobin. Then, for a given tension of CO_2 the chain of reactions is limited by the buffering power of the haemoglobin. Now at this time, when the blood is in the tissue capillaries, oxygen is also being given off to the tissues, and the removal of oxygen from the iron atoms of haemoglobin renders this molecule a weaker acid, and hence a better proton acceptor. The blood is therefore able to carry more carbon-dioxide as bicarbonate ion in the reduced, as opposed to the oxygenated, form.

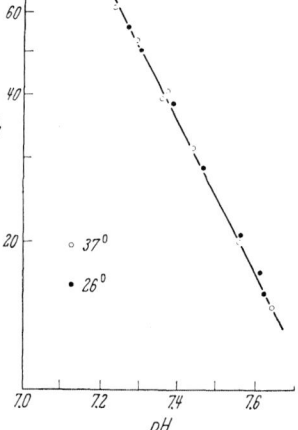

Now when the temperature of blood is reduced, the degree of disso-ciation of haemoglobin to give hy-drogen ions, that is, its strength as an acid, is also reduced. So in a

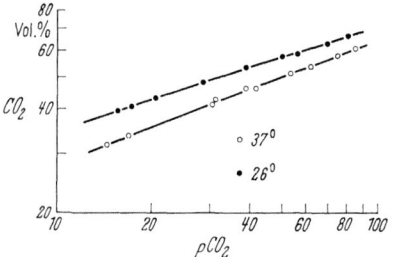

Fig. 1. Left: Dissociation lines of human blood at 37° C and 26° C. The CO_2 content (vol. %) is plotted against the CO_2 tension, each on a logarithmic scale. Note that the carrying power of the blood for CO_2 is increased at the lower temperature. Right: Log pCO_2/pH graph of human blood. The points obtained by equilibration at 37° C lie on the same line as those obtained by equilibration at 26° C. (By kind permission of the Editor of the Guy's Hospital Reports)

manner similar to that of reduced blood, cooled blood is able to carry more carbon-dioxide as bicarbonate ion, for a given tension of CO_2, than is blood at normal temperature.

The result of this theoretical discussion is that in order to assess metabolic acidosis in hypothermia, the bicarbonate content of the hypothermic blood must be compared with that of normal blood equilibrated at the same temperature, for a given CO_2 tension.

Fig. 1 illustrates this point: CO_2 dissociation curves are plotted logarithmically from samples of the same blood at two different temperatures. It can be seen that the cooler blood has a greater carrying power for carbon-dioxide than the warm — to the extent of 8 vol. % (just under 4 mEq.) at $pCO_2 = 40$ mm./Hg.

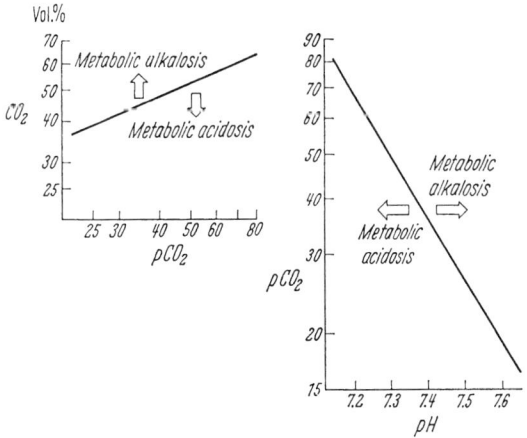

Fig. 2. The figure on the left illustrates that on a dissociation line graph, for any given temperature, metabolic acidosis will cause the line to shift downwards, metabolic alkalosis shifting the line upwards. These shifts indicate respectively decrease and increase in CO_2 carrying power. The figure on the right shows that in a log pCO_2/pH graph, metabolic acidosis shifts the line to the left, metabolic alkalosis to the right. The relationship is independent of temperature

The other relationship shown in this diagram is most interesting. It is a logarithmic plot of CO_2 tension against hydrogen ion concentration, that is, essentially a buffer slope, showing (logarithmically) the change in pH with increments of acid. It can be seen that the relationship is linear and, what is more, independent of temperature, as we first showed (BREWIN et al., 1955). That is to say, if samples of the same blood are equilibrated at different temperatures (e. g. 26° C and 37° C), determinations lie on the same line. However, metabolic acidosis shifts this slope bodily to the left, and alkalosis to the right. This is a convenient relationship, being independent of temperature; it does not give the quantitative picture seen in the dissociation lines, however, which is valuable in treatment.

Assessment of the degree of metabolic acidosis, then, should be made by construction of dissociation curves and log pCO_2/pH plots, the equilibrations for which are all done at the same temperature, no matter what the temperature of the patient at the time.

Change in acid-base equilibrium is then estimated as in Fig. 2.

Summary

The value of hypothermia in the treatment of shock is discussed. The evidence in support of its usefulness as a prophylactic measure is convincing, although it is not often that opportunity arises for it to be used in this way. More commonly, hypothermia must be induced when shock is already established, and the evidence for its value in these circumstances is not quite so good.

Shock appears to pass into an irreversible phase through the effects of the tissue anoxia which is the sequel of reflex vasoconstriction and the consequent reduction in tissue perfusion. One result of this tissue anoxia is a metabolic acidosis. When circulatory arrest is induced to permit open cardiac surgery, or when, for a similar purpose, artificial body perfusion at low flow rates is employed, metabolic acidosis is again produced. Surgical experience has shown that assessment and correction of the acidosis in open cardiac surgery leads to improved results.

It is suggested that hypothermia should be employed in the treatment of shock since it gives a measure of protection against anoxia. However, the condition of a reduced body temperature will make the assessment of the metabolic acidosis more difficult because of physico-chemical changes associated with reduced temperature; the method of assessment in these circumstances is described.

References

ALLEN, J. M., J. ESTES, and A. MANSBERGER: Amer. Surgeon 26, 11 (1960). — BLALOCK, A., and M. F. MASON: Arch. Surg. (U.S.A.) 42, 1054 (1941). — BREWIN, E. G., R. P. GOULD, F. S. NASHAT, and E. NEIL: Guy's Hosp. Rep. (G.B.) 104, 177 (1955). — FEDOR, E. J., B. FISHER, and E. R. FISHER: Surgery (U.S.A. 43, 807 (1958). — MEDINS, G., and H. LAUFMAN: Ann. Surg. U.S.A. 148, 747 (1958). — NEIL, E.: Personal Communication. — OVERTON, R. C., and M. E. DE BAKEY: Ann. Surg. U.S.A. 143, 439 (1956). — POSTEL, A. H., L. C. REID, and J. W. HINTON: Ann. Surg. (U.S.A.) 145, 311 (1957). — RICHARDS, D. W.: Harvey Lect. Series (U.S.A). 39, 217 (1943—44).

Discussion

KROG: I would like to draw attention here to the "sham-death" phenomenon. It is well known that certain animals, like the opossum, and even snakes and beetles, lie down and pretend to be dead if they are attacked by an enemy. This reaction has been interpreted as a protective mechanism designed to fool the attacker, thereby enabling the victim to save itself from being killed.

During my stay in Alaska a few years ago, I had an opportunity of investigating a mountain goat which was brought to the laboratory by the Fishing and Wildlife Service for treatment. The agency was at that time trying to transfer mountain goats from the mainland to Kodiak Island. These animals showed a tendency to go into a shock-like state, I was told, and many of them would die without recovering from that state. When I examined the goat, I found that it had a low blood pressure and a very soft pulse, with a low pulse pressure and all the signs of shock. Injections of vasoconstrictor substances were tried, such as adrenaline, but without success. However, the animal recovered spontaneously after a few hours.

There are also records referring to instances in which humans claim to have shammed death in order to deceive an attacker, such as a bear, or in order to escape death at the hands of their enemies in war time. Unfortunately, there are no records of the pulse pressure or pulse from humans during such states.

I would like to stress that such a mechanism as the "sham-death" phenomenon, which is considered protective, may under certain circumstances, as in the case of the mountain goat, be so severe as to endanger the life of the animal. I should also think that investigation of this curious phenomenon might be of some value to those interested in the causes and the different mechanisms of shock, quite apart from its basic interest to the physiologist concerned with circulatory functions.

BACQ: This introduces us to problems of comparative physiology. I should think that animals which might prove very interesting to study are the normal, non-hibernating, hypothermic mammals, including notably the sloths of South and Central America. They have a normal temperature of 29° to 34° C and they can withstand surgical shock in an absolutely amazing fashion.

KROG: I should like to comment on the sloth, because I have had an opportunity of working on this animal during an expedition to Panama in 1956 to study counter-current heat exchange systems in their brachial vessels. The sloth, of course, takes to experimentation without much of a struggle, but I would not agree that the sloth is very resistant to trauma. I think it is a rather delicate animal. It also has a wonderful temperature-regulation system — like an adjustable thermostat, with which it can regulate its body temperature up and down according to its needs. From a circulatory point of view it is a very interesting animal and should certainly be studied further.

NEIL: I am tempted to announce myself as HIPPOCRATES of Cos! I might just add a note of irrelevancy about the sloth; it hangs upside down all the time and is the only animal which shows decerebrate flexor rigidity.

KROG: Another thing which might be mentioned while discussing the sloth: I found a hardened aortic arch in a sloth in Panama — a rare disease in animals and one which, as far as I know, has only been reported as occurring in the baboons of East Africa.

ADAMS-RAY: May I ask my friend BREWIN whether he has done any experimental work treating irreversible haemorrhagic shock by hypothermia and paying attention to the acidosis?

BREWIN: No, I haven't done this on dogs specifically.

HALPERN: With regard to CO_2, I would like to mention an observation made in my department, showing that intact tissues are very permeable to carbonic acid, whereas they are not at all permeable to other acids, whether organic or inorganic. Am I allowed to use the black-board to make a little drawing to show how we did it? Two receptacles containing Tyrode solutions are separated by a living membrane: intestine, bladder, etc. If we feed CO_2 into one of the receptacles, the pH level will drop in the adjacent compartment. But if we add an organic acid here, to reduce the pH to the same level as when carbonic acid is used, no changes occur in the other compartment. This shows that the living membrane is permeable to CO_2 but not to the H^+ ion. If the membrane is killed or poisoned, this selective permeability disappears.

MIGONE: I should like to ask Dr. BREWIN about the mechanisms underlying two opposite effects of hypothermia: one mechanism serving to prevent shock and the other, on the contrary, operating in the experimental procedure of cold shock. Cold shock reveals many metabolic and circulatory aspects which are very similar to those encountered in other kinds of shock.

BREWIN: I don't think I can throw any light on this at all. I know that this appears and I know that people have been curious in the past as to whether the temperature comes down as a compensatory reaction or as an ill effect of shock, but I don't know the answer.

MIGONE: There are certain "vegetative-lytic" drugs which in human subjects are often used during hypothermia to counteract the more dangerous autonomic nervous and adrenergic reactions, but I believe that in animals these drugs are not given to afford protection against cold shock.

BREWIN: I am unconvinced about this. I have never used any of these "lytic cocktails," because I think the experimental situation is complicated by the obscure pharmacology of these drugs. When these drugs are used alone, as they were for instance in the French battle casualties in Indo-China, I understand that the reduction in body temperature was never more than a degree or two, and I wouldn't like to call this hypothermia. What their action is, then, I don't know. If the drugs are combined with hypothermia, then I think the situation is very complex, and I have kept away from it on this account. I prefer a simple situation which I can control and understand a little.

FINE: The case reports on the wounded men in shock in Indo-China treated with LABORIT's "lytic cocktail" were very few and brief. I read them. As I remember them, only some ten patients were fully reported on, and I guessed that the surgeons dropped the use of the cocktail because they were not enthusiastic about its benefits.

We have had some experience with acidosis in experimental haemorrhagic shock. We tested the role of acidosis by using the artificial kidney in order to maintain ionic equilibrium from the onset of shock. We succeeded in maintaining ionic equilibrium, but we did not alter the outcome of the experiment. Consequently, we concluded that the acidosis was in itself not the lethal mechanism. Of course, as Dr. SENNING says, a patient with a blood pH of 6.9 is probably irreversible. But the irreversibility lies in something causing that pH rather than in the acidosis itself.

Hypothermia, as Dr. BREWIN surmised, does have a protective action if induced before shock. We could define this protection in terms of the functional behaviour of the antibacterial defence systems. We found that if you put the hypothermic dog in shock for two hours and then transfuse him, he will dispose of a dose of bacteria that is lethal in the uncooled dog otherwise treated in the same way. But we did not get this protection if hypothermia was induced after the onset of shock.

SENNING: I have been able to observe a few cases of hypothermia used in shock. If you wish to treat shock, what you try to do is either to make the tissues more resistant to the bad circulation or to increase the circulation through the tissues. But these patients I saw had a very bad peripheral circulation before treatment, and when they were put into hypothermia, they had no peripheral circulation at all. And when you saw the fingers and arms afterwards, they were rigid like a "rigor mortis", and as far as I could see the hypothermia had no beneficial effect at all. With regard to acidosis, if I say that a patient is in irreversible shock when he has a pH of 6.9, I don't mean that it's the pH which makes the shock irreversible; I merely think this low pH is a sign that the patient has such enormous tissue damage, due to anoxia, that he cannot recover.

IMHOF: I would like to make a remark on Dr. MATTHES's paper presented this morning. According to his experience, the activation of fibrinolysis in shock due to myocardial infarction seems to be a valuable measure. However, there is a certain danger in as much as definite hypercoagulability can be observed when maximum fibrinolysis occurs. This is reflected in a shortening of the reaction time as measured by thrombelastography. This potential danger can easily be overcome by administering anticoagulants.

GREGERSEN: I have a question which has never been answered satisfactorily for me and which I would like to raise in this distinguished company. What is the cause of mental depression in shock ? When you see the dramatic effect of giving some bicarbonate, as observed already in World War II, I believe by Dr. CANNON, also by others later, it seems one should be able to find the key. Is it CO_2? Is it pH ? Has it anything to do with the observations of FEMOX and GIBBS, I believe, that subjects can retain consciousness even when breathing 5% O_2 if sufficient CO_2 is added to the inspired air ?

NEIL: KETY and SCHMIDT in 1946 and 1948 did show that CO_2 had a marked quantitative effect on the cerebral blood flow. Low arterial pCO_2 reduced cerebral blood flow from 55 ml./100 g./min. to 35 ml./100 g./min. High arterial pCO_2 increased it to 95 ml./100 g./min. No one has ever examined the effects of altering $[H^+]$ on the cerebral blood flow, unless the $[H^+]$ was altered by changing the pCO_2. There is a wearisome argument that infests every text-book except mine as to whether CO_2 exerts its effects on neurons — particularly of the respiratory centre — as CO_2 itself or whether it acts only as a source of intracellular H^+, which it could do by virtue of its ready diffusibility if there were carbonic anhydrase in the cell accompanied by protein hydrogen acceptors. No one will ever answer this question except by recording intracellular pH with a micro-electrode. However, if we put this problem on one side, we do know perfectly well that pCO_2 changes do profoundly affect synaptic transmission in both spinal and upper brain-stem reflexes. Ascending reticular relays are less responsive in hypercapnia; conversely, they are more easily affected in hypocapnia. The same sort of thing has been shown for the spinal reflex, and I should think that this is part of a very complicated story. I should like to ask Dr. GREGERSEN a question in return: there is something that puzzles me as a physiologist — who fortunately is always kept away from patients except to take samples of blood and such like. I had got the impression from my own clinical days long ago that, in early or what you might call incipient shock, the patient was an agitated, restless, sort of individual, and Dr. BULL said something very similar this morning. Now, as I pointed out yesterday, there are many reasons why, because of the discharges into the reticular formation affecting corticohypothalamic impulse activity, that would be expected to be the case. But of course this is eventually superseded by sheer depression of the higher centres as you get reduced blood flow and such like. But I should have thought it would be really quite a complicated picture. It also bears upon Dr. MIGONE's remarks, I think, on the phenomenon of cold shock, where after all, if the body temperature gradually falls away, you convert the hypothalamus — which is ordinarily a temperature regulator — into virtual inactivity, and the body becomes like a poikilotherm; then the temperature drops steadily, because the temperature regulating centre is virtually paralysed; the metabolic rate of all the tissues inevitably goes down. Physiologists and cardiac surgeons have assumed with a picturesque naivety that all the metabolic rates seem to be affected at about the same level. Well, I do not think that it is true; but no one could dispute that at a body temperature of 25° C the metabolic rate — over-all — would only be about a third of normal. And that would contribute in a no uncertain manner to failure of the peripheral circulation in the subject in question.

GREGERSEN: I recall some heated discussions years ago in the Physiological Meetings over cooling versus heating in shock, led by the late Dr. BAZETT of the University of Pennsylvania, who believed cold was beneficial. He cited instances from World War I of wounded men in shock believed to be beyond resuscitation, who were left to die in the cold outside the casualty station, but who survived, whereas less severe cases treated meanwhile inside did not. BAZETT also talked of the characteristic behaviour of severely injured animals, which crawl away, hide, and lie motionless as the body temperature falls. Maybe we should pay more attention to nature in this matter.

FINE: Yes, we should, and we do. When I was a student, shock was treated with hot-water bottles. Today, we consider the application of heat bad therapy; we uncover the patient and prefer cool environmental temperatures. The keen observations of BAZETT during World War I on the advantages of a cool environment need re-emphasis.

It is not correct to say that the patient's state of mind is a guide to the presence or absence of shock. People are extremely variable. Most of them are dull and subdued in shock. Others are alert and interfere with efforts to treat them.

GREGERSEN: That is, as we have heard, a challenging problem, Dr. FINE. It also strikes me that there is a remarkable, unexplained difference in the mental state associated with stagnant anoxia as compared with the effects of anoxic anoxia (breathing low oxygen). Patients in advanced stages of shock (stagnant anoxia) are mentally depressed, dull, and insensitive to pain, but still rational, however slowly they answer or respond; and they are also seemingly remote, as though nothing had any emotional content for them.

FINE: Some of them answer quite rationally, and some of them are severely obtunded.

GREGERSEN: But is that in the phase of shock when they have really reached the stage of nervous depression before they go into coma ? We had the best opportunity to observe this depressed state and follow it to the end in traumatic and haemorrhagic shock in dogs where it was not interrupted by resuscitation. They, too, seemed "remote", with slowed and diminished responses, but the responses were otherwise normal in pattern and character. Now that is in sharp contrast to the irrational behaviour and obviously confused mental state of individuals breathing low oxygen in a high-altitude chamber and as also described in the stories of bomber crews getting into fights and knocking each other over the head when flying at high altitude. This difference in effect of the two forms of anoxia is presumably well known, but how is it to be explained ? The answer may lie partly at least in the questions raised by Dr. NEIL. I might also add that it is a problem to which I have wanted to apply certain analytic procedures we have developed which can account for 99.5% of the total mass of small, anatomically localised, brain samples in terms of water, lipid, protein, the major electrolytes, etc. We found that the chemical composition of brain tissue is remarkably difficult to alter. Even drastic changes in fluid balance had little effect on the water content. Nevertheless, this approach might reveal some differential effects of the two forms of anoxia on the chemical composition of certain parts of the brain and perhaps indicate the basis of the dramatic beneficial effects of bicarbonate mentioned earlier.

Fluid substitution in shock

By

L.-E. GELIN

It is the purpose of this paper to discuss capillary-flow changes in traumatic shock and the question of fluid substitution under these conditions. No reference will be made to metabolic problems and their treatment.

Neurogenic shock calls for treatment with vagus-blocking and sympathetic-stimulating agents, in addition to which the position of the body must be lowered. Fluid substitution is indicated only where the shock is of prolonged duration.

Acute haemorrhagic shock is in principle chiefly a mere problem of volume and time. In this respect it differs from:

Traumatic and toxic shock — although this category also includes delayed haemorrhagic shock — a condition associated with changes in the flow properties of blood which cannot be offset by simple volume replacement. Hence, the therapeutic aspects and the requirements which the substitute must fulfil differ in various kinds of shock.

Substitutes

Whole blood is the ideal substitute in acute haemorrhagic shock. When substituted in amounts equal to those lost at zero time it completely reverses shock.

Cell-free colloidal solutions have been used to restore volume in different types of shock, including even haemorrhagic shock, in cases where whole blood was not immediately available. Plasma and serum, as well as blood, have both practical and biological disadvantages; this accounts for the great interest that has been aroused by *artificial colloids* for volume replacement. In haemorrhagic shock, volume replacement is often sufficient to ensure adequate tissue perfusion. In traumatic and toxic shock, however, owing to disorders affecting capillary flow, adequate tissue perfusion cannot be achieved simply by volume replacement.

In most studies on shock an increasing amount of evidence has underlined the importance of the reduced blood volume, arteriolar constriction, and lowered blood pressure resulting in a diminishing cardiac output and cessation of capillary flow. However, deaths still occur as the result of shock or the consequences of shock which are not related to the above-mentioned factors. This brings us back to the question as to how we should define the term "shock". I have not been able to accept the definitions of shock generally used; the definition I would propose is the following: "Shock is any acute haemodynamic disturbance which causes such a degree of reduced capillary blood flow that tissue hypoxia of a degree leading to functional and/or morphological changes occurs."

Shock is thus not always merely a problem of blood volume, blood pressure, and anaemia, but essentially a problem of flow. Hence, though blood volume and blood pressure must be maintained, this in itself affords no guarantee that the tissues will be adequately perfused with blood, i.e. that the aim of fluid substitution in shock, viz. the passage of red cells through the true capillaries, will be achieved.

Flow properties of blood in traumatic shock

I should like first to present some data and experiments showing what we consider to be the main blood changes resulting from

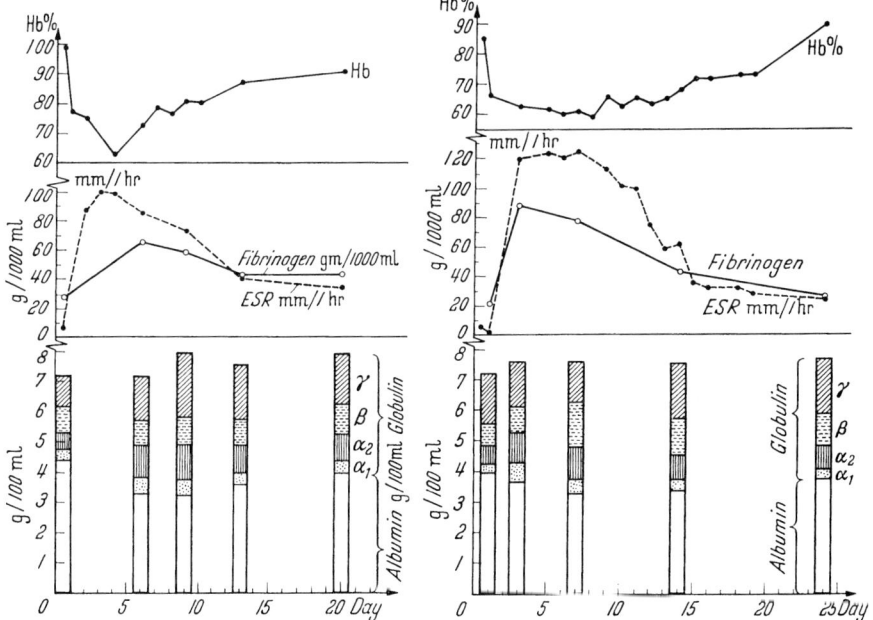

Fig. 1. Changes in haemoglobin, suspension stability, and plasma protein pattern in two patients with compound fractures of the lower leg

injury — changes which have an important bearing on the problem of substitution treatment for traumatic shock.

Figure 1 shows changes in the haemoglobin, erythrocyte sedimentation rate, and plasma protein patterns of two patients with compound fractures of the lower leg. They were only treated for their local injuries and received no intravenous therapy. In both cases there was a decrease in the haematocrit, an increase in the sedimentation rate, a decrease in albumin, an increase in globulins, including especially the α_2 fraction, and an increase in fibrinogen.

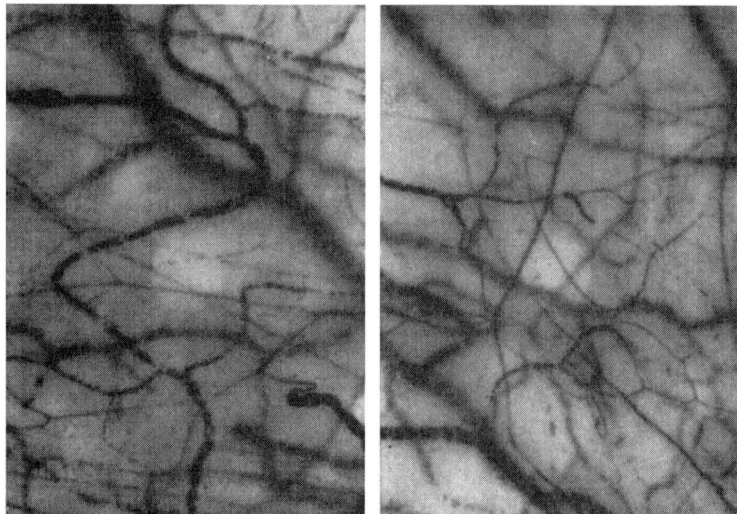

Fig. 2. Capillary flow in the bulbar conjunctiva 18 hours and 2 days after the injury
(from the first patient in Fig. 1)

This accumulation of large protein molecules at the expense of albumin leads to an increase in the viscosity of the plasma and a decrease in the suspension stability of the blood, with consequent aggregation of cells. These changes vary in degree depending upon the severity of the injury.

Figure 2 shows the capillary flow in the bulbar conjunctiva of one of these patients. Aggregation and stasis of cells in the venules is visible, and blood is being shunted through arteriolo-venular anastomoses eighteen hours after the injury. In the second picture occlusive aggregates are seen in post-capillary venules. Later the stasis is less marked and the flow improves.

Figure 3 shows the capillary flow in the bulbar conjunctiva of a rabbit with an untreated ten percent third-degree burn injury of the back. In the top picture aggregated cells are visible in the smallest capillary venules four hours after burning. In the middle picture, we see larger aggregates occluding the venules twelve hours after burning. The bottom picture illustrates the flow characteristics three days after the injury. Marked changes in the blood flow are apparent, with obstructing aggregates in larger collecting venules as well as arteriolo-venular shunting of blood.

Figure 4 lists the changes in the haematocrit, E.S.R., urinary output, and blood volume of the same burned animal. After primary haemoconcentration, a progressive decrease is observed in the haematocrit, together with oliguria and a diminution in the circulating red-cell volume, but a spontaneous restoration of blood volume occurs.

The viscosity of whole blood and plasma are altered in response to tissue injury. The variations occurring in the viscosity of whole blood and plasma at different time intervals following a contusion injury are reported in the discussion on page 99.

In order to study the effect of the above-mentioned disturbances occurring in the flow properties of blood in pathophysiology, we have

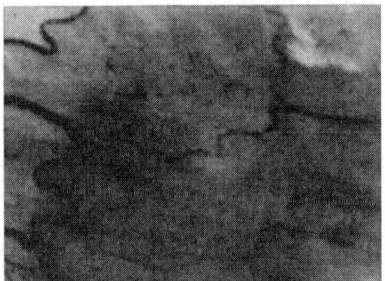
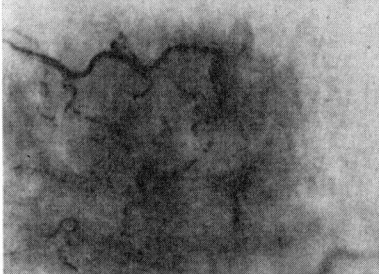
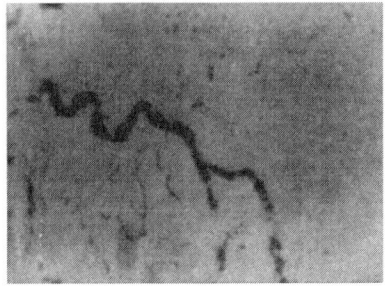

Fig. 3. Capillary flow in the bulbar conjunctiva of a rabbit with an untreated burn injury

induced them experimentally by a variety of means: injury of various kinds, hypothermia, intravenous infusion of thrombin, thromboplastin, fat, and large macromolecules in solution. Critical experiments designed to demonstrate the significance of these disturbances must, however, also meet the requirement of reversibility. For this reason, dextran of high molecular weight was used to produce the desired changes and dextran of low molecular weight to reverse them. Thus, one and the same substance used as plasma expander was employed both to produce and to reverse aggregation by varying its molecular properties. In this way, changes in the flow characteristics of blood in capillaries can be graded by varying the amounts and properties of the macromolecules infused.

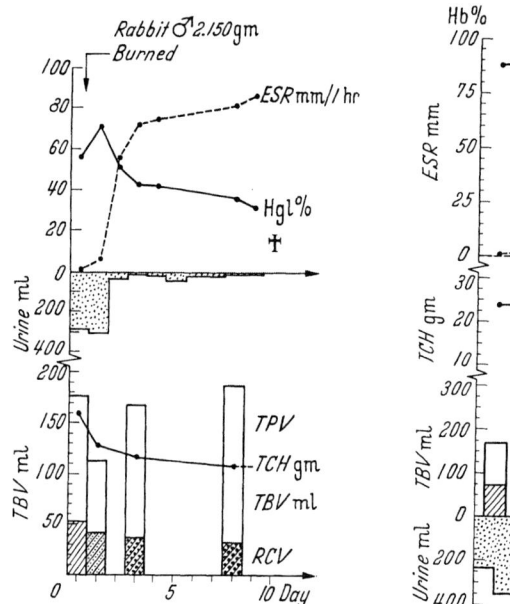

Fig. 4. Blood volume and blood changes in the same rabbit as in Fig. 3

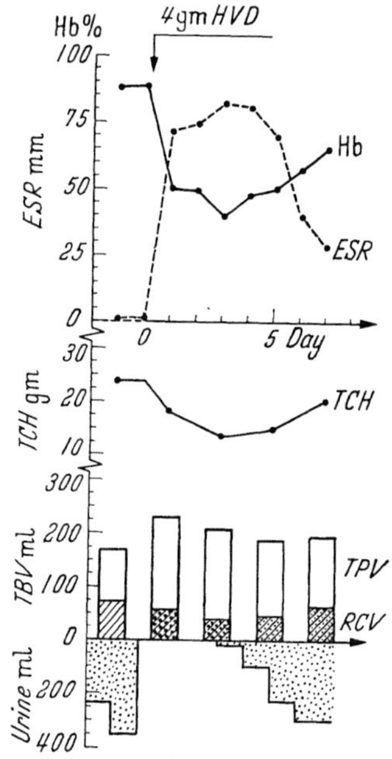

Fig. 5. Plasma volume, red-cell volume, and urinary output in a rabbit given high-viscosity dextran

Effects of dextrans with high and low viscous properties

Figure 5 shows an experiment on a rabbit which had been given highly viscous dextran in order to produce increased plasma viscosity and red-cell aggregation, i. e. to imitate the accumulation of large and viscidising protein molecules such as takes place after injury.

Following administration of high-viscosity dextran, a drop in the haematocrit occurs, together with an increase in the E.S.R., oliguria or anuria, and an increase in blood volume, but a decrease in the red-cell volume. These changes are thus quite similar to those following untreated burn injuries, even though there is no trauma and despite a slight increase in blood volume.

Figure 6 illustrates the changes which occur in the capillary flow in the bulbar conjunctiva of the rabbit after the administration of highly viscous dextran.

The upper picture shows slight changes in flow with aggregation in the venules and occlusion by small aggregates of red cells in the

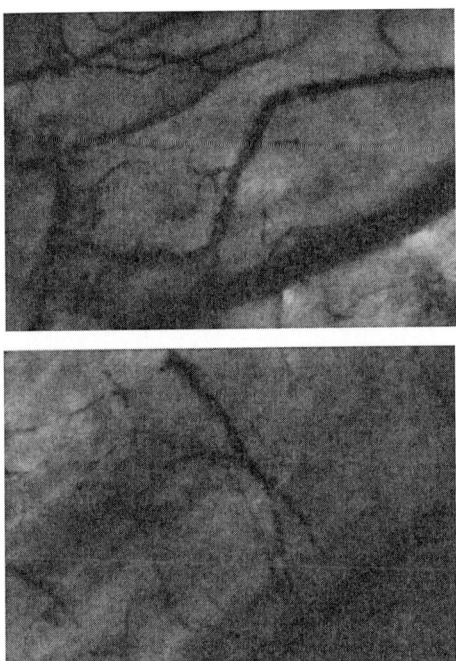

Fig. 6. Capillary flow in the bulbar conjunctiva of a rabbit given high-viscosity dextran

smallest post-capillary venules after administration of 0.5 g. high-viscosity dextran per kg. body-weight. The lower picture reveals stasis of cells in the larger venules and arteriolo-venular shunting after further administration of 1 g. high-viscosity dextran per kg. body-weight.

Figure 7 shows pictures of the capillary flow in the bulbar conjunctiva of the rabbit, as well as blood smears. On the left can be seen aggregation and stasis of cells in the venules and pronounced aggregation of cells in smears following administration of H.V.D.[1]

[1] H.V.D.: mean molecular weight 1,000,000; intrinsic viscosity 0.7

(high-viscosity dextran). On the right are pictures from the same rabbit after subsequent administration of L.V.D.[1] (low-viscosity dextran), showing disaggregation of aggregated cells previously accumulated in the venules as well as a more even suspension of the cells in the smears. The influence of dextran-induced intravascular

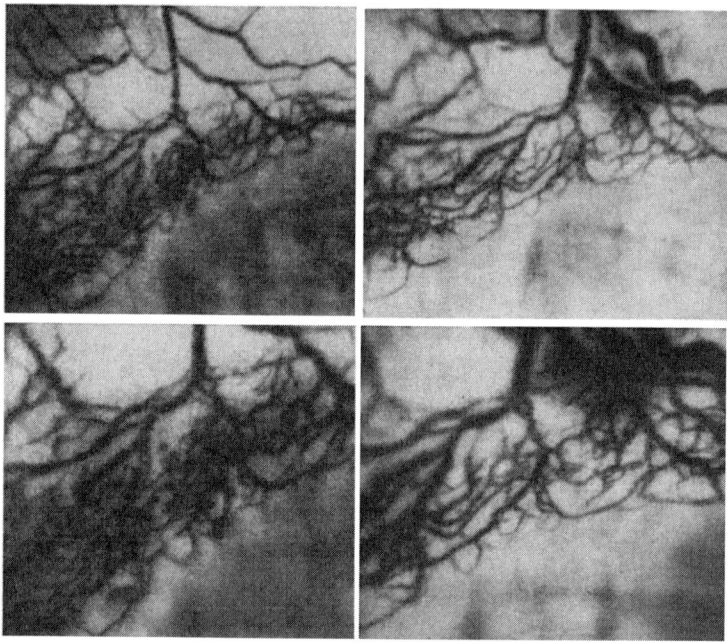

Fig. 7. Capillary flow in the bulbar conjunctiva of a rabbit given first high-viscosity dextran (left) and subsequently low-viscosity dextran (right)

aggregation has been investigated by measuring cardiac output, peripheral resistance, hind-limb blood flow, and renal and hepatic blood flow before and after administration of H.V.D. and subsequent treatment with L.V.D. The experiment shows that despite increased blood pressure (and increased blood volume) administration of H.V.D. is followed by a decrease in flow, whereas subsequent infusion of L.V.D. is followed by an increase in flow to pre-experimental values without any further rise in blood pressure.

Figure 8 shows changes in cardiac output determined with the cardio green method in control and experimental dogs. The ex-

---

[1] L.V.D.: mean molecular weight 39,000; intrinsic viscosity 0.18

perimental dogs were given 1 g. H.V.D. to produce aggregation, followed by 2 g. L.V.D. per kg. body-weight to obtain disaggregation. During aggregation, cardiac output decreased progressively but returned to control values after disaggregation with L.V.D.

In a study on the acid-base balance in dogs in which intravascular aggregation and disaggregation were induced with H.V.D. and L.V.D., we have found during aggregation a normal pH, a decrease in pCO_2, an increase in lactic acid, and a decrease in oxygen consumption and carbon dioxide elimination. After reversal of the

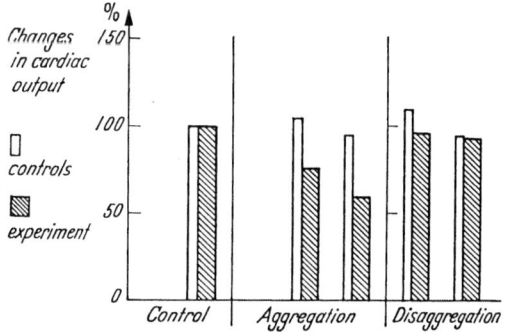

Fig. 8. Changes in cardiac output during a period with intravascular aggregation and during disaggregation in control and experimental dogs

aggregation, in response to infusion of L.V.D., the dogs show a transient increase in acidosis with a lowering of the pH and an increase in pCO_2 and lactic acid, which points to an accumulation in the tissue of acid material which is not released until the flow improves.

Microscopic examination of organs from animals which were subjected to standardised contusion, burning, or cold injury, or to administration of H.V.D., and sacrificed during a period when capillary flow was markedly changed owing to intravascular aggregation of cells, revealed anatomical damage in the liver, kidneys and heart, the intravascular aggregation being due either to injury or to infusion of H.V.D. Animals subjected to the same standardised injury but treated with L.V.D. to counteract the flow changes did not present signs of damage to the organs.

The influence of traumata and induced intravascular aggregation on wound healing as a parameter of effective nutritive blood flow has been studied by Dr. ZEDERFELDT using a method based on the determination of tensile strength. Figure 9 gives the main results of this study. In the figure are seven groups of animals, with ten rabbits in each group, subjected to three different experimental procedures: femoral fracture, induced intravascular aggregation with H.V.D., and withdrawal of blood. Femoral fracture, administration of H.V.D., and withdrawal of blood were all followed by a diminution in the rate of healing. This decreased rate of healing could not be explained by the accompanying anaemia, since withdrawal of blood, if substituted with commercial dextran (Macrodex), did not cause any reduction in the rate of healing. Nor could the decreased rate of healing be ascribed to the reduction in blood

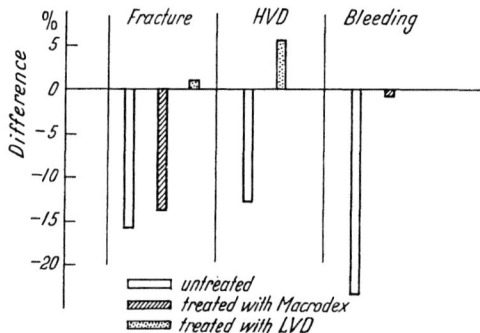

Fig. 9. Difference in rate of healing of pre- and post-experimental wounds in seven groups of rabbits under the following experimental conditions: femoral fracture without treatment, after treatment with commercial dextran (Macrodex), and after treatment with L.V.D.; administration of H.V.D. without and with treatment with L.V.D.; withdrawal of blood without and with treatment with commercial dextran (Macrodex)

volume in the case of femoral fracture, since in this instance substitution with commercial dextran did not significantly improve the rate of healing. The decreased rate of healing can, however, be counteracted by reversing intravascular aggregation with the aid of L.V.D. infusions; hence the intravascular aggregation must be due either to injury, such as a femoral fracture, or to the presence of large and viscidising molecules as after the infusion of H.V.D.

We therefore conclude that volume replacement is not sufficient to restore capillary flow and that after tissue injury the disordered capillary flow is due to disturbances in the flow properties of the blood.

Dextran with low viscous properties

The fundamental requirements of a fluid suitable both for volume expansion and for improving the blood flow are that it should be able to maintain an effective blood volume and blood pressure and to counteract the disturbances in blood flow arising from the above-mentioned qualitative alterations in the blood. To meet these requirements the fluid must have a low viscosity and must be capable of counteracting aggregation of the formed elements of blood.

Saline and glucose solutions, though adequate in this respect, have a very limited duration of effect.

The properties of colloidal solutions vary depending on molecular size, weight, shape, and concentration. Gelatine and polyvinyl pyrrolidone (P.V.P.) have molecular properties which induce physical alterations in the blood at lower concentrations and lower

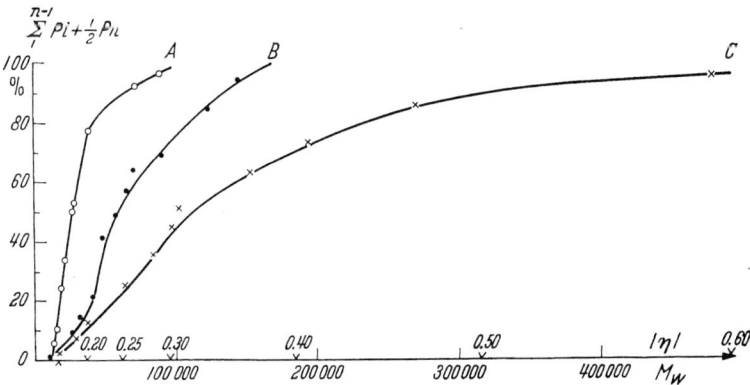

Fig. 10. Integral molecular weight and intrinsic viscosity distribution curves for: *A*, low viscous dextran; *B*, Swedish and American dextran plasma expanders (Macrodex); and *C*, British dextran plasma expander

molecular weights than dextran. This superiority of dextran is attributable to special intramolecular linkages which to some extent can also be varied depending upon the purpose for which the dextran is used.

Many years of experimental and clinical investigation have proved that dextran is a suitable colloid for infusion as a plasma expander. The British type of dextran plasma expander has much higher molecular weights and intrinsic viscosity than the Swedish and American dextran plasma expanders (Figure 10).

For several years now, Dr. INGELMAN and I have been working in an attempt to produce a dextran fraction suitable for the treatment of impaired capillary flow.

The dextran fraction which has so far yielded the best results as a flow improver has a very narrow band of molecules with a mean molecular weight of about 40,000 and an intrinsic viscosity of 0.18 — 0.19.

Infusion of this new dextran solution into healthy subjects expands the plasma volume to a greater extent but for a shorter period of time than Macrodex, which mainly depends on a more rapid excretion in the urine. Saline has no expanding effect, as is apparent from Figure 11.

Low-viscosity dextran increases the peripheral blood flow more effectively than

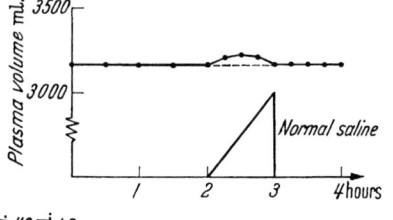

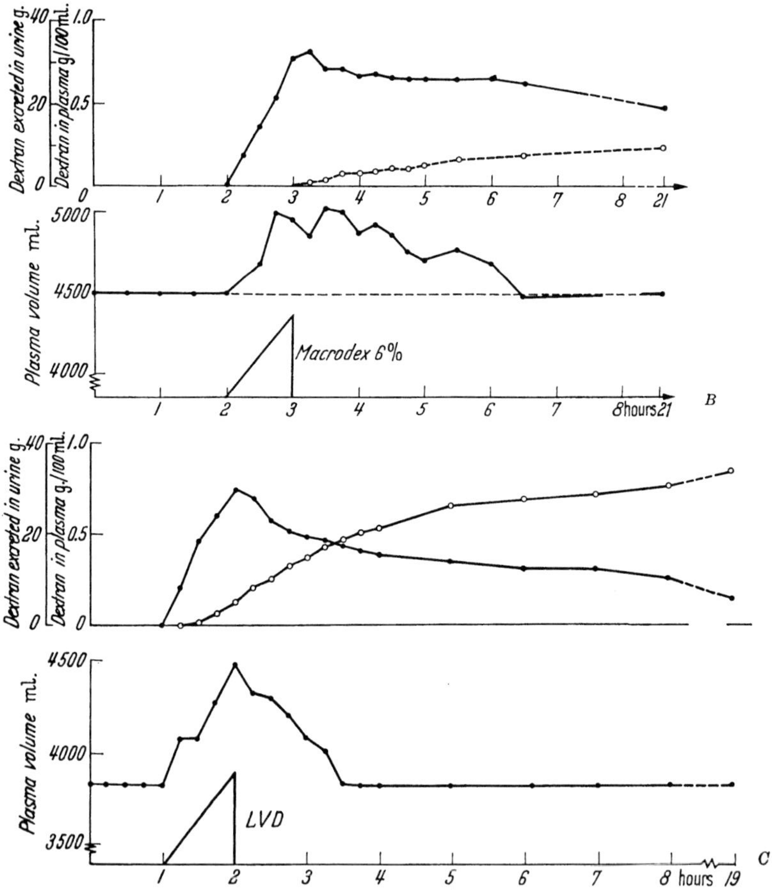

Fig. 11. Plasma volume expansion after infusion of: *A*, 500 ml. normal saline; *B*, 500 ml. Macrodex; and *C*, 500 ml. low-viscosity dextran

Macrodex when the same amounts of L.V.D. and Macrodex are administered.

The coagulation process — which is disturbed by all colloidal substitutes with high molecular weights owing to intravascular clotting — is not affected by this dextran; the dilution results in a

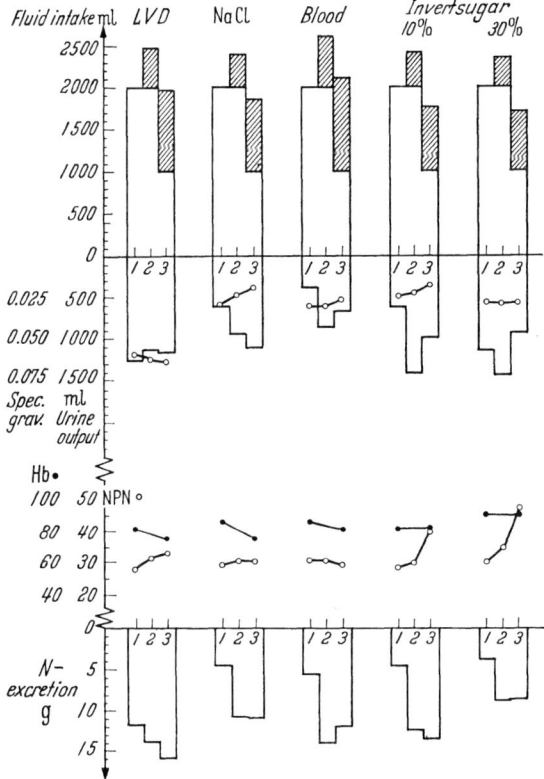

Fig. 12. Effects of low-viscosity dextran, normal saline, blood, and invert sugar in the early post-operate period

transient drop in the number of platelets and a transient prolongation of the bleeding time, though the latter remains within normal limits.

This dextran preparation has been administered to comparable groups of cholecystectomised patients in the early post-operative period in order to compare its effect with that of saline, blood, and invert sugar. I will not discuss the results given in Figure 12 in detail but will merely sum up by pointing out that the urinary output and nitrogen excretion are increased after L.V.D. — an effect which must be ascribed both to osmotic diuresis and to an increase in the renal blood flow.

Infusion of this dextran solution in patients with intravascular aggregation of blood cells and impaired capillary flow reverses or reduces the aggregation, increases the fluidity of the blood, and improves the capillary flow.

Figure 13 shows the influence of this dextran solution on the viscosity of whole blood and plasma in a patient with shock due to

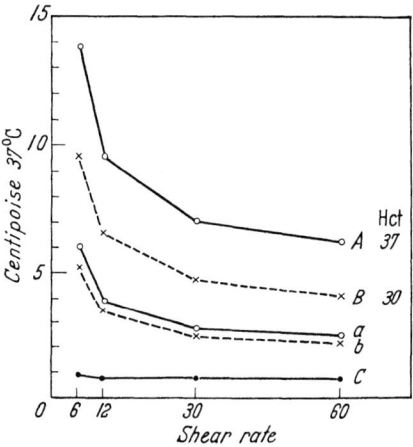

Fig. 13. Viscosity of whole blood (A) and plasma (a) before and after (B and b) the infusion of 500 ml. 15% L.V.D. in a patient with bile peritonitis. C: viscosity of water

bile peritonitis. In this case, the infusion clearly diminished the viscosity of the blood, i.e. enhanced its fluidity. This increased fluidity is most pronounced at low rates of shear, a fact of the utmost importance for the flow of blood in the sinusoids and venules, where the flow rate is low even under normal circumstances and may be very low in the presence of disease.

Figure 14 illustrates the effect of this dextran fraction on the viscosity of blood, peripheral resistance, and blood flow in a patient suffering from a 40% burn injury. It shows that prior to the infusion the viscosity of whole blood was high at all rates of shear (curve A), that the haematocrit was high, that the perfusion pressure was 110 mm. Hg, and that the volume flow was about 10 ml. per 100 ml. tissue per min. After infusion of 1,000 ml. low-viscosity. dextran the haematocrit dropped and the whole-blood viscosity decreased at all rates of shear, especially at lower rates (curve B). The perfusion pressure was unchanged, but the blood flow increased to about 14 ml. per 100 ml. tissue per min. This means that the peripheral resistance decreased by about 35%. Curve C gives the viscosity of whole blood 24 hours later under continuous infusion of L.V.D. Despite an increased haematocrit, the viscosity remained low.

These cases thus demonstrate that this dextran preparation increases the fluidity of the blood.

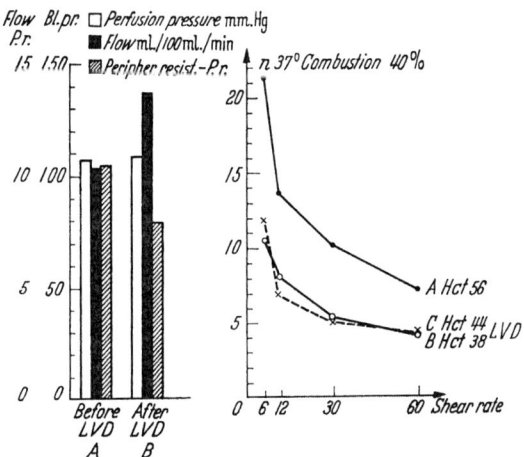

Fig. 14. Flow of blood (after 5 minutes arterial occlusion) recorded with a forearm plethysmograph and whole blood viscosity in a case with 40% burned area before and after infusion of 1,000 ml. 15% L.V.D. *A*: before, *B*: 1 hour after the infusion, *C*: 24 hours later during continued infusion. The infusion was followed by unchanged perfusion pressure (open columns), increased flow (black columns), decreased peripheral resistance (shaded columns), and decreased viscosity of whole blood

The value of this dextran fraction when employed in patients suffering from irreversible shock, despite adequate volume replacement of blood, is illustrated by the following case.

52-year-old woman weighing 55 kg. Advanced peritonitis from perforated intestinal tumour. Admitted to hospital in poor condition with severe shock. Blood pressure 70 mm. Hg; pulse rate 140. Pre-operative treatment with Macrodex and blood. Massive haemorrhage occurred during the operation. Operative and post-operative shock was combated with whole blood and with Aramine as a pressor agent. Despite copious transfusion of whole blood, increasing doses of Aramine were necessary to maintain blood pressure. Blood volume was determined during this period and showed normal values: P. V. 2,670 ml. and R.C.V. 1,670 ml., haematocrit 44%. Microscopy revealed a very poor capillary flow in the bulbar conjunctiva, standstill of aggregated blood cells in the venules, arteriolo-venular shunting, and marked constriction of the arterioles. There were persistent pale pressure marks on the skin. The patient was considered to be in "irreversible shock".

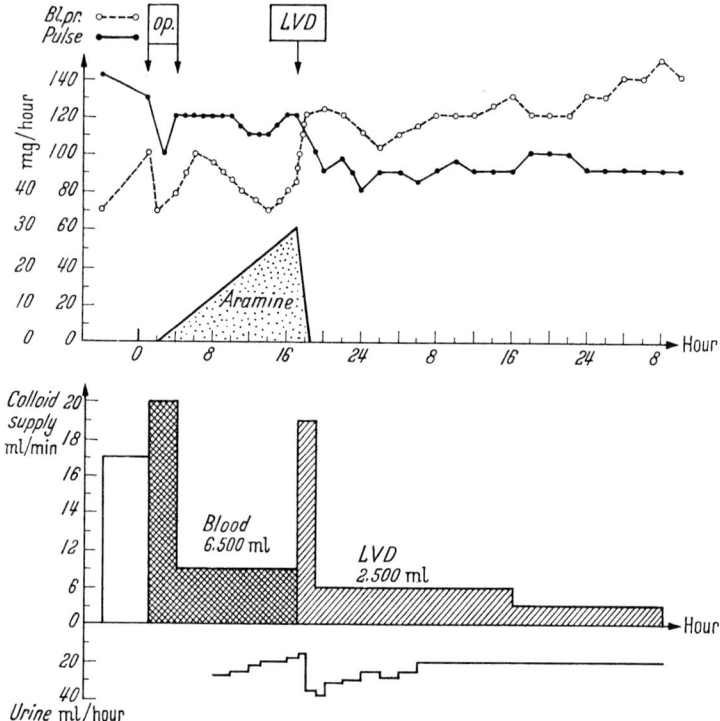

Fig. 15. Case report of so-called "irreversible shock"

500 ml. of 10% L.V.D. in dextrose was now rapidly infused, followed by continuous infusion of 2,000 ml. L.V.D. for two days. Within one hour after the start of the L.V.D. infusion administration of Aramine was stopped. The response of the blood pressure, pulse rate, and urine flow is recorded in Figure 15. The patient's general condition improved rapidly and the cold, cyanotic skin became warm and red. The capillary flow in the bulbar conjunctiva accelerated and cell stagnation disappeared. The blood pressure and pulse rate were maintained at adequate levels without the need for any extra drugs. The urine flow increased. In short, the "irreversible shock" had been reversed.

Summary

Our work on fluid therapy in shock has underlined the importance of differentiating between the various types of shock when selecting the appropriate substitute.

Whole blood is the ideal substitute in acute haemorrhagic shock.

Plasma or artificial plasma expanders in routine use are capable of restoring volume and pressure. In traumatic and toxic shock, however, where disorders in the flow properties of the blood impair the blood flow, they are unable to restore an adequate flow. To meet this additional requirement, a *new dextran fraction*[1] has been elaborated as a substitute, which is able to counteract these disturbances in blood flow.

References

1. BERGENTZ, S.-E.: Acta Chir. Scand. Suppl. 282 (1961). — 2. FAJERS, C.-M. and L.-E. GELIN: Acta Path. Microbiol. Scand. **46**, 97 (1959). — 3. GELIN, L.-E.: Acta Chir. Scand. Suppl. 210 (1956). — 4. GELIN, L.-E.: Bull. Soc. Int. Chir. **18**, 4 (1959). — 5. GELIN, L.-E.: Acta Chir. Scand. **122**, 287 (1961). — 6. GELIN, L.-E. and B. INGELMAN: Acta Chir. Scand. **122**, 294 (1961). — 7. THORSEN, G. and H. HINT: Acta Chir. Scand. Suppl. 154 (1950).— 8. ZEDERFELDT, B.: Acta Chir. Scand. Suppl. 224 (1957).

---

[1] This new dextran solution with low viscous properties will be commercially available under the name Rheomacrodex.

Further aspects of fluid substitution

By

M. I. GREGERSEN

Other things being equal the ideal therapy would appear to be to restore the volume that has been lost. But, as we know, other things are not the same after a period of stagnant anoxia. The purpose must then be to increase capillary blood flow adequately to reverse the metabolic acidosis and to meet the functional demands of the tissues. In this symposium "irreversible shock" has repeatedly been defined as the state in which volume replacement fails to achieve survival and recovery. It has also been stated or implied that the defect lies in the microcirculation. Dr. GELIN's investigations with high and low molecular dextran provide rather good evidence that this is indeed the crux of "irreversibility", at least in hypovolemic stagnant anoxia. Further, Dr. GELIN's correlations of changes in fluidity of the plasma and whole blood at low sheer rates with changes in capillary flow, directly observed, and with the reversal of the metabolic acidosis, show that the influence of plasma substitutes on the physical properties of the perfusing blood can be of critical importance. This appears to me to be a valuable contribution, and it serves to remind us that when we use the term "irreversible shock" we only mean that we have not yet found the cure. Here, then, the studies on LMD may very well be what is popularly referred to as a "break-through". This work may also have useful applications in some forms of peripheral vascular occlusive disease.

In connection with the problem of fluid substitution, it may not be amiss to bring up the possibility of "autotransfusion", that is to say, mobilizing the extravascular body fluids by manipulating the neuro-humoral control of the small vessels. We know that the transcapillary fluid exchange is rapid and large in volume and that the steady state by which plasma volume is normally maintained is readily disturbed by alterations in osmotic and hydrostatic forces (e.g. exercise, gravity, hypertonic solutions, etc.) (1). Therefore, the relative constancy of the plasma volume, normally, must mean that the overall capillary pressure is rather strictly controlled, despite fluctuations in arterial and venous pressures, cardiac output, and regional distribution of the blood in accordance with varying functional demands. Let me give a specific illustration. Some years ago I found in the unanesthetized dog, as well as in dogs anesthetized with Nembutal, that when both common carotids were clamped for periods up to an hour during which the mean arterial pressure was far above the control value, there was no change whatsoever in plasma protein concentration, in hematocrit value, or in the slope of the time-concentration curve of T-1824 (2). Since this sizable change in mean arterial pressure is achieved without alterations in plasma volume, it must be concluded that the overall capillary pressure was unchanged. The mechanism may hold a clue to "autotransfusion". Earlier we had probed the effects of adrenaline, acetylcholine, and Pituitrin. The latter seems to retard the escape of solutes from the blood stream, and you will recall that KROGH (1922) long ago suspected that the posterior lobe secretion had some role in regulating capillary permeability. In the dog, the effect of moderate doses of adrenaline on plasma volume is variable and quite small. In the cat, adrenaline increases plasma volume (3). In both cat and dog, plasma volume is permanently increased by total sympathectomy.

At my suggestion my young colleague Dr. SHU CHIEN undertook a quantitative evaluation of the circulatory adjustment of unanesthetized splenectomized dogs to hemorrhage (4). Single bleedings ranging from 5 to 49% of the measured blood volume were done and the blood later returned. Comparable tests were also made on sympathectomized-splenectomized dogs with single bleedings up to 32% of the blood volume. I believe Dr.RUSHMER will find in Dr. CHIEN's report the factual answer to the question he raised on the first day of this symposium, namely: that circulatory changes appear when volume reduction exceeds 10%.

What is of special interest to the present discussion is the fact that Dr. CHIEN found that hemodilution was slower and of lesser magnitude in sympathectomized dogs than in normal dogs. So far as I know, this is the first definitive evidence we have that sympathetic activity can promote compensatory dilution, although we have suspected that vasomotion has something to do with it.

The precision with which replacement can occur is astonishing. In quiescent, conscious dogs subjected only to withdrawal of 5—10 ml. samples at 10-minute intervals, Dr. T. H. ALLEN in my laboratory observed some years ago that replacement by compensatory hemodilution kept pace exactly with the sampling for several hours. This and other evidence speaks for the existence of sensitive receptor feed-back mechanisms still beyond our ken. We have suggested that the ultimate volume control is in metabolic processes and that the mechanism for adjustment and control of volume may be activated by chemo-receptor mechanisms that monitor discrepancies between supply and demand (*5, 6*). As we learn more about these control mechanisms perhaps "autotransfusion" can become a practical reality to supplement present methods of fluid substitution.

The importance of precise blood volume determinations in abnormal circulatory states has been stressed by some members of this symposium. I heartily agree that the values obtained in some shock-like states, such as anaphylaxis, endotoxin or histamine shock, and in severe stagnant anoxia, should always be critically examined. In these conditions the mixing-time may be very much prolonged, and arterial rather than venous samples may be required.

In the United States there is renewed interest in reviving systematic studies of shock in man and I, for one, have been keenly interested in the reports of the excellent clinical investigations presented at this symposium. We are hoping that plans now in the making for setting up a research unit in Taiwan may soon be realized in order, at long last, to verify reports received from the India-Burma-China Theater during World War II that the clinical and physiological response to injury and blood loss in native soldiers was in several respects different from that seen in the West.

References

1. Gregersen, M. I., and R. A. Rawson: Physiol. Rev. (U.S.A.) **39**, 307 (1959). — 2. Gregersen, M. I.: Amer. J. Physiol. **129**, 369 (1940). — 3. Hamlin, E., and M. I. Gregersen: Amer. J. Physiol. **125**, 713 (1939).— 4. Chien, S.: Amer. J. Physiol. **193**, 605 (1958). — 5. Gregersen, M. I., and R. A. Rawson: Physiol. Rev. (U.S.A.) **39**, 337 (1959). — 6. Gregersen, M. I.: Chin. Med. J. **6**, 171 (1959).

Discussion

NICKERSON: I would like to introduce one problem which has not yet come out in this discussion. This arises from work done by Dr. ARNOLD BURGEN and his collaborators in Montreal (HUTCHISON et al., 1960[1]). Following their studies on plasma incompatibility in dogs, they studied autologous and non-autologous plasma transfusions in man. A group of normal subjects was bled to obtain plasma, which was administered a few days later to the same individual or to another subject of the same erythrocyte blood group. Blood volume determinations before and shortly after the plasma infusion showed that autologous plasma expanded the circulating volume by the calculated amount. However, non-autologous plasma usually gave an expansion of the circulating volume considerably less than anticipated, and in some subjects caused a net loss of plasma volume. Obviously, non-autologous plasma may not stay in the circulation. I think this is an extremely important point. I do not know all of its implications, but I think it may be a factor in some of our unfavourable responses to transfusion.

SELKURT: I would like to comment on an investigation not yet published, done by HANSON and JOHNSON in our laboratory, which has a bearing on the opening remarks of Dr. GREGERSEN relating to the constancy of capillary filtration during carotid compression hypertension. In isolated intestinal loops of the dog they found that, with reduction of arterial perfusion pressure by partial clamping of the arterial supply, there was evidence of venular and small venous vessel constriction so that filtration pressure in the capillaries appeared to be quite well maintained, as evidenced by maintenance of an isogravimetric state. This persisted with acute denervation of the loop, but was blocked by Dibenzyline and other blocking agents — which suggests an intrinsic reflex (arterio-venous) perhaps of an axon type. Capillary filtration pressure would therefore be maintained as arterial inflow pressure was reduced. It is conceivable that the decrease in pressure in the distal segments of the arterial tree, beyond the point of more central vasoconstriction resulting from the carotid reflex, might activate this "arteriolar-venous" reflex.

BACQ: I would like to put a question to Dr. GELIN. There are spontaneous cases — very interesting in man — of macroglobulinaemia, in which the plasma is exceedingly viscous owing to the presence of a kind of SS polymer macroglobulin. Does one find in these cases the changes that Dr. GELIN has observed after injecting dextran of high molecular weight?

ALLGÖWER: There is a ghost haunting many surgical circles called fat embolism. I wonder whether Dr. GELIN in his fascinating flow studies has made any observations relevant to this problem. Every year I have around 600 fractures coming to the hospital. We make it a point to carry out immediate transfusion in all cases involving a larger injury, and fat embolism has not constituted any problem so far. Any femur fracture, for example, coming to the clinic, even when combined with other fractures, including

---

[1] HUTCHISON, J. L., S. O. FREEDMAN, B. A. RICHARDS, and A. S. V. BURGEN: J. Laborat. Clin. Med. (U.S.A.) **56**, 734 (1960).

352   Discussion

those of the pelvis, is treated by operation within a few hours after hospitalisation — as soon as circulation is considered adequate. In about 30 cases we never had cause to regret this "aggressive" approach, but many surgeons take a much more conservative attitude for fear of fat embolism. This conservative attitude — I am afraid — is very often accompanied by insufficient blood volume replacement, jeopardising the circulation and facilitating fat embolism at or after secondary repair procedures or even during "bedside trauma".

Another point I would like to raise is the comparison between dextran and gelatin. I did not quite understand whether Dr. GELIN prefers dextran to gelatin, and if so, whether he has flow studies or expander studies which show dextran to be superior to gelatin. How would dextran compare with gelatin in relation to thrombopenic effect?

FOLKOW: I would like to comment on what Dr. GREGERSEN said about the influence of the sympathetic vasoconstrictor fibres on capillary pressure. Dr. MELLANDER in our laboratory has worked out a technique by which one can estimate independently shifts in the pre- and post-capillary resistances in cats. In Dr. MELLANDER's study it was found that direct stimulation of the sympathetic vasoconstrictor fibres always increased the pre-capillary flow resistance relatively more than the post-capillary flow resistance. Therefore, if other factors are unchanged, such a constrictor fibre activation lowers mean capillary pressure, resulting in an inward transcapillary fluid shift so that the blood becomes diluted. If at the same time arterial blood pressure is also decreased, this inward fluid filtration at the capillary level will be correspondingly increased. However, as I mentioned before, local accumulation of so-called vasodilator metabolites will predominantly affect the pre-capillary resistance vessels, which of course tends to counteract this effect of the constrictor fibres. What will be the net outcome in a given situation is a matter of the competitive balance in the two vascular sections mentioned — a competitive balance between the released constrictor fibre transmitter and the locally produced dilator agents. In addition, another locally controlled mechanism affects the mean capillary pressure, i.e. the so-called "autoregulation" of vascular tone, which is independent of the vasomotor nerves. If pressure (and flow) is increased, the smooth muscles of the pre-capillary resistance vessels respond with a constriction, which — other factors being unchanged — tends to counteract the increase in capillary pressure which would otherwise have taken place. Thus, there are several important local and nervous factors affecting the relationship between the pre- and post-capillary flow resistance, and the net outcome with respect to the mean capillary pressure depends on the interaction of these factors in any given situation[1].

BULL: I would like to comment on Dr. GREGERSEN's point. Haemodilution in man is, I believe, different from that in dogs. We have studied this in many patients, and we did not find haemodilution to be as quick or as complete as described in experimental animals. The haemodilution after injury and blood loss in man is not complete over a period even of one day, and the low haemoglobin resulting does not fully represent the loss; this we have found in many cases. The follow-up blood volumes that we used in our studies were genuine convalescent values and checked well with those expected. However, there is a blood volume change due to bed rest which has to be brought into the picture sometimes. We did a number of blood

MELLANDER: Acta physiol. Scand. 50, Suppl. 176 (1960); FOLKOW, B., and B. ÖBERG: Acta physiol. Scand. (in press).

volume studies on patients admitted just for the operation of meniscectomy, where one would not expect any blood loss at all at operation, and there was a drop in blood volume of about 5% due to bed rest.

NEIL: I'd like to make some suggestions at the front, using the board. There is something terribly interesting in what Dr. GREGERSEN reports about the oriental shock cases showing hypotension with bradycardia and vaso-dilated extremities. This seems to be a very good example of the importance of the influence of pulse pressure amplitude on the baroreceptor reflex responses. It is still not properly realised that the afferent activity of the baroreceptors is much more influenced by an amplitude and a rate of rise of pulse pressure than by any given mean pressure maintained steadily, unless of course such a mean pressure be over 200 mm.Hg. I think, however, that a very simple experiment, such as I did with DALY and SCHWEITZER years ago, demonstrates what 1 mean very conclusively. If you record the pressure simultaneously in the external and common carotid arteries, ordinarily of course the two pressure values are virtually the same. Now if both common carotid arteries are clipped, as everyone knows, the pressure in the external carotid artery (which is similar to that in the carotid sinus) falls, and mean-while there is a rise in systemic pressure which is always ascribed to the fall in sinus pressure. However, if the clips be left *in situ* on the common carotid arteries, the reflex rise in systemic pressure is well maintained for many minutes. Meanwhile, recording of the external carotid artery pressure shows that it steadily rises towards its initial normal value, owing to back-flow from anastomotic channels. Indeed, the external carotid artery pressure may exceed the normal mean pressure (which was registered prior to occlusion), although it remains of course below the reflexly raised mean pressure in the rest of the arterial system. As the external carotid mean pressure becomes the same as before occlusion, one can hardly argue that the sustained reflex systemic hypertension is engendered by the effects of mean pressure on the sinus receptors. It *is* due to the feeble pulsatile pressure which affects the sinus region, for the anastomotic channels cannot transmit the normal full pulse pressure to the sinus region.

Returning to the vasodilatation in the oriental subjects who are shocked, I think that the bradycardia which occurs in these subjects — for what reason I do not know — would at least secure a wide pulse pressure which may well be responsible for vasodilation reflexly engendered from the arterial baroreceptors. One further point about these subjects — I am terribly inter-ested that there should be no change in blood volume. It does suggest what Dr. FOLKOW was saying, that there might be venular constriction as well as, or instead of, arteriolar constriction. Medical students have great difficulty in understanding that the loss of fluid from the capillary is more or less in-dependent of the mean arterial blood pressure, but is ordinarily much more fundamentally related to the state of constriction of the arterioles. Vasomotor discharge which particularly affects the arterioles must reduce the hydro-static pressure transmitted to the capillaries and must inevitably increase the fluid uptake from the tissues. On the other hand, if — as Dr. FOLKOW and Dr. MELLANDER have suggested — there is a preponderant venular constriction, then more fluid is likely to be lost from the capillaries than is ordinarily the case — resulting of course in haemoconcentration. So I feel that we must further examine the small vessel response to sympathetic dis-charge provoked by baroreceptor reflexes. One must not forget, nevertheless, that some of the baroreceptor reflexes in haemorrhage and shock must concern cardiac output and venous capacity as well as altering the vascular resistance.

KRAMER: Dr. GREGERSEN, may I just mention something about the spleen ? The spleen in dogs has a red-cell store that is virtually plasma-free; so that when it contracts, plasma volume increases very little, but the haemoglobin concentration rises. Of course in man the red-cell storage function of the spleen is not significant and can be neglected.

GELIN: First a remark to Dr. BACQ. The macroglobulinaemia cases really show a very disturbed capillary flow and, as you know, they have an increased tendency to form thrombi and to develop petechial bleeding and gangrene — which in itself indicates that their peripheral flow is very poor. If you look at them during crises, you will find standstill of blood in the venules and open arteriolo-venular shunts. So macroglobulinaemia is a condition in which this disturbance of flow plays an important role. Such patients also have liver lesions, kidney lesions, and myocardial lesions. It is a kind of a "chronic shock" that is involved.

Concerning gelatin and the bleeding tendency, I should like to remark on the bleeding tendency first of all. We have studied this. Dr. BERGENTZ and Dr. NILSSON have particularly stressed the importance of molecular distribution, because the bleeding tendency following infusion of artificial colloids is due to the size and symmetry of the molecules. The large molecules induce intravascular clotting and consume all coagulation factors, but these changes can be prevented by large doses of heparin in the dog, indicating that it is really an intravascular clotting which is induced by the macromolecules. The difference between gelatin and dextran in this respect is that gelatin is a much more asymmetric molecule. In gelatin preparations used for infusion purposes, the molecular weights have been brought down to about 25,000, and that is just the limit at which these changes start to develop. It is at molecular weights of gelatin above about 30,000 and of dextran about 90,000 that these physical disturbances start. To express it in other terms, gelatin has a much higher intrinsic viscosity than dextran at the same molecular weights.

Regarding the problem of fat emboli, this is of very great interest to us at the moment, because it is the very first event following injury. Fat embolism is regularly found after tissue injury and starts with the formation of white aggregates, and if you look at these aggregates, formed within the first few minutes of injury, you will find that they contain platelets and chylomicrons. Fluorescence microscopy reveals fat droplets generated within them.

Finally, just a word about blood volume determinations. I think that it is important to point out that, when the flow is very poor and stagnation is present in the venules, the equilibration of marked cells in our experiments is prolonged, and this prolonged equilibration can give rise to an error with regard to the red-cell mass of about 10—15%.

GREGERSEN: The comments and questions from Dr. BULL, Dr. FOLKOW, Dr. NEIL, and Dr. GELIN show that I seem to have achieved my aim of raising problems for discussion. The evidence of difference in speed and magnitude of compensatory haemodilution in man and dog is, of course, an interesting point, but perhaps the explanation is to be found in the fact that the experimental conditions are not strictly comparable. Dr. CHIEN hopes to repeat the haemorrhage experiments on volunteers in order to find out whether or not there is a species difference. Now as for the convalescent blood volume, Dr. BULL, until we had finished the Bellevue studies, we — that is to say Dr. NOBLE and I — did not know that bed rest alone lowers the blood volume as shown by the ANCEL KEYS group. In the review RAWSON and I published two years ago, we emphasised that the size of the circulatory system as well as blood volume are primarily determined by the functional demands of the tissues and are hence dependent upon physical activity and training, as shown for example by SJOSTRAND. Dr. NEIL's comments on the carotid clamping experiments are welcome, because attention to pulse pressure as well as level of mean pressure may indeed be important in the further study which, I hope, will be made of this problem. Dr. KRAMER's remarks on the spleen I understand, and it is interesting that the spleen can contract without any change in plasma volume. I agree entirely with Dr. GELIN's warning about the importance of mixing time. It is sometimes so long that it is hard to believe. Thank you very much.

Drug therapy of shock

By

M. NICKERSON

In shock, as in so many other pathological conditions, the development of effective therapy depends to a large extent on knowledge of etiology. Consequently, questions of treatment and of etiology cannot be discussed entirely in isolation. Our understanding of the shock process is still very inadequate, but one of the few points on which there is general agreement is that a decrease in effective circulating blood volume is a major contributing factor in most cases. This knowledge has made it possible for treatment by blood transfusion and other fluid volume replacement to develop much more rapidly and successfully than any other type of therapy of shock. This presentation will not cover the use of blood or other fluid and electrolyte preparations except as this relates to the use of "drugs" in a more restricted sense. However, I should like to begin my discussion by re-emphasizing that proper attention to intravascular volume should be the first consideration in the management of all cases of shock, and that it is the only type of treatment necessary in the majority. This principle is applicable to shock due to many different precipitating factors, but it obviously excludes shock associated with myocardial infarction. Cardiogenic shock will not be included in the following discussion because it involves etiological factors sufficiently different from those responsible for other types to require that all aspects of its treatment be considered separately.

Innumerable types of therapy in addition to circulating volume replacement have been proposed for the treatment of shock, but, for most, the theoretical basis is still very inadequate. The present discussion will be limited, perhaps somewhat arbitrarily, to three types of agents which have received major attention in recent years.

Adrenal steroids

Interest in the effects of adrenal steroids in shock undoubtedly arose from the known important role of the adrenal cortex in responses to a variety of stressful situations, and the extreme sensitivity of adrenalectomized animals to any shock-inducing procedure. There is no question but that the administration of a relatively small dose of adrenal steroid can increase dramatically the survival of adrenal-deficient animals, but it is not equally clear that adrenal deficiency exists during the development of shock in either animals or man, unless the adrenals are specifically compromised by disease, surgery or the prior administration of exogenous adrenal steroids.

Measurements of adrenal steroids under conditions of protracted stress, including lethal shock of varying etiology, both in experimental animals and in man (FRANK et al., 1955a; HUME and NELSON, 1955; MELBY and SPINK, 1958), have demonstrated increased plasma levels, increased rates of secretion, and a good response to ACTH. Output may decrease somewhat when adrenal blood flow becomes very low, but the gland is still capable of responding when the blood flow is again increased. The basic question, then, is whether an even greater increase in adrenal steroids can increase resistance to shock above the normal level.

In spite of many earlier attempts, protection of animals with normal adrenals against shock of any etiology by the administration of exogenous adrenal steroids has been demonstrated only recently (LILLEHEI and MACLEAN, 1959; WEIL, 1961). Convincing evidence of protection is limited to experiments on acute endotoxin toxicity. This is frequently referred to as "endotoxin shock", and although the cardiovascular collapse and the pathological picture produced by endotoxin from gram-negative bacteria are very similar to those seen in hemorrhagic or traumatic shock, the available data do not allow a clear evaluation of the relation of this condition to other types of "shock". Doses of steroid many times higher than the usual maintenance level are required to antagonize endotoxin toxicity. Indeed, maximum protection is observed with doses just below the toxic level for the steroid itself — in mice at a weight equivalent of over 15 grams of prednisolone in a man. Prednisolone appears to be somewhat more effective than hydrocortisone, which might suggest some correlation between protection and glucocorticoid activity. However, aldosterone is many times more potent than either (BEIN and JAQUES, 1960), and at present there is little evidence to correlate the protection with either gluco- or mineralocorticoid activities as usually measured.

The protective effects of massive doses of adrenal steroids have been adequately tested only in endotoxin shock. However, these agents appear to have been uniformly ineffective in traumatic and hemorrhagic shock under the conditions reported to date (INGLE,

1943; SWINGLE et al., 1944; FRANK et al., 1944; FRANK et al., 1955 b).

Little progress has as yet been made in elucidating the mechanism or mechanisms by which adrenal cortical steroids suppress the lethal effects of endotoxin. The toxin itself has been reported to potentiate several vascular responses to catecholamines (THOMAS, 1956; ZWEIFACH et al., 1956; GOURZIS et al., in press), but BEIN and JAQUES (1960) observed inhibition or reversal of pressor responses to adrenaline and noradrenaline following administration of lethal doses of endotoxin to anesthetized cats. Both augmentation (BEIN and JAQUES, 1960) and inhibition (LILLEHEI and MacLEAN, 1959) of responses to catecholamines have been suggested as mechanisms of the steroid protection. The latter possibility receives some support from the observation that large doses of hydrocortisone provide considerable protection against the lethal effect of infused adrenaline (LILLEHEI and MacLEAN, 1959) and from accumulated evidence of the involvement of excessive adrenergic vasoconstriction in the genesis of lethal shock (NICKERSON, 1955 a), but a general pharmacological antagonism between the steroids and catecholamines has not been demonstrated. It has been suggested that endotoxin may be detoxified by some direct interaction with the steroid (BEIN and JAQUES, 1960; WEIL, 1961). If this explanation is correct, only limited beneficial effects might be expected in other types of shock. In any case, it is apparent that the processes involved in this protection are quite different from those associated with the actions of the adrenal cortical hormones at maintenance levels.

The adrenal steroids have been utilized in a somewhat haphazard fashion in a very large number of cases of clinical shock without convincing results. In addition to the usual problems of interpreting therapeutic results in a heterogeneous group of patients, evaluation of the role of this type of therapy is complicated by the generalized suppression of inflammatory processes and the non-specific feeling of well-being produced. Attention should be called specifically to the well-known ability of adrenal steroids to suppress the signs and symptoms of inflammation and to decrease resistance to the spread of infection. These effects can greatly complicate the overall management of cases of clinical shock, which usually involve a variety of etiological factors, among which infection is not uncommon.

Sympathomimetic amines

Agents of this type are probably the most commonly utilized in the clinical treatment of shock or suspected shock, but evidence regarding their efficacy is conflicting. The popularity of this type of treatment is undoubtedly related to the physician's preoccupation with the patient's blood pressure. This attitude is quite understandable, because blood pressure is one of the few criteria of shock which can be measured and recorded quantitatively. However, it should be noted that it is one of the least reliable. The significance of a given level of hypotension is entirely dependent on the status of the cardiac output and regional blood flows, which in turn are dependent on the processes inducing the hypotension. Hemorrhagic shock can be standardized effectively on the basis of bleeding animals to a given pressure, but comparable pressures induced by procedures such as spinal cord section or depressor nerve stimulation are tolerated for extended periods of time without the development of progressive cardiovascular failure if an adequate fluid balance is maintained (PHEMISTER, 1943; WIGGERS et al., 1943).

Many clinical reports provide testimonials to the value of vasopressor therapy in that the blood pressure is elevated in a high percentage of patients and many of them look and feel better, at least temporarily. However, there is little reliable evidence that survival is equally favorably affected. It appears that much of the data on this subject is well summarized by two quotations from a report on the use of noradrenaline in the treatment of shock associated with epidemic hemorrhagic fever (YOE, 1954): "That continuous l-arterenol infusion is a useful procedure in the management of severe primary shock in hemorrhagic fever is demonstrated by its initial prompt and beneficial effect on clinical appearance, pulse and blood pressure" and ". . . the mortality rate in the shock phase for this group (treated with the vasopressor) was not significantly different from the control group with equally severe shock". A similar lack of prognostic significance of vasopressor-induced changes in blood pressure and clinical appearance has been observed in animal experiments. Administration of a pressor amine to dogs during the development of hemorrhagic shock can raise the blood pressure and improve alertness and activity, although the survival rate is not increased (FRANK et al., 1945).

The significance of symptomatic improvement during vasopressor therapy must be evaluated in the light of the demonstrated ability of sympathetic nervous system overactivity (FREEMAN, 1933), adrenaline (BAINBRIDGE and TREVAN, 1917; ERLANGER and GASSER, 1919), or noradrenaline (YARD and NICKERSON, 1956) to decrease plasma volume and cardiac output and induce typical shock in experimental animals. Similarly, milder adrenergic vasoconstriction due to infusion of adrenaline, noradrenaline or other sympathomimetics, or to section of buffer nerves or stimulation of sensory nerves can increase the lethality of hemorrhage (OVERMAN and WANG, 1947; REMINGTON et al., 1950; CLOSE et al., 1958) or endotoxin (LILLEHEI and MacLEAN, 1959). Related findings include increased histological evidence of hepatic, renal and cardiac damage in patients and animals who had received sympathomimetic vaso-pressor therapy for shock (BOUGHTON and SOMMERS, 1957; LILLEHEI and MacLEAN, 1959).

Many attempts have been made to anticipate the effects of vaso-pressor therapy in shock on the basis of hemodynamic studies, but the reported observations are very difficult to relate to effects on survival. Factors which contribute to this difficulty include: 1) Most hemodynamic studies are of much shorter duration than the shock process to which they are compared. 2) Reports of significant drug-induced changes in mortality frequently do not adequately distinguish between deaths occurring during the shock-inducing procedure, attributable to acute trauma or exsanguination, and later "shock" deaths. (Vasoconstrictors may temporarily prevent death in the former by maintaining circulation to the respiratory centers.) 3) Alterations in blood flow or peripheral resistance are infrequently analyzed with respect to specific vascular beds. 4)When regional blood flows are considered, the cerebral, renal and coronary beds receive major attention, although the splanchnic area appears to be most intimately involved in the development of irreversibility in shock (LILLEHEI, 1957). It is of interest that noradrenaline, administered to hypovolemic dogs under conditions in which an increase in cardiac output is induced, decreases portal blood flow (LEVY, 1958).

This difficulty of relating hemodynamic events to the develop-ment of lethal shock is exemplified by the effects of metaraminol (Aramine) in shock due to the administration of endotoxin. A major component of the hemodynamic response to endotoxin appears to be venous pooling, which can be largely corrected by the infusion of metaraminol (WEIL et al., 1956). However, under very similar conditions this agent has been shown to increase the lethality of endotoxin (LILLEHEI and MacLEAN, 1959).

Improvement in the survival rate of shocked animals has been demonstrated in a few experiments in which noradrenaline was administered relatively late in the shock process in doses which had little or no effect on the blood pressure (LANSING et al., 1957; LANSING and STEVENSON, 1958). Although the mechanism involved in this protection has not been evaluated fully, it appears probable that it involves a cardiac rather than a vasoconstrictor action. The heart and other organs above the diaphragm do not appear to be limiting in the earlier stages of the shock process, when irreversibility to transfusion ordinarily is determined (NICKERSON, 1955 b; SMITH et al., 1957), but it is quite possible that myocardial inadequacy may develop during late deterioration (WIGGERS and WERLE, 1942; SARNOFF et al., 1954).

Agents inducing vasodilatation

This type of treatment represents the exact opposite of the pressor, vasoconstrictor therapy discussed above. It is predicated on the concept that blood flow through certain critical areas, rather than blood pressure, is the main determinant of survival. Observations which may be considered to contribute to a theoretical basis for this type of treatment include: 1) Most of the more reliable clinical signs of shock (pallor, cold skin, sweating, tachycardia, low pulse pressure, slow capillary filling, etc.) are also signs of vasoconstriction and of sympathetic nervous system overactivity. 2) In groups of animals subjected to a standard shocking procedure, those with evidence of greater initial sympathetic nervous system activity (higher blood pressures and heart rates) have the higher mortality (Table 1). 3) In the presence of vasodilatation due to procedures

Table 1. *Initial blood pressures and heart rates of untreated dogs subjected to a standard hemorrhagic shock procedure*

Outcome	No. of animals	Initial blood pressure	Heart rate	
			Initial	At reinfusion
Survived . . .	16	126 ± 3	138 ± 5	222 ± 7
Died	52	143 ± 3	170 ± 5	230 ± 5

All values are mean ± S. E.

such as high spinal cord section and an adequate blood volume, prolonged survival at very low blood pressure is possible. 4) Excessive vasoconstriction, due either to exogenous sympathomimetic amines or to sympathetic nervous system overactivity, can produce or accentuate shock. 5) Elimination of reflex vasoconstriction by deafferentation of traumatized areas can increase survival at a given level of residual circulating blood volume.

A significant increase in the survival rate of animals subjected to traumatic, hemorrhagic or endotoxin shock has been demonstrated by many workers using many different agents and procedures to induce vasodilatation or limit vasoconstriction. These include sympathectomy (FREEMAN, 1938), deafferentation by nerve section or local anesthetics (EVERSOLE et al., 1944; WANG, 1947), adrenergic blocking agents (REMINGTON et al., 1950; WIGGERS et al., LOTZ et al., 1955; OVERTON and DEBAKEY, 1956; BAEZ et al., 1958; KOVACH et al., 1958; LILLEHEI and MACLEAN, 1959; NICKERSON and CARTER, 1959), ganglionic blocking agents (GLASSER and PAGE, 1948; LEVY et al., 1954; ROSS and HERCZEG, 1956) and direct-acting vasodilators (NICKERSON and CARTER, 1959; ZINGG et al., 1960).

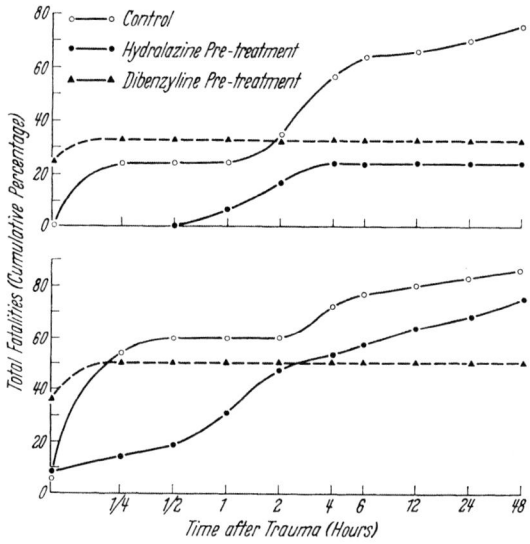

Fig. 1. Cumulative mortality of rats subjected to 400 (upper) and 450 (lower) turns in a Noble-Collip drum with 2 shelves. Note the somewhat greater susceptibility of animals treated with Dibenzyline to acute trauma (deaths in the drum or within 15 minutes after the end of the drumming), and the complete absence of late "shock" deaths in this group. (NICKERSON and CARTER, Canad. J. Biochem. Physiol., 1959)

In interpreting these results it is important to distinguish between effects on resistance to "shock" and those on resistance to "acute hemorrhage or trauma". Inhibition of compensatory vasoconstriction may increase sensitivity to acute trauma or hemorrhage, probably by allowing a more marked acute fall in blood pressure, which may cause respiratory arrest due to inadequate perfusion of medullary centers. This is particularly apparent when an agent such as phenoxybenzamine (Dibenzyline) is administered to hypovolemic animals or patients. In this situation, an amount as small as 2% of the usual blocking dose may cause a sudden fall in blood pressure and respiratory arrest. Differences between effects on responses to acute trauma and to "shock" have been clearly demonstrated also in drum-trauma experiments (Fig. 1), where the number of acute deaths during the drumming period may be unaltered or even increased by a dose of blocking agent which protects completely against later "shock" deaths (LEVY et al., 1954; NICKERSON and CARTER, 1959).

Table 2. *Bleeding volumes and survival of control and Dibenzyline pre-treated dogs subjected to a standard hemorrhagic shock procedure*

Group		No. of animals	Bleeding volume (ml./kg.)		Blood rein-fused[1] (ml./kg).	Sur-vival %
			Initial	Maximal		
Control	Survived	7	38.3 ± 1.6	55.6 ± 3.7	2.7	22
	Died	25	41.9 ± 1.8	56.9 ± 1.9	12.8	
Dibenzyline	Survived	7	36.7 ± 3.1	52.7 ± 3.1	0	88
pre-treatment	Died	1	35.6	41.3	13.0	
1.0 mg./kg.						

[1] During the period when the connection between the animal and the bleeding reservoir was clamped, small amounts of blood were reinfused when necessary to prevent the blood pressure from falling below 40 mm. Hg.
All values are mean ± S. E.

Although it is generally accepted that agents inhibiting sympathetic vasoconstriction can protect against a fatal outcome in animals subjected to various shock-inducing procedures, interpretation of the significance of these observations is controversial. In many of the reported hemorrhagic shock experiments, loss of blood has been less in the treated than in the control series, and it has been suggested by several authors that the observed protection is due only to a reduction in the degree of stress applied in bleeding to a standard pressure, or to loss of a smaller volume of fluid into damaged tissues. However, marked protection can be induced by appropriate doses of a blocking agent such as Dibenzyline (REMINGTON et al., 1950; BAEZ et al., 1958), particularly if administered several hours before the animal is subjected to the shock-inducing procedure, without any appreciable change in bleeding volume (Table 2). In addition, protection has been demonstrated in experiments in which a vasodilator agent (hydralazine, Apresoline) was administered after bleeding had been completed (ZINGG et al., 1960). Similarly, KOVACH et al. (1958) found the protective effect of Dibenamine in tourniquet shock in dogs not to be dependent on a reduced fluid loss into the involved extremities.

In evaluating the circulatory status of animals subjected to a stress such as bleeding, it is important to distinguish between alterations in the volume lost to an external reservoir and in the residual intravascular volume. It has been observed that severe sympathetic vasoconstriction (FREEMAN, 1933) or infusion of a sympathomimetic amine (LILLEHEI and MACLEAN, 1959) can reduce markedly the circulating volume. This probably involves both loss of fluid from the vascular compartment and trapping of blood in poorly circulated areas, because both the plasma and erythrocyte volumes may decrease, although changes in the former are always the greater. Conversely, we have recently demonstrated that administration of Dibenzyline to dogs can induce a prompt increase in plasma volume (Fig.2), a considerable part of which may persist

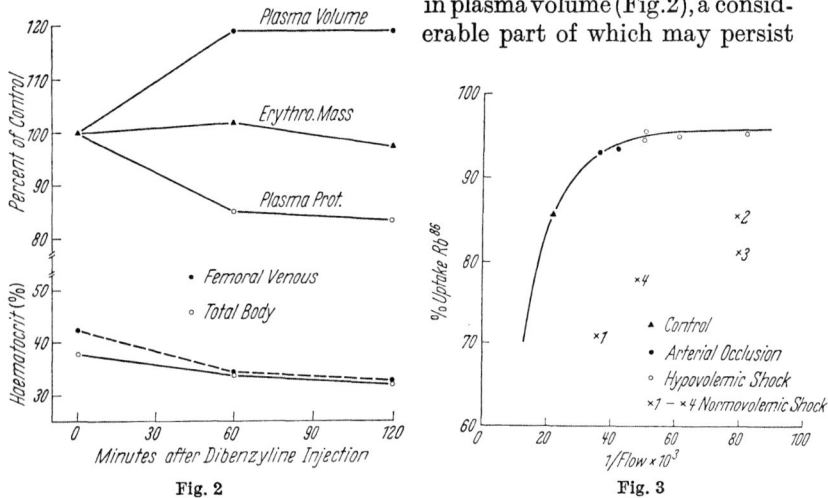

Fig. 2

Fig. 3

Fig. 2. Response of a control dog, lightly anesthetized with pentobarbital, to the intravenous administration of 1.0 mg./kg. of Dibenzyline at 0 time. Simultaneous measurements of plasma volume with I[131]-tagged albumin and of erythrocyte mass with Cr[51]-tagged cells. Note particularly that the venous and whole-body hematocrits are almost identical after two hours

Fig. 3. Simultaneous measurements of total blood flow and Rb[86] uptake in a vascularly-isolated loop of ileum of a dog lightly anesthetized with pentobarbital, before and during the development of hemorrhagic shock. Total blood flow was reduced to varying degrees before hemorrhage by application of a clamp to the mesenteric artery supplying the ileal segment. X_1, X_2 and X_3 are determinations 5, 15 and 35 minutes after reinfusion respectively; X_4 is 60 minutes after reinfusion and immediately following intravenous infusion of 100 ml. of 6% dextran in saline, which increased flow in the loop from 12.5 to 20 ml./min. but did not improve Rb[86] extraction

for 18 to 24 hours. The blocking agent may thus reverse the loss of intravascular volume which is induced by vasoconstriction and is characteristic of cardiovascular decompensation during the development of shock. An observation of even greater interest, demonstrated by simultaneous independent measurements of plasma volume and total erythrocyte mass, is that the venous hematocrit falls more markedly than the whole-body hematocrit after administration of Dibenzyline, and the two may become almost identical. This change appears to indicate a considerable opening of the microcirculation and an equalization of the rates of passage of erythrocytes and of plasma.

An additional factor which may contribute to protection by agents that inhibit sympathetic vasoconstriction is a local redistribution of blood flow. Simultaneous measurements of total regional blood flow and of the extraction of rubidium[86], introduced by close intra-arterial injection, show that during the development of shock there may be a considerable decrease in the percentage extraction at a given flow rate. In our experiments to date, this change appears to be particularly marked in the intestinal circulation and during the post-reinfusion period (normovolemic shock) (Fig. 3). Infusion of relatively small doses of noradrenaline produces changes similar to those observed in hemorrhagic shock, and, conversely, they are largely prevented in hemorrhaged animals by pre-treatment with Dibenzyline. We believe the observed decrease from the normal level of Rb[86] extraction indicates that an increased precentage of the total flow is passing through channels which do not exchange readily with tissue cells, a deleterious shift in the local distribution of blood flow which is promoted by adrenergic vasoconstriction and inhibited by the adrenergic blocking agent.

On the basis of the considerable protection observed in animals treated with agents which block sympathetic vasoconstriction, and the availability of at least a partial theoretical basis for this protection, we have initiated a trial of Dibenzyline in the treatment of clinical shock of varying etiology. The logic of this step has been questioned by some on the basis that the major protection observed in laboratory studies involves pre-treatment, i. e. administration of the blocking agent before subjecting the animal to a shock-inducing procedure. However, a significant increase in survival can be induced by a vasodilator agent administered at an intermediate point during the hemorrhagic stress (LOTZ et al., 1955; ZINGG et al., 1959), although no protection is obtained if the agent is administered at a time when reinfusion of shed blood is itself inadequate to allow survival. It is obviously impossible to treat clinical cases before the development of "shock". However, this "shock" is quite different from the point of irreversibility to retransfusion in controlled laboratory experiments. The major clinical problems are presented by cases in which there is continuing insult due to extensive tissue damage or infection. In this situation the distinction between pre- and post-treatment largely disappears and, in many clinical cases, therapy at the time the patient is first diagnosed as "in shock" probably represents pre-treatment for most of the shock-inducing stress.

Cases of severe shock resulting from mechanical trauma, burns, extensive surgery and sepsis, most involving more than one factor, have been studied to date. Shock due to uncomplicated hemorrhage is not included, as we have encountered no cases in this category

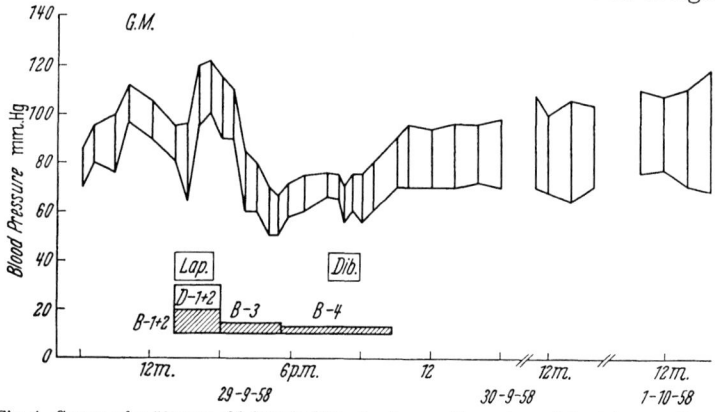

Fig. 4. Course of a 50-year-old female following traumatic rupture of the jejunum. During operative repair (Lap.) rapid administration of blood and 6% dextran in saline caused a considerable increase in blood pressure. However, the pulse pressure remained low and the clinical signs of shock, which had been present since admission, were unaltered. After a total of 1,000 ml. of 6% dextran in saline and almost 2,000 ml. of blood, the circulation and clinical status were not improved. Administration of 1.0 mg./kg. of Dibenzyline over a period of 40 minutes produced little immediate change in the blood pressure, indicating that circulating volume replacement had been at least adequate. During the next hour the pulse pressure widened and the systemic pressure began to rise, and 2 hours after the beginning of Dibenzyline administration all clinical signs of shock were gone. The patient maintained an adequate circulation without further specific shock therapy

which did not respond to adequate transfusion alone. In each case, an attempt was first made to manage the patient with adequate blood and other fluid volume replacement, and only when such therapy appeared to have failed was Dibenzyline administered. This sequence was utilized both because it facilitated interpretation of responses to the vasodilator agent, and because hypovolemic patients are extremely sensitive to vasodilatation and respond to very small doses of the blocking agent with a precipitous fall in blood pressure, as was noted above for laboratory animals during the hypovolemic phase of hemorrhagic shock.

Although it still is too early to evaluate accurately the results of this form treatment in the highly heterogeneous group of cases characterized as "clinical shock", they are most encouraging. A considerable number of patients who had failed to respond to blood volume replacement began to improve within 1 to 4 hours after the administration of Dibenzyline (Fig. 4), and others who had failed to maintain improvement induced by one or more large transfusions did so after administration of the blocking agent (Fig. 5). The most common pattern has been a relatively small (10 to 15 mm). fall in blood pressure during the administration of Dibenzyline, which was given in a dose of 1.0 mg./kg. over a period of $^1/_2$ to 1 hour, followed

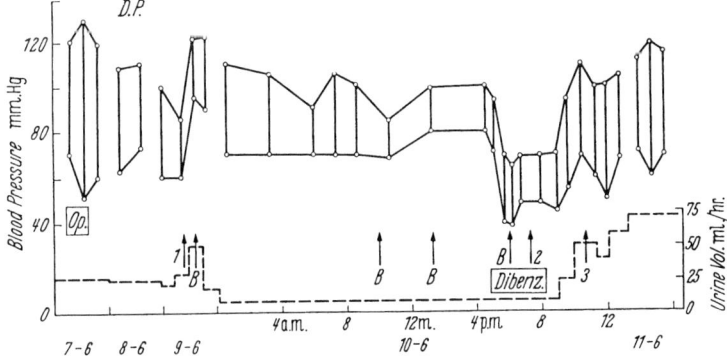

Fig. 5. Course of a 65-year-old male following partial gastric resection (Op.) complicated by leakage of gastro-intestinal contents and peritonitis. Clinical shock and oliguria were first noted on the second post-operative day (1). Transfusion of 1,000 ml. of blood (B) caused transient improvement of the clinical condition and urine output. However, the patient's condition again deteriorated and transfusions of 500 and 1,000 ml. of blood (B) produced only limited improvement. Blood pressure fell rather sharply when Dibenzyline infusion was started, indicating that the effective circulating volume was still somewhat inadequate. However, the pressure stabilized after the administration of only 500 ml. of blood. Definite clinical improvement was apparent by the time the Dibenzyline infusion (1.0 mg./kg. over 2 hours) was completed (2). Three hours later all clinical signs of shock had disappeared and diuresis was well established (3). The patient maintained a satisfactory cardiovascular status for 3 days without further specific therapy, but died seven days later from uncontrolled peritonitis

by improvement in clinical condition, widening of the pulse pressure, and a subsequent gradual rise in mean blood pressure without additional specific shock therapy. In many cases, even in patients who had been severely oliguric for 24 hours or more, a marked increase in the urine output began shortly after the blood pressure reached the level necessary for glomerular filtration.

Observations on this series of patients have reinforced our conviction that systolic or mean blood pressure is an unreliable criterion of clinical status (Fig. 6), although pulse pressure and particularly the ease with which systolic and diastolic pressures can be determined (indices of pulse or stroke volume) are often quite significant. In most cases the classical clinical picture of shock, a complex of signs associated with peripheral vasoconstriction and sympathetic nervous system hyperactivity, has proved to be the most sensitive and reliable criterion of the status of the patient. We feel that cases presenting with a low blood pressure, but without the classical peripheral signs of sympathetic nervous system hyperactivity, should not be classified as "shock". We have treated a small number of such cases with Dibenzyline without any obvious favorable or deleterious effects on their clinical course.

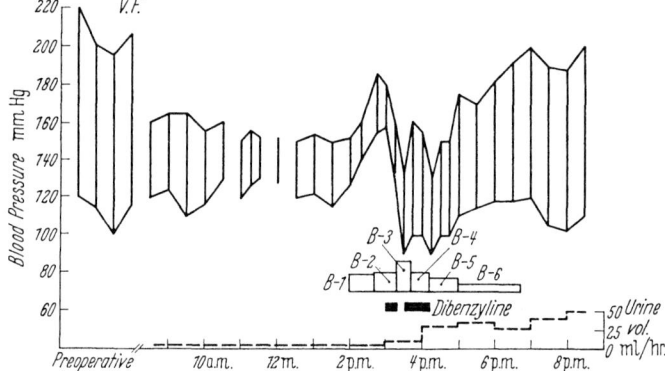

Fig. 6. Course of a 50-year-old male during shock associated with acute regional ileitis complicated by peritonitis following bowel surgery. The patient had been hypertensive for many years and had previously experienced two myocardial infarcts. Clinical signs of shock had been present for nearly 24 hours and were very marked prior to initiation of specific shock therapy. Urine output had been less than 10 ml./hr throughout this period. Systolic pressure ranged between 160 and 180 mm. Hg, but was difficult to determine, and several entries in the clinical chart indicated the blood pressure as "unobtainable". Circulating volume obviously was quite inadequate, but moderately slow administration of 500 ml. of blood (B—1) caused initial signs of pulmonary congestion. Because of the hypovolemia, the first 7 mg. of Dibenzyline induced a sharp fall in blood pressure, but a full dose of 1.0 mg./kg. was well tolerated when balanced by a total of 2,000 ml. of blood. At this time pressure was 130/85, all clinical signs of shock were gone, pulse was full and systolic and diastolic pressures easily determined. Urine output began to increase by the time the Dibenzyline infusion was completed. Note particularly the marked improvement associated with a fall in systolic pressure of about 50 mm. Hg during the period of vasodilator administration

Summary

The use of adrenal cortical steroids, sympathomimetic pressor amines, and vasodilator agents in the treatment of shock of varying etiology has been discussed. The adrenal steroids, administered in doses much larger than those employed for other purposes, appear to provide effective protection against endotoxin "shock", but their value in other types of shock has not been demonstrated. The protection does not appear to be well correlated with either gluco- or mineralocorticoid properties as usually measured.

Vasoconstrictor agents are commonly employed clinically in the treatment of shock, and frequently improve blood pressure and clinical appearance. However, they have not been clearly demonstrated to improve survival. Indeed, excessive vasoconstriction due to sympathetic nervous system activity or exogenous sympathomimetic amines can itself induce shock, and milder adrenergic vasoconstriction may accentuate the development of traumatic, hemorrhagic or endotoxin shock. Vasoconstrictor agents may temporarily prevent death in acute exsanguination or other acute hypovolemic hypotension by maintaining circulation to the respiratory centers, and reports of beneficial effects of these agents in experimental shock are frequently complicated by failure to distinguish acute cardiovascular collapse from more protracted "shock". Administration of a sympathomimetic amine during the late, decompensatory phase of shock in a dose which has little vasoconstrictor effect, may have some beneficial effect attributable to myocardial stimulation.

Even severe hypotension is well tolerated for extended periods if it is associated with generalized vasodilatation, and drugs inducing vasodilatation by various mechanisms have been shown by many workers to increase survival in haemorrhagic, traumatic and endotoxin shock. Although such agents increase sensitivity to acute hypovolemia, and may decrease the hemorrhage volume required to induce a given level of hypotension, their protective action is not necessarily dependent on decreasing the hemorrhagic or traumatic stress to which the experimental animal is subjected. Evidence has been presented to suggest that protection by blockade of sympathetic vasoconstrictor activity may involve both a hemodynamic effect promoting the movement of fluid into the vascular system, and a redistribution of blood flow to channels from which exchange with tissue cells occurs readily. Observations on the treatment of clinical shock of varying etiology indicate that blockade of adrenergic vasoconstriction with Dibenzylene may have a beneficial effect in patients who have responded poorly to adequate blood and other fluid volume replacement.

Acknowledgements

The author is indebted to JAMES T. GOURZIS for several contributions to the unpublished work presented, including that shown in Figs 2 and 3. Various aspects of the experimental work reported in this paper have been supported by grants-in-aid from the National Reserach Council of Canada, the Defence Research Board of Canada, and the Life Insurance Medical Research Fund.

References

BAINBRIDGE, J. A., and J. W. TREVAN: Brit. Med. J. 1917/I 382. — BAEZ, S., S. G. SRIKANTIA, and B. BURACK: Amer. J. Physiol. 192, 175 (1958). — BEIN, H. J., and R. JAQUES: Experientia (Switz.) 16, 24 (1960). — BOUGHTON, G. A., and S. C. SOMMERS: Amer. J. Clin. Path. 27, 29 (1957). CLOSE, A. S., J. A. WAGNER, R. A. KLOEHN Jr., and R. C. KORY: Surg. Forum (U.S.A.) 8, 22 (1958). — ERLANGER, J., and H. S. GASSER: Amer. J. Physiol. 49, 345 (1919). — EVERSOLE, W. J., W. KLEINBERG, R. R. OVERMAN, J. W. REMINGTON, and W. W. SWINGLE: Amer. J. Physiol. 140, 490 (1944). — FRANK, H. A., M. D. ALTSCHULE, and N. ZAMCHECK: J. Clin. Invest. (U.S.A.) 24, 54 (1945). — FRANK, H. A., E. D. FRANK, H. KORMAN, I. A. MACCHI, and O. HECHTER: Amer. J. Physiol. 182, 24 (1955a). — FRANK, H. A., S. JACOB, H. A. E. WEIZEL, L. REINER, R. COHEN, and J. FINE: Amer. J. Physiol. 180, 282 (1955b). — FREEMAN, N. E.: Amer. J. Physiol. 103, 185 (1933). — FREEMAN, N. E., S. A. SHAFFER, A. E. SCHECTER, and H. E. HOLLING: J. Clin. Invest. (U.S.A.) 17, 359 (1938). — GLASSER, O., and I. H. PAGE: Amer. J. Physiol. 154, 297 (1948). — GOURZIS, J. T., M. W. HOLLENBERG, and M. NICKERSON: J. Exper. Med.

(U.S.A.) 1961 (in press). Hume, D. M., and D. H. Nelson: Surg. Forum
(U.S.A.) 5, 568 (1955). — Ingle, D. J.: Amer. J. Physiol. 139, 460 (1943). —
Kováсн, A., J. Manyhárt, A. Erdélyi, G. Molnár, and E. Kováсн:
Acta physiol. Acad. sc. Hungaricae 13, 5 (1957). — Lansing, A. M., and
J. A. F. Stevenson: Amer. J. Physiol. 193, 289 (1958). — Lansing, A.
M., J. A. F. Stevenson, and C. W. Gowdy: Canad. J. Biochem. 35, 93
(1957). — Levy, E. Z., W. C. North, and J. A. Wells: J. Pharmacol.
Exper. Therap. (U.S.A.) 112, 151 (1954). — Levy, M. N.: Circulation Res.
(U.S.A.) 6, 587 (1958). — Lillehei, R. C.: Surgery (U.S.A.) 42, 1043
(1957). — Lillehei, R. C., and L. D. MacLean: Arch. Surg. (U.S.A.) 78,
464 (1959). — Lotz, F., L. Beck, and J. A. F. Stevenson: Canad. J.
Biochem. 33, 741 (1955). — Melby, J. C., and W. W. Spink: J. Clin. In-
vest. (U.S.A.) 37, 1791 (1958). — Nickerson, M.: J. Michigan Med. Soc.
54, 45 (1955a). — Nickerson, M.: In: Shock and Circulatory Homeostasis,
p. 260. Ed. Green, H. D. New York: Josiah Macy Jr. Foundation 1955b. —
Nickerson, M., and S. A. Carter: Canad. J. Biochem. 37, 1161 (1959). —
Overman, R. R., and S. C. Wang: Amer. J. Physiol. 148, 289 (1947). —
Overton, R. C., and M. E. DeBakey: Ann. Surg. (U.S.A.) 143, 439
(1956). — Phemister, D. B.: Ann. Surg. (U.S.A.) 118, 256 (1943). —
Remington, J. W., W. F. Hamilton, G. H. Boyd,W. F. Hamilton Jr., and
H. M. Caddell: Amer. J. Physiol. 161, 116 (1950). — Ross, C. A., and S.
A. Herczeg: Proc. Soc. Exper. Biol. Med. (U.S.A.) 91, 196 (1956). — Sar-
noff, S. J., R. B. Case, P. E. Waithe, and J. P. Isaacs: Amer. J. Physiol.
176, 439 (1954). — Smith, J. J., A. A. Pandazi, and R. A. Grace: Proc.
Soc. Exper. Biol. Med. (U.S.A.) 95, 104 (1957). — Swingle, W. W., R. R.
Overman, J. W. Remington, W. Kleinberg, and W. J. Eversole: Amer.
J. Physiol. 139, 481 (1943). — Thomas, L.: J. Exper. Med. (U.S.A.) 104,
865 (1956). — Wang, S. C.: Amer. J. Physiol. 148, 547 (1947). — Weil, M.
H.: Amer. Practitioner 12, 162 (1961). — Weil, M. H., L. B. Hinshaw,
M. B. Visscher, W. W. Spink, and L. D. MacLean: Proc. Soc. Exper.
Biol. Med. (U.S.A.) 92, 610 (1956). — Wiggers, C. J., and J. M. Werle:
Amer. J. Physiol. 136, 421 (1956). — Wiggers, H. C., G. H. Glaser, K.
de. S. Canavarro, and A. E. Treat: Amer. J. Physiol. 139, 217 (1943). —
Wiggers, H. C., H. Goldberg, F. Roemhild, and R. C. Ingraham: Circu-
lation (U.S.A. 2, 179 (1950). — Yard, A. C., and M. Nickerson: Fed. Proc.
(U.S.A.) 15, 502 (1956). — Yoe, R. H.: Amer. J. Med. 16, 683 (1954). —
Zingg, W., M. Nickerson, and S. A. Carter: Surg. Forum (U.S.A.) 9, 22
(1959). — Zweifach, B. W., A. L. Nagler, and L. Thomas: J. Exper.
Med. (U.S.A.) 104, 881 (1956).

Some aspects of treatment in shock

By

G. Ström

Drug treatment in shock should be evaluated against the background of our general concept and classification of shock (Table 1). A meeting such as this provides an overwhelming tide of detailed analyses relating firstly to nomenclature and classification, secondly to aetiological factors, thirdly to those pathophysiological mechanisms which accompany or follow each other in a time order and combination that certainly varies depending on the different aetiological types of shock involved but which ultimately produce irreversibility, and fourthly to the immediate causes of death. When the tide has ebbed away, our previous concept is changed in detail and emphasis but not in general outline.

The following should be stressed. Tissue hypoxia, a low cardiac output, increased capillary permeability, invasion of endotoxins or release of vasoactive substances, intravascular red-cell aggregation, myocardial depression, or changes in the vasomotor control of blood distribution and capillary blood flow to key organs, etc. (Table 1) may all be relevant mechanisms to consider in the patient, but there seems to be no main mechanism as a common denominator for the different types of clinical shock. Death may ensue rapidly owing to one mechanism, or slowly owing to another. For instance, during clinical shock of a certain type, acute pain or emotional stress may provoke sudden vasovagal syncope or extreme hypotension with secondary ventricular fibrillation; in another case involving the same type of shock, renal dysfunction may cause delayed death.

The mortality rate in experiments, although serving as the index of success in treatment, therefore does not provide any direct information as to which mechanisms have been modulated. A drug may have a favourable effect on one mechanism without necessarily changing the mortality rate.

In many aetiologically clarified conditions of shock, there exist specific remedies (Table 1). Uncertainty arises mainly from diagnostic difficulties *in casu* or from doubts as to the value of additional treatment of a preventive or curative nature, e.g. with vasoconstrictor or vasodilator drugs.

24*

Table 1

Specific aetiology	Specific therapy
* Blood loss	Blood transfusion
* Trauma, tissue destruction	Surgical repair
* Burn	Excision, transplantation
Water-electrolyte imbalance	Water-electrolyte adjustment
* Infection (bact. toxaemia)	Antibact. agents, glucocorticoids
* Pain	Analgesics
Pulmonary dysfunction	Free airways, mech. ventilation, oxygen
Cerebral oedema	Hyperosmotic solutions
* Irradiation (ionising)	—
Anaphylactic reaction	Antihistaminics, glucocorticoids, vasoconstrictors
Cardiac dysfunction	Myocardial anaesthetics, pos. inotropic agents, etc.
Hormonal dysfunction: adrenocortical insufficiency . .	Glucocorticoids
adrenomedullary overactivity, or	Adrenergic blockade
post-op. underactivity (phaeochr.).	Noradrenaline
hyperthyroid crisis	Iodine, etc.
hypothyroid coma	Thyroxine
Hepatic coma	Various
Chemical toxaemia (barbiturates, etc.)	Various
* Emotional stress	Various
Hyper- and hypothermia	Temperature equilibration
Orthostatic stress	Recumbency

When considering the effect of vasoactive drugs, one must bear in mind not only the dosage and the chronological pattern of the effect — including possible post-excitatory depression or tachyphylaxis — but also the geometry within the vascular tree and the effect on capillary exchange; in addition, the natural function of the vasoconstrictor nervous system and its transmitters may be influenced. Our knowledge on these points is certainly incomplete, especially with regard to man and clinical shock. Vasoconstrictor agents, such as noradrenaline or angiotensin, may prove specific

Table 1

General mechanisms	Therapy against mechanisms
Low cardiac output	Various
Tissue hypoxia	Various
Low intravascular blood volume	Blood or plasma transfusion
Vasodilatation (low vasoconstr. tone)	Vasoconstrictors
Abnormal distribution of cardiac output, blood volume, and body fluids	Various
Vasoconstriction (high vasoconstr. tone)	Adrenergic blockade
Endotoxin invasion	—
Histamine (-serotonin) release	Antihistaminics, glucocorticoids
Intravasc. red-cell aggregation	Low-molecular dextran
Increased capillary permeability	Various
Myocardial dysfunction	Pos. inotropic agents
Renal dysfunction	Dialysis
Hepatic dysfunction	Various
Respiratory dysfunction	Oxygen, free airways, etc.
Acidaemia	Metabolic adjustment, alkaline solutions, etc.

Text to Table 1

Reversible and irreversible clinical shock. Examples of specific aetiology and corresponding specific therapy in clinical conditions, most of which may ultimately result in irreversible shock with either a slow or a rapid course. Some pathophysiological mechanisms which are known to, or thought to, play a role in different types of shock are also listed, together with their corresponding therapy (* indicates types of shock of special importance under war-time conditions).

The outward signs of clinical shock include tachycardia, hypotension, lowered urinary output or anuria, cold and pale skin with sweat and collapsed veins, restlessness, or a tendency to coma. These are accompanied by a low cardiac output, a lowered oxygen uptake with a tendency to generalised tissue hypoxia and acidosis, impaired detoxification by the liver, and reduced glomerular filtration and tubular function. There is a characteristic chronological course for the different mechanisms, including spontaneous deterioration and a tendency to irreversibility.

in unusual cases, e.g. noradrenaline in the short-term post-operative treatment of a case of constantly secreting phaeochromocytoma; in other instances they are used as additional therapy for short periods in order to save such key organs as the heart, kidneys, and brain because an element of insufficient vasoconstrictor tone, which might possibly prove fatal, is judged to be present.

Contra-indications to the use of noradrenaline include: already existing critical vasoconstriction in key organs promoting irreversibility in shock, e.g. such vasoconstriction affecting the visceral circulation; and serious cardiac arrhythmia. If vasodilatation occurs in the course of shock because of tissue hypoxia, vasoconstrictor drugs should not be administered; on the other hand, if dilatation occurs owing to the release of histamine, such drugs might be used. Hypoxia of most tissues appears to develop sooner or later in all types of shock, but release of histamine as a common mechanism is disputed. The trend of experimental evidence therefore favours Dr. Nickerson's general standpoint.

The question of whether to use sympathetic blockade in clinical shock, as raised by the results of research on experimental animals, cannot be answered with certainty until a carefully controlled clinical evaluation has been made. Such an evaluation is difficult, because clinical shock often has a multiple aetiology, and because the chronological course and severity of the ensuing mechanisms can seldom be expressed in quantitative terms, e. g. in terms of reversibility or irreversibility. Cases of traumatic injury, of burns, and of myocardial infarction appear to be best suited for such clinical trials; so many functions should then be studied that active pathophysiological mechanisms can be specified and their chronological course described. Cardiac, renal, and hepatic functions seem to be of special interest — but neurohumoral control of the vascular tree, and hormonal and humoral modulation of vascular responsiveness are also of cardinal importance, and the changes they undergo in shock need further clarification.

Discussion

GILBERT: We, too, found a drop in cardiac output in response to *prolonged* infusions of norepinephrine, but it disappointed me that we were not able to correct this to any appreciable degree by increasing the blood volume. Instead, this produced only minor changes in cardiac output and arterial pressure with a rise in atrial pressure.

SPINK: I would like to clear up some of the confusion that has been created by two different approaches employed at the University of Minnesota in attempts to reverse endotoxin shock. LILLEHEI and his associates in the Department of Surgery have evaluated therapeutic agents by *pre-treating* dogs, whereas our group has made an evaluation by treating *after* the onset of shock. We have found in dogs that a vasopressor drug used alone *after* the onset of shock will not protect them. However, when a pressor agent and a steroid, such as cortisol, are both employed, survival does occur. Why exogenous adrenal steroid should have a satisfactory additive effect with a pressor drug we do not know. The *post-treatment* of the dog having endotoxin shock has served as a good model in an attempt to evaluate what we are doing in the human subject. Again, clinical evaluation is very difficult in critically ill patients, and one must be cautious in transposing the results of animal experiments to human beings.

LILLEHEI: I would like to emphasise the critical need for increasing the blood volume concomitantly with the use of adrenergic blocking agents, such as phenoxybenzamine (Dibenzyline), whether this be in the clinical patient or the experimental animal. Our own studies, as well as those of others, have shown that these agents increase the capacity of the vascular space by at least 15%. If the vascular space is not filled up with blood, plasma, or low molecular weight dextran, the mean blood pressure may fall to levels such that coronary flow is markedly reduced and cardiac standstill or ventricular fibrillation is the inevitable result. This replacement of blood volume concomitant with the use of adrenergic blocking agents is, of course, in addition to the blood volume replacement already accomplished to match losses occurring as a result of the original stress causing the shock, whether it be haemorrhage, trauma, infection, or combinations of these three.

Latterly, in the laboratory we have worked on the problem of post-treatment of shock. Most of these experiments have dealt with the post-treatment of shock due to the endotoxins of gram-negative bacteria (*Escherichia coli* in this instance). Following the induction of the shock, we have found that a combination of phenoxybenzamine (Dibenzyline) and low molecular weight ("Swedish") dextran or plasma is more effective than either agent given separately. Hydrocortisone is also being added to this cocktail. The beneficial effects of such a post-treatment regimen are mirrored in the increased blood flow to the viscera, and particularly the bowel, which can be monitored by the electromagnetic flow-meter. Thus, not only can we measure qualitatively the benefits of such post-treatment by increased numbers of survivors but also quantitatively by recording the increased blood flow to vital organs resulting from such combinations of fluids, adrenergic blocking agents, and cortisone.

In contrast, post-treatment of dogs suffering from endotoxin shock with combinations of vasopressors (1-norepinephrine or metaraminol) and fluids gives the same results as pre-treatment with these substances. Almost all the animals die, and prior to death electromagnetic measurements of blood flow to vital organs, including the bowel, show even further decreases in blood flow over and above the decrease already resulting from the shock itself.

NICKERSON: I will try to be very brief and would like to comment only on one point made by Dr. STRÖM, which is a bit dangerous, because it is a positive statement. He mentioned that it is necessary to induce vaso-constriction with a noradrenaline infusion after removal of a phaeochromo-cytoma. We felt that the very common post-operative hypotension seen in these patients was secondary to the vasoconstriction which occurred during removal of the tumour. We now have a series of 9 cases which were blocked effectively with Dibenzyline prior to the operation, and in none of them has there been any post-operative hypotension. Even in this condition there may not be a clear indication for the use of noradrenaline.

I think the best summary is to again thank CIBA Limited and Prof. VON EULER for what to me has been an extremely interesting and profitable symposium.

Closing remarks

By

U. S. von Euler

Such an overwhelming mass of new and interesting data has been presented here that to give a summary of it all would be exceedingly difficult and might in some respects even be superfluous. I would, however, like to comply with Dr. Gross's request and say just a few words if you can summon up the patience to listen to me for a moment or two.

First of all, it seems to be extremely important to differentiate between reversible and irreversible shock, as pointed out in the highly informative papers read by Dr. Rushmer and especially by Dr. Fine. We have, of course, to apply quite a different mode of thinking when we try to evaluate what happens during the reversible state and what happens during the irreversible state. I would also like to spotlight a few of the different functions in regard to which the pathophysiological events might give us some more information if they are properly studied and on which so much fine work has been presented here at this symposium. I am thinking firstly of the cardiovascular events, concerning which careful studies and measurements have been presented by many of the participants. In this connection, I should like to mention particularly the papers by Dr. Gregg, Dr. Rushmer, Dr. Folkow, Dr. Ström, Dr. Takács, and Dr. Bein, who by many different means have shown us that it is possible to analyse these events in such a way as to provide us with more information of use in the understanding of shock. The nervous system, I feel, has been somewhat neglected with regard to the pathogenesis of shock. Dr. Neil has presented a lot of hought-provoking concepts and ideas on this subject, and I believe that what he has said is very important. What we need is more precise knowledge as to how the nervous system affects the initiation and the development of shock. Dr. Ossipov has also been arguing along these lines and has stressed in particular the importance of the sympathetic autonomic outflow.

Endocrinological factors as well have been mentioned in certain contexts, particularly by Dr. Hökfelt, and I think that this is another aspect on which more work has to be done. The role played by the kidney in shock is of course obvious, and it has been a great pleasure to listen to the important contributions by Dr. KRA-MER, Dr. SELKURT, Dr. BING, and Dr. HOWARD, who have presented us with a vast amount of new and most interesting information. Blood volume, blood aggregation, and viscosity are other factors whose importance is becoming increasingly apparent, as borne out in the papers by Dr. GREGERSEN, Dr. GELIN, and Dr. NICKERSON. We must also pay more attention to the biochemical events occurring during shock. I was especially pleased that Dr. MIGONE was able to come here and present his data. Several papers have referred to the occurrence and development of acidosis during shock. This is another point which, I feel, requires to be studied in even greater detail. The data presented by Dr. BREWIN, Dr. BJURSTEDT, and Dr. MATTHES have been particularly elucidating in this respect and will no doubt lead to further studies.

The endotoxins and other toxic products are certainly of the utmost significance, and it was therefore especially interesting to hear the reports and results presented by Dr. FINE in the first place, as well as by Dr. GILBERT, Dr. SPINK, Dr. LILLEHEI, and Dr. ALLGÖWER. If we can obtain more knowledge about the nature of these substances, we might also have a better idea as to how to combat their effects. I should also like to refer in particular to Dr. SPINK's report on the mechanism of action of endotoxins, which, I think, indicates a new field of very great interest. The effects of allergy and of irradiation, as outlined by Dr. HALPERN and Dr. BACQ, are also highly important for many reasons, and here again much remains to be done.

From the therapeutic point of view I think this symposium has afforded convincing proof of the importance of preventing irrevers-ible shock — especially by the use of drugs which prevent sympa-thetic overactivity, since the latter may be said to act as a kind of internal tourniquet and is therefore, of course, highly undesirable. The effects of Dibenzyline, as outlined by Dr. NICKERSON, are certainly most revealing in this respect, although we must not forget that the use of conventional pressor drugs may be indicated in certain stages. Here, I am thinking of the case of falling blood pressure cited by Dr. HALPERN, where of course fluid substitution would not be of any good; for such a case it is essential to raise the blood pressure in order to restore flow. The effect of cortical hormones also requires further study, since we still know far too little about their real effects in low and high doses.

Finally, I would like to refer in particular to the comments made by Dr. GREGERSEN and by Dr. RUSHMER, who have presented us with concepts of more general significance, just as Dr. STRÖM's list has given us an overwhelming picture of the many factors encountered in any study of shock. However, if we are to make further progress in this field, I think we must face up to the complexity of the situation and try, by means of well-planned experiments, to obtain more and more exact data. In closing, I should like to express to you my very sincere thanks for your contributions and for your co-operation; I must say that it has been a very special pleasure for me to act as chairman at this meeting.

The editor acknowledges with special gratitude the valuable assistance of Mr. H. D. PHILPS, M. A., Dr. W. HATZINGER, Miss S. R. NAEGELI, and Miss B. PFEIFER.

List of authors

Subject index

REPRINT FROM
SHOCK
AN INTERNATIONAL SYMPOSIUM
CHAIRMAN
U. S. von EULER · STOCKHOLM
EDITED BY
K. D. BOCK · BASLE

SPRINGER-VERLAG / BERLIN · GÖTTINGEN · HEIDELBERG / 1962
PRINTED IN GERMANY
NOT IN CIRCULATION

DEFINITION AND CLASSIFICATION
OF VARIOUS FORMS OF SHOCK
BY
R. F. RUSHMER, R. L. VAN CITTERS, AND D. FRANKLIN
WITH 6 FIGURES

Diuresis and Diuretics - Diurese und Diuretica

An International Symposium — Ein Internationales Symposion
Herrenchiemsee, June 17th—20th, 1959. Sponsored by CIBA. Chairman
H. SCHWIEGK, Munich. Edited by E. BUCHBORN, Munich and K. D. BOCK
Basle
With 88 figures. XII, 382 pages (290 pages in German and 92 pages in
English) 8vo. 1959.   Cloth DM 25,50

"The entire gamut of Diuresis and Diuretics is covered from the cellular
level of renal Physiology to the uses of diuretics in Clinical Medicine. Not
only the practicing physician, but also the medical research men, the
physiologists, and the biochemists, should make every possible effort to
acquire and study this book."   *Westchester Medical Bulletin*

Essential Hypertension

An International Symposium
Berne, June 7th—10th, 1960. Sponsored by CIBA. Chairman F. C. REUBI,
Berne. Edited by K. D. BOCK, Basle, and P. T. COTTIER, Berne
With 81 figures. VIII, 392 pages 8°. 1960.   Cloth DM 33,80

The book is available in an English and in a German edition

The subjects covered by prominent experts ranged from the nature, course,
and prognosis of untreated essential hypertension to topical problems
relating to electrolyte metabolism, endocrinology, pathophysiology, and
experimental research on high blood pressure. Following papers dealing
with experimental and clinical aspects of the pharmacology, mode of action,
and therapeutic effect of the newer anti-hypertensive substances it was
possible to review the influence of such treatment on the prognosis of
essential hypertension.

Shock

Pathogenesis and Therapy — An International Symposium
Stockholm, June 27th—30th, 1961. Sponsored by CIBA.
Chairman U. S. VON EULER, Stockholm. Edited by K. D. BOCK, Basle
With 120 figures. VIII, 387 pages 8°. 1962.   Cloth DM 37,50

The book is available in an English and in a German edition

Besides questions relating to the definition and classification of shock,
topics discussed at length includ the pathogenesis of traumatic, haemorrhagic, infectious, toxic, cardiogenic, allergic, and irradiation shock and
their corresponding animal-experimental equivalents. Considerable attention
is also devoted to the treatment of shock, with particular reference to
pharmacotherapy.

SPRINGER-VERLAG · BERLIN · GÖTTINGEN · HEIDELBERG

REPRINT FROM

SHOCK

AN INTERNATIONAL SYMPOSIUM

CHAIRMAN

U. S. VON EULER · STOCKHOLM

EDITED BY

K. D. BOCK · BASLE

SPRINGER-VERLAG / BERLIN · GÖTTINGEN · HEIDELBERG / 1962
PRINTED IN GERMANY

NOT IN CIRCULATION

COMPARISON OF VARIOUS FORMS
OF EXPERIMENTAL SHOCK
(WITH SPECIAL REFERENCE TO EXPERIMENTAL DESIGN)

BY

J. FINE

REPRINT FROM
SHOCK
AN INTERNATIONAL SYMPOSIUM
CHAIRMAN
U. S. von EULER · stockholm
EDITED BY
K. D. BOCK · basle

SPRINGER-VERLAG / BERLIN · GÖTTINGEN · HEIDELBERG / 1962
PRINTED IN GERMANY
NOT IN CIRCULATION

POSSIBLE ROLE OF ENDOTOXIN
IN THE PERPETUATION OF SHOCK

BY

R. P. GILBERT

WITH 1 FIGURE

REPRINT FROM

SHOCK

AN INTERNATIONAL SYMPOSIUM

CHAIRMAN

U. S. von EULER · stockholm

EDITED BY

K. D. BOCK · basle

SPRINGER-VERLAG / BERLIN · GÖTTINGEN · HEIDELBERG / 1962
PRINTED IN GERMANY
NOT IN CIRCULATION

HEMODYNAMIC FACTORS IN SHOCK

BY

D. E. GREGG

WITH 6 FIGURES

REPRINT FROM
SHOCK
AN INTERNATIONAL SYMPOSIUM
CHAIRMAN
U. S. von EULER · stockholm
EDITED BY
K. D. BOCK · basle

SPRINGER-VERLAG / BERLIN · GÖTTINGEN · HEIDELBERG / 1962
PRINTED IN GERMANY
NOT IN CIRCULATION

NERVOUS ADJUSTMENTS OF THE VASCULAR BED
WITH SPECIAL REFERENCE TO PATTERNS
OF VASOCONSTRICTOR FIBRE DISCHARGE

BY

B. FOLKOW

WITH 6 FIGURES

REPRINT FROM

SHOCK

AN INTERNATIONAL SYMPOSIUM

CHAIRMAN

U. S. von EULER · STOCKHOLM

EDITED BY

K. D. BOCK · BASLE

SPRINGER-VERLAG / BERLIN · GÖTTINGEN · HEIDELBERG / 1962
PRINTED IN GERMANY

NOT IN CIRCULATION

METABOLIC ASPECTS OF SHOCK

BY

L. MIGONE

WITH 8 TABLES

REPRINT FROM

SHOCK

AN INTERNATIONAL SYMPOSIUM

CHAIRMAN

U. S. von EULER · stockholm

EDITED BY

K. D. BOCK · basle

SPRINGER-VERLAG / BERLIN · GÖTTINGEN · HEIDELBERG / 1962
PRINTED IN GERMANY

NOT IN CIRCULATION

MICROSCOPIC OBSERVATIONS
OF THE MESENTERIC CIRCULATION IN RABBITS
SUBJECTED TO REVERSIBLE
AND IRREVERSIBLE HAEMORRHAGIC SHOCK

BY

S. BELLMAN, P. B. LAMBERT, AND J. FINE

REPRINT FROM

SHOCK

AN INTERNATIONAL SYMPOSIUM

CHAIRMAN
U. S. von EULER · STOCKHOLM

EDITED BY
K. D. BOCK · BASLE

SPRINGER-VERLAG / BERLIN · GÖTTINGEN · HEIDELBERG / 1962
PRINTED IN GERMANY

NOT IN CIRCULATION

THE NATURE OF IRREVERSIBLE SHOCK: ITS RELATIONSHIP TO INTESTINAL CHANGES

BY

R. C. LILLEHEI, J. K. LONGERBEAM, AND J. C. ROSENBERG

WITH 8 FIGURES

REPRINT FROM

SHOCK

AN INTERNATIONAL SYMPOSIUM

CHAIRMAN

U. S. VON EULER · STOCKHOLM

EDITED BY

K. D. BOCK · BASLE

SPRINGER-VERLAG / BERLIN · GÖTTINGEN · HEIDELBERG / 1962
PRINTED IN GERMANY

NOT IN CIRCULATION

RENAL FAILURE IN SHOCK

BY

K. KRAMER

WITH 11 FIGURES

REPRINT FROM

SHOCK
AN INTERNATIONAL SYMPOSIUM
CHAIRMAN
U. S. von EULER · STOCKHOLM
EDITED BY
K. D. BOCK · BASLE

SPRINGER-VERLAG / BERLIN · GÖTTINGEN · HEIDELBERG / 1962
PRINTED IN GERMANY
NOT IN CIRCULATION

RENAL BLOOD FLOW AND RENAL CLEARANCES
DURING HEMORRHAGE AND HEMORRHAGIC SHOCK

BY

E. E. SELKURT

WITH 2 FIGURES